THE THERAPEUTIC
REVOLUTION

THE THERAPEUTIC REVOLUTION · Essays in the Social History of American Medicine ·

edited by MORRIS J. VOGEL ·
CHARLES E. ROSENBERG

University of Pennsylvania Press · 1979

Most of the essays in this volume were presented, in preliminary form, to a conference on the history of medicine sponsored by Temple University and the University of Pennsylvania. Held in December 1976, the conference was supported in part by funding from the National Endowment for the Humanities, RM21516-75-685.

Library of Congress Cataloging in Publication Data

Main entry under title:

The Therapeutic revolution.

    Bibliography: p. 267
     1. Medicine—United States—History—Congresses.
2. Social medicine—United States—History—
Congresses. 3. Therapeutics—United States—
History—Congresses. I. Vogel, Morris J.
II. Rosenberg, Charles E.
R151.T5   362.1'0973   79-5043
ISBN 0-8122-7773-2

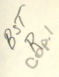
CONTENTS

v

INTRODUCTION

MORRIS J. VOGEL

Contemporary analyses of medicine are usually complaints. They argue that we have trusted too strongly in the healing power of the profession and that we have been wrong to idealize the achievements of medical science. The history of medicine itself is suspect, recounting, it is said, one glorious triumph after another, and the path-breaking insights of great doctors. These are not unfounded charges; while exaggerated, they balance a too often uncritical story.

Decades of medical progress and improvements in the level of health in industrialized nations have made modern medicine the most completely fulfilled of all the promises of the twentieth century. The evidence is everywhere: American life expectancy at birth has more than doubled between 1800 and the present; antibiotics control infection; surgery dramatically relieves pain and prolongs life; smallpox and plague have all but disappeared; medical foundations and fund raisers have promised to conquer, first, tuberculosis and polio, and now, cancer and heart disease.

As might be expected, histories of medicine from the late nineteenth century until nearly the present reflected the optimism of the science and profession which they studied. Since progress was cumulative, the historian's role was to identify and chronicle the ideas and events which brought medicine ever closer to the secrets of disease and health.

Two distinct strains characterized this teleology. One strain, often focusing on the Classical Age, or the Renaissance, celebrated the emergence of a rational medicine. Freeing itself from superstition, theological dogma, and metaphysical speculation, medicine established an identity distinct from the magic and ritual in which it had originated. The realization that disease was not of supernatural origin led to the examination of bodily structure and function. While historians could ascribe only minimal therapeutic consequence to this awakening, they have emphasized the building of the intellectual tradition on which modern medicine would be based.

The other strain did not deal with gestalt, but traced the appearance of still valid ideas about disease processes, and still acceptable drugs. A minor theme here has been locating the historic antecedents of contemporary therapies in remote times and places. Digitalis and cinchona bark have done heroic service in this tradition, as one early culture after another has been credited with developing a cardiac stimulant or a prophylaxis against malaria. But the major theme generally starts with the breakthroughs of the mid-nineteenth century. The concept of disease specificity, the introduction of anesthesia, and the acceptance of germ theory revolutionized medical knowledge and practice. The pace of the march of progress accelerated, as causes of long-baffling diseases were uncovered and new procedures in diagnosis, surgery, and public health were adopted. This medical revolution coincided neatly with the observed fall in death rates and the increase in life expectancy. Cause and consequence were clear. Problems remained, but they were merely unfinished business for medical researchers and practitioners.

The premise of medical progress generally has a corollary: the emergence of the medical profession. Medicine's heroes were both clinicians and researchers. In periods when most healers thrashed about, harming patients as often as helping them, a farsighted and often heroic few redeemed their brethren and kept alive, or added to the store of knowledge. Within the past century or so, collective professional endeavor began to overshadow individual activity. While some physicians continued to devote their lives to lonely searches for microbes or other pathogens, the focus shifted to a profession seeking to upgrade the standards of all its practitioners and to translate research progress into therapeutic benefits and a better quality of life for all. No longer would an army of barely competent empirics and sectarians detract from the efforts of dedicated and skilled physicians. No longer would economic competition and backbiting among physicians mar the profession's record of achievement. A unified profession emerged, one that successfully identified itself with the welfare of the public, while at the same time setting itself off from the society at large as a self-conscious elite with a special competence to understand matters which affected all. The profession established its own code of ethics and standard of practice. Doctors aggressively practiced the arcane skills and techniques made possible by the expansion of science. An increasingly rational and bureaucratic age provided an appreciative public, grateful for the expert ministrations of thoroughly professional medical practitioners.

This is the account of medical advance that has come under attack as medicine itself has come under scrutiny. Contemporary scholars and polemicists have raised questions about the march of medical progress on several grounds: Has modern medicine wrongly assumed credit for the undeniable fall in morbidity and mortality rates? Perhaps the rise in living standards, and especially the improvement of nutrition has made a more substantial contribution to the increase in life expectancy, and the better health levels of the population, than medicine has. It has been argued that the decline of certain once devastating diseases preceded the introduction of effective therapeutic regimens. We are also beginning to ask if we have overvalued the professional attitude of clinical detachment. Though it has enabled physicians to closely study and scientifically manage the sick, modern professionalism has deprived patients of supportive care addressed to their emotional needs. Treatment has become an occasion for the exercise of formal knowledge; it is no longer an existential process. Have medical experts assumed control over too much of human life? Many experiences—birth and death, for example—have been redefined as medical events and drained of meaning. And as life has become increasingly medicalized, individuals have forfeited responsibility for their own health and well-being, relying instead on doctors and drugs. Have physicians used their scientifically sanctioned authority to regulate and control personal behavior? Perhaps sickness is just another socially defined form of deviance. Perhaps medicine is just another institution of social control, its hospitals and asylums duplicating schools and prisons. The critique minimizes the benefits which we have derived from scientific medicine and medical professionalization, and demands that these benefits be weighed against staggering personal, cultural, and social costs.

How broadly this medical iconoclasm has spread, and how deeply it has penetrated, remains a question. But we can speculate about why it now seems so fashionable. A century of significant medical progress has generated the expectation of continuing triumph over disease. But contemporary breakthroughs tend to be more discrete in their impact and less dramatic than earlier victories, such as the conquest of infectious disease. The residuum of sickness may not yield as readily to investigation, prevention, and therapy as smallpox or infant mortality appeared to have. Spokesmen for medicine have emphasized its promises; the limits which now, apparently, check progress call into question the achievements which medicine has claimed in the past. On another level, there is concern—in science in general, and in medicine in particular—for the unintended consequences of innovations which appear, at first, to be for the better. Concern about iatrogenic disease, and complaints that physicians have abandoned their caring function as they have become more technically competent parallel the sensitivity displayed by segments of the public to environmental issues. Finally, it is said that there is a general "crisis of confidence" in contemporary institutions, and that we are troubled by the "shape of the future." These oft-repeated phrases are imprecise in their meaning, but they make it clear that medicine has not been singled out for criticism. Given the hostility directed at science and technology, the attack on the legitimacy of medicine is understandable.

Contemporary criticism has made us increasingly aware that medicine, far from tending toward absolute truth, reflects and interacts with culture, society, and politics. But some of today's complaints are so shrill in rejecting the benefits of modern medicine that they obscure its history as much as did the panegyric. The essays in this volume are neither worshipful nor condemnatory. Rather, they examine American medicine within its multiple contexts, sensitive to the role of medical knowledge, practitioners, and institutions in the nineteenth and twentieth centuries.

The title essay, Charles E. Rosenberg's "The Therapeutic Revolution," explores the gradual modernization of world-view, as reflected in the nineteenth-century history of medicine. At the beginning of the century, a holistic view of the body dominated. Organism and environment were understood to be in a constant state of interaction, and this interactive process was visible in the body's intake and output: food, perspiration, feces, urine, secretions, and the like. Equilibrium, rather than the absence of a particular disease, constituted health. The physician's role was to aid, through his knowledge of the patient, and his use of drugs or other therapeutic regimens with perceptible physiological consequences, in the maintenance or restoration of this harmonious balance. Therapy "worked" because doctor and patient alike could observe the predictable physiological effects of treatment. Insights gained from medical science over the course of the century moderated, but did not destroy traditional therapeutics.

Practitioners resisted the notion of specificity: the identification, that is, of diseases as discrete clinical entities with unique causes, courses, and pathologies. The conflict between science and therapeutics intensified during the course of the century, as medicine gradually shifted from a holistic view of the body to a more mechanistic and reductionist understanding of its functions. This, according to Rosenberg, paralleled general shifts in social attitudes.

Robert E. Kohler, Gerald L. Geison, and Russell C. Maulitz illuminate aspects of the interplay between clinical medicine and the emerging medical sciences in the late nineteenth and early twentieth centuries. They take issue with the long-standing assumption that medical practitioners eagerly reoriented their healing art, embracing scientific medicine. At the same time, they dispute the contemporary critique of the profession which explains the increasing scientific content of medicine as an economic or political ploy, designed to exclude marginal groups from medical practice.

Kohler examines the newly independent discipline of biochemistry. Turn-of-the-century agitation for the reform of medical education sprang from diverse groups with varied agendas. Medical school instructors of the sciences were part of this coalition and were the first to benefit from reform. Higher standards for student admission and a lengthened curriculum allowed for the expansion and specialization of science. Biochemists exploited this opportunity by creating new courses; in the process, they lent the legitimacy of their science to the movement to upgrade medical practice. Kohler argues that employment opportunities, first in medical schools, and then in hospitals, industry, and government, were at least as important as scientific breakthroughs in establishing biochemistry.

Clinical consequences of another science, physiology, specifically concern Geison. In his tentative essay, he wonders whether doctors integrated into their practice the physiology of their medical school curricula. Physicians were skeptical of the utility of the science in their therapeutics even as physiologists boasted that their work would create a scientific medicine. Geison suggests that physiology's major contribution to medicine may actually be cultural: while its application to practice has been minimal, it has vested medicine with the special authority which science has commanded for much of the twentieth century.

Noting the central role of bacteriology in the late nineteenth century's new understanding of disease, Maulitz argues that clinicians were especially fearful that this science might subvert their healing art. Elite physicians, more exposed to bacteriology than their less educated professional colleagues, took the lead in proclaiming a rigorously scientific clinical medicine which they hoped would forestall the reorientation of medicine as a laboratory science. Maulitz, like Kohler and Geison, is concerned with how physicians and medical scientists defined their professional roles as medicine assumed its modern form.

Five essays in this volume treat medicine against the backdrop of broader social phenomena. James Reed studies the influence of social mores upon medical policy and practice in the birth control controversy. He notes that physicians generally avoided the subject of family limitation until the 1960s, even though effective birth control techniques had been widely available since the mid-nineteenth century. In refusing to inform their patients of these methods, doctors were not making abstract medical decisions; rather, they were acting as stewards of respectable society. Dependent on community support, and sharing community values, physicians left birth control activity to lay reformers, until the public perception of a world population crisis made such activity socially desirable.

Gerald N. Grob argues that the polarized interpretations of the rise of the mental hospital are both simplistic and misleading. Never simply a therapeutic institution, the asylum should not be understood as a milestone on the march of progress, an enlightened application of humane thought about insanity. Nor has social control been the primary purpose of the mental hospital. Mental illness is not, as some contemporary polemicists would have it, a set of labels designed to penalize socially disruptive behavior. The asylum must rather be viewed in the light of the multiple roles it filled in a modernizing society.

Another medical institution, the public municipal hospital, is the focus of my own essay. In the late nineteenth century, city hospitals witnessed the clash between two urban groups assertively seeking to redefine their roles and identities. Elite physicians sought to transform the hospital, until then very much an undifferentiated welfare institution, into an arena for the practice of their professional craft. Immigrant groups, exercising their new political power, demanded an institution that would be more responsive to the needs of patients, as they themselves defined those needs. The result was a creative tension in which the city hospital flourished.

Ronald L. Numbers explores the health insurance controversy. Though favorably inclined to health insurance when the issue was introduced seriously in the 1910s, American medicine—motivated by economic fears— soon took the lead in opposition. To quiet demands for compulsory federal insurance during the Great Depression, organized medicine approved both voluntary group hospitalization and medical service plans which physicians controlled. Until the 1960s, further campaigns for national health insurance were answered by the medical profession's successful advocacy of voluntary coverage. Ironically, the health benefit to patients covered by most plans, whether Blue Cross or Medicare, is less clear than the financial benefits of those plans to physicians.

A feminist perspective contributes to Janet Wilson James's examination of nursing. Concentrating biographically on Isabel Hampton, who headed the pioneer Training School for Nurses at Johns Hopkins Hospital in the late nineteenth century, James notes the difficulties encountered by nurses as they sought to establish professional standards in a context—medicine, and the hospital—within which women had very little authority. Physicians provided professional role models, but nurses had to cope with tensions generated by their attempt to create a modern occupation while not abandoning their traditionally nurturing feminine identities.

In a retrospect and prospect, Edmund D. Pellegrino considers the consequences of modern therapeutics and suggests strategies for resolving some of the dilemmas of contemporary medicine. The reductionist conceptualization of disease and treatment in terms of specificity, and the genuine curative power of many therapeutic regimens has created a very narrow and technical style of medical practice. Shunning supportive care in favor of the display of technical expertise, highly professionalized physicians may evade the moral and social responsibilities of their healing art. Further, doctors and patients are more likely to hold conflicting expectations for their encounters. We must thus recognize that the physician's role has become more ambiguous even as it has been more narrowly defined.

Medicine is not an abstraction. It is more than the sum of its intellectual content and its institutional structure. Its meaning as well as its significance to its time and place must be sought through the examination of its contextual reality. The history of medicine, as the essays in this volume demonstrate, can share in this task. By recapturing the texture of the medical past, we can formulate questions about what we expect from medicine in the present.

THE THERAPEUTIC
REVOLUTION

1 THE THERAPEUTIC REVOLUTION: Medicine, Meaning, and Social Change in Nineteenth-Century America

CHARLES E. ROSENBERG

Medical therapeutics changed remarkably little in the two millennia preceding 1800; by the end of the century, traditional therapeutics had altered fundamentally. This development is a significant event, not only in the history of medicine, but in social history as well. Yet historians have not only failed to delineate this change in detail; they have hardly begun to place it in a framework of explanation which would relate it to all those other changes which shaped the twentieth-century Western world.

Medical historians have always found therapeutics an awkward piece of business. On the whole, they have responded by ignoring it.[1] Most historians who have addressed traditional therapeutics have approached it as a source of anecdote, or as a murky bog of routinism from which a comforting path led upward to an ultimately enlightened and scientifically-based therapeutics. Isolated incidents such as the introduction of quinine or digitalis seemed only to emphasize the darkness of the traditional practice in which they appeared. Among twentieth-century students of medical history, the generally unquestioned criterion for understanding prenineteenth-century therapeutics has been physiological, not historical: did a particular practice act in a way that twentieth-century understanding would regard as efficacious? Did it work?

Yet therapeutics is after all a good deal more than a series of pharmacological or surgical experiments. It involves emotions and personal relationships, and incorporates all of those cultural factors which determine belief, identity, and status. The meaning of traditional therapeutics must be sought within a particular cultural context; and this is a task more closely akin to that of the cultural anthropologist than the physiologist. Individuals become sick, demand care and reassurance, and are treated by designated healers. Both physician and patient must necessarily share a common framework of explanation. To understand therapeutics in the opening decades of the nineteenth century, its would-be historian must see that it relates, on the one hand, to a cognitive system of explanation, and, on the other, to a patterned interaction between doctor and patient, one which evolved over centuries into a conventionalized social ritual.

Instead, however, past therapeutics has most frequently been studied by scholars obsessed with change as progress and concerned with defining such change as an essentially intellectual process. Historians have come to accept a view of nineteenth-century therapeutics which incorporates such priorities. The revolution in practice which took place during the century, the conventional argument follows, reflected the gradual triumph of a critical spirit over ancient obscurantism. The increasingly aggressive empiricism of the early nineteenth century pointed toward the need for evaluating every aspect of clinical practice; nothing was to be accepted on faith, and only those therapeutic modalities which proved themselves in controlled clinical trials were to remain in the physician's arsenal. Spurred by such arguments, increasing numbers of physicians grew sceptical of their ability to alter the course of particular ills, and by mid-century (this interpretation continues), traditional medical practice had become far milder and less intrusive than it had been at the beginning of the century. Physicians had come to place ever-increasing faith in the healing power of nature and the natural tendency toward recovery which seemed to characterize most ills.

This view of change in nineteenth-century therapeutics constitutes accepted wisdom, though it has been modified in recent years. An increasingly influential emphasis sees therapeutics as part of a more general pattern of economically motivated behavior which helped to rationalize the regular physician's place in a crowded marketplace of would-be healers.[2] Thus the competition offered by sectarians to regular medicine in the middle third of the century was at least as significant in altering traditional therapeutics as a high-culture based intellectual critique; the sugar pills of homeopathic physicians or baths and diets of hydropaths might possibly do little good, but could hardly be represented as harmful or dangerous in themselves. The often draconic treatments of regular physicians—the bleeding, the severe purges and emetics—constituted a real handicap in competing for a limited number of paying patients, and were accordingly modified to fit economic realities. Indeed, something approaching an interpretive consensus might be said to prevail in historical works of recent vintage, a somewhat eclectic, but not illogical position which views change in nineteenth-century therapeutics as proceeding both from a high-culture-based shift in ideas and the sordid realities of a precarious marketplace.

Obviously, both emphases reflect a measure of reality. But insofar as they do, they serve essentially to identify sources of instability in an ancient system of ideas and relationships; they do not explain these ideas and relationships. For neither deals with traditional therapeutics as a meaningful question in itself. As such, therapeutic practices must be seen as a central component in a particular medical system, a system characterized by remarkable tenacity over time.[3] The system must, that is, have worked, even if not in a sense immediately intelligible to a mid-twentieth-century pharmacologist or clinician. I hope in the following pages to suggest, first, the place of therapeutics in the configuration of ideas and relationships which constituted medicine at the beginning of the nineteenth century, and then the texture of the change which helped to create a very different system of therapeutics by the end of the century.

The key to understanding therapeutics at the beginning of the nineteenth century lies in seeing it as part of a system of belief and behavior participated in by physician and laymen alike. Central to the logic of this social subsystem was a deeply assumed metaphor—a particular way of looking at the body and of explaining both health and disease. The body was seen, metaphorically, as a system of dynamic interactions with its environment. Health or disease resulted from a cumulative interaction between constitutional endowment and environmental circumstance. One could not well live without food and air and water; one had to live in a particular climate, subject one's body to a particular style of life and work. Each of these factors implied a necessary and continuing physiological adjustment. The body was always in a state of becoming—and thus always in jeopardy.

Two subsidiary assumptions organized the shape of this lifelong interaction. First, every part of the body was related inevitably and inextricably with every other. A distracted mind could curdle the stomach; a dyspeptic stomach could agitate the mind. Local lesions might reflect imbalances of nutrients in the blood; systemic ills might be caused by fulminating local lesions. Thus the theoretical debates which have bemused historians of medicine over local, as opposed to systemic models of disease causation, solidistic versus humoral emphases, models based on tension or laxity of muscle fibres or blood vessels—all served the same explanatory function relative to therapeutics; all related local to systemic ills; they described all aspects of the body as interrelated; they tended to present health or disease as general states of the total organism. Second, the body was seen as a system of intake and outgo—a system which had, necessarily, to remain in balance if the individual were to remain healthy. Thus the conventional emphasis on diet and excretion, perspiration, and ventilation. Equilibrium was synonymous with health, disequilibrium with illness.

In addition to the exigencies of everyday life which might destabilize the equilibrium which constituted health, the body also had to pass through several developmental crises inherent in the design of the human organism. Menstruation and menopause in women, teething and puberty in both sexes—all represented points of potential danger, moments of structured instability, as the body established a new internal equilibrium.[4] Seasonal changes in climate constituted another kind of recurring cyclical change which might imply danger to health and require possible medical intervention: thus the ancient practice of administering cathartics in spring and fall to help the body adjust to the changed seasons. The body could be seen, that is—as in some ways it had been since classical antiquity—as a kind of stewpot, or chemico-vital reaction, proceeding calmly only if all its elements remained appropriately balanced. Randomness was minimized, but at a substantial cost in anxiety; the body was a city under constant threat of siege, and it is not surprising that early nineteenth-century Americans consumed enormous quantities of medicines as they sought to regulate assimilation and excretion.

The idea of specific disease entities played a relatively small role in such a system. Where empirical observation pointed unavoidably toward the existence of a particular disease state, physicians still sought to preserve their accustomed therapeutic role. The physician's most potent weapon was his ability to "regulate the secretions"—to extract blood, to promote the perspiration, or the urination, or defecation which attested to his having helped the body to regain its customary equilibrium. Even when a disease seemed not only to have a characteristic course, but (as in the case of smallpox) a specific causative "virus," the hypothetical pathology and indicated therapeutics were seen within the same explanatory framework.[5]

The success of inoculation and later of vaccination in preventing smallpox could not challenge this deeply internalized system of explanation. When mid-eighteenth and early nineteenth-century physicians inoculated or vaccinated, they always accompanied the procedure with an elaborate regimen of cathartics, diet, and rest. Though such elaborate medical accompaniments to vaccination might appear, from one perspective, as a calculated effort to increase the physician's fees, these preparations might better be seen as a means of assimilating an anomalous procedure into the physician's accustomed picture of health and disease.

The pedigree of these ideas can be traced to the rationalistic speculations of classical antiquity. They could hardly be superceded, for no information more accurate or schema more socially useful existed, to call them into question. Most importantly, the system provided a rationalistic framework in which the physician could at once reassure the patient and legitimate his own ministrations. It is no accident that the term "empiric" was pejorative until the mid-nineteenth century, a reference to the blind cut and try practices which regular physicians liked to think characterized their quackish competitors. The physician's own self-image and his social plausibility depended on the creation of a shared faith—a conspiracy to believe —in his ability to understand, and rationally manipulate the elements in this speculative system. This cognitive framework and the central body metaphor about which it was articulated provided a place for his prognostic, as well as his therapeutic skills; prognosis, diagnosis, and therapeutics had all to find a consistent mode of explanation.

The American physician in 1800 had no diagnostic tools beyond his senses, and it is hardly surprising that he would find congenial a framework of explanation which emphasized the importance of intake and outgo, the significance of perspiration, of pulse, of urination and menstruation, of defecation, and of the surface eruptions which might accompany fevers or other internal ills. These were phenomena which he as physician, the patient, and the patient's family could see, evaluate, and scrutinize for clues to the sick man's fate. These biological and social realities had several implications for therapeutics. Drugs had to be seen as adjusting the body's internal equilibrium; in addition, the drug's action had, if possible, to alter these visible products of the body's otherwise inscrutable internal state. Logically enough, drugs were not ordinarily viewed as specifics for particular disease entities; materia medica texts were generally arranged not by drug or disease, but in categories reflecting the drug's physiological effects: diuretics, cathartics, narcotics, emetics, diaphoretics. Quinine, for example, was ordinarily categorized as a tonic and prescribed for numerous conditions other than malaria.[6] Even when it was employed in "intermittent fever," quinine was almost invariably prescribed in conjunction with a cathartic; as in the case of vaccination, a drug with a disease-specific efficacy ill-suited to the assumptions of the physician's underlying cognitive framework was assimilated to it. (Significantly, the advocacy of a specific drug in treating a specific ill was ordinarily viewed by regular physicians as a symptom of quackery.)

The effectiveness of the system hinged to a significant extent on the fact that all the weapons in the physician's normal armamentarium worked: "worked," that is, by providing visible and predictable physiological effects; purges purged, emetics vomited, opium soothed pain and moderated diarrhoea. Bleeding, too, seemed obviously to alter the body's internal balance, as evidenced both by a changed pulse and the very quantity of the blood drawn.[7] Blisters and other purposefully induced local irritations certainly produced visible effects—and presumably internal consequences proportional to their pain, location, and to the nature and extent of the matter discharged.[8] Not only did a drug's activity indicate to both physician and patient the nature of its efficacy (and the physician's competence) but it provided a prognostic tool, as well; for the patient's response to a drug could indicate much about his condition, while examination of the product elicited—urine, feces, blood, perspiration—could shed light on the body's internal state. Thus, for example, a patient could report to her physician that

> the buf on my blood was of a blewish Cast and at the edge of the buf it appeared to be curded something like milk and cyder curd after standing an hour or two the water that came on the top was of a yellowish cast.[9]

The patient's condition could be monitored each day as the doctor sought to guide its course to renewed health.

The body seemed, moreover, to rid itself of disease in ways parallel to those encouraged or elicited by drug action. The profuse sweat, diarrhoea, or skin lesions often accompanying fevers, for example, all seemed stages in a necessary course of natural recovery. The remedies he employed, the physician could assure his patients, only acted in imitation of nature:

> Blood-letting and blisters find their archtypes in spontaneous haemmorrhage and those sero-plastic exudations that occur in some stage of almost every acute inflammation; emetics, cathartics, diuretics, diaphoretics, etc. etc. have each and all of them effects in every way similar to those arising spontaneously in disease.[10]

Medicine could provoke or facilitate, but not alter, the fundamental patterns of recovery inherent in the design of the human organism.

This same explanatory framework illuminates as well the extraordinary vogue of mercury in early nineteenth-century therapeutics. If employed for a sufficient length of time and in sufficient quantity, mercury induced a series of progressively severe and cumulative physiological effects: first, diarrhoea, and ultimately, full-blown symptoms of mercury poisoning. The copious involuntary salivation characteristic of this toxic state was seen as proof that the drug was exerting an "alterative" effect—that is, altering the fundamental balance of forces and substances which constituted the body's ultimate reality. Though other drugs, most prominently arsenic, antimony, and iodine, were believed able to exert such an "alterative" effect, mercury seemed particularly useful because of the seemingly unequivocal relationship between varying dosage levels and its consequent action (and the convenient fact that it could be administered either orally or as a salve).[11] Moderate doses aided the body in its normal healing pattern, while in larger doses, giving mercury could be seen as a forceful intervention in pathological states which had a doubtful prognosis. Mercury was, in this sense, the physician's most flexible, and, at the same time, most powerful weapon for treating ailments in which active intervention might mean the difference between life and death. In such cases he needed a drug with which he might alter a course toward death—one stronger than those with which he routinely modified the secretions and excretions in less severe ailments.

Both physician and layman shared a similar view of the manner in which the body functioned, and the nature of available therapeutic modalities reinforced that view. The secretions could be regulated, a plethoric state of the blood abated, the stomach emptied of a content potentially dangerous. Recovery must, of course, often have coincided with the administration of a particular drug and thus provided an inevitable post hoc endorsement of its effectiveness. A physician could typically describe a case of pleurisy as having been "suddenly relieved by profuse perspiration" elicited by the camphor he had prescribed.[12] Fevers seemed, in fact, often to be healed by the purging effects of mercury or antimony. Drugs reassured insofar as they acted, and their efficacy was inevitably underwritten by the natural tendency toward recovery which characterized most ills. Therapeutics thus played a central role within the system of interaction between doctor and patient; on the cognitive level, therapeutics confirmed the physician's ability to understand and intervene in the ongoing physiological processes which defined health and disease; on the emotional level, the very severity of drug action assured the patient and his family that something was indeed being done.

In the medical idiom of 1800, "exhibiting" a drug was synonymous with administering it (and the administration of drugs so routine that "prescribing for" was synonymous with seeing a patient). The use of the term *exhibit* was hardly accidental. For the therapeutic interaction we have sought to describe was a fundamental cultural ritual, in a literal sense—a ritual in which the legitimating element was, in part at least, a shared commitment to a rationalistic model of pathology and therapeutic action. Therapeutics served as a pivotal link in a stylized interaction between doctor and patient, encompassing organically (the pun is unfortunate but apposite) the cognitive and the emotional within a framework of rationalistic explanation.[13] To "exhibit" a drug was to act out a sacramental role in a liturgy of healing. The analogy to religious ritual is not exact, but it is certainly more than metaphorical. A sacrament, after all, is conventionally defined as an external, visible symbol of an invisible, internal state. Insofar as a particular drug caused a perceptible physiological effect, it produced phenomena which all —the physician, the patient, and the patient's family—could witness (again the double meaning, with its theological overtones, is instructive), and in which all could participate.

This was a liturgy calculated for the sickroom, of course, not for church. And indeed, the efficacy and tenacity of this sytem must be understood in relation to its social setting. Most such therapeutic tableaux took place in the patient's home, and thus the healing ritual could mobilize all of those community and emotional forces which anthropologists have seen as fundamental, in their observations of medical practice in traditional, non-Western societies. Healing, in early nineteenth-century America, was in the great majority of cases physically and emotionally embedded in a precise, emotionally resonant context. The cognitive aspects of this system of explanation, as well, were appropriate to the world view of such a community. The model of the body, and of health and disease, which we have described was all-inclusive, antireductionist, capable of incorporating every aspect of man's life in explaining his physical condition. Just as man's body interacted continuously with his environment, so did his mind with his body, his morals with his health. The realm of causation in medicine was not distinguishable from the realm of meaning in society generally.

There was no inconsistency between this world of rationalistic explanation and traditional spiritual values. Few Americans in the first third of the century felt any conflict between these realms of reassurance. If drugs failed, this expressed merely the ultimate power of God, and constituted no reason to question the truth of either system of belief. Let me quote the words of a pious mid-century physician who sought in his diary to come to terms with the dismaying and unexpected death of a child he had been treating; "the child seemed perfectly well," the troubled physician explained,

> till it was attacked at the tea table. Remedies, altho' slow in their action, acted well, but were powerless to avert the arm of death. The decrees of Providence . . . cannot be set aside. Man is mortal, and tho' remedies often seem to act promptly and effectually to the saving of life—they often fail in an unaccountable manner! "So teach me to number my days that I may apply my heart unto wisdom."[14]

The Lord might give and the Lord take away—but until he did, the physician dared not remain passive in the face of those dismaying signs of sickness which caused his patient anxiety and pain.

The physician's art, in the opening decades of the nineteenth century, centered on his ability to employ an appropriate drug, or combination of drugs and bleeding, to produce a particular physiological effect. This explains the apparent anomaly of physicians employing different drugs to treat the same condition; each drug, the argument followed, was equally legitimate, so long as it produced the desired physiological effect. The selection of a proper drug or drugs was no mean skill, authorities explained, for each patient possessed a unique physiological identity, and the experienced physician had to evaluate a bewildering variety of factors, ranging from climatic conditions to age and sex, in the compounding of any particular prescription. A physician who knew a family's constitutional idiosyncracies was necessarily a better practitioner for that family than one who enjoyed no such insight—or even one who hailed from a different climate, for it was assumed that both the action of drugs and reaction of patients varied with season and geography.[15] The physician had to be aware, as well, that the same drug in different dosages might produce different effects. Fifteen grams of ipecac, a young Southern medical student cautioned himself, acted as an emetic, five induced sweating, while smaller doses could serve as a useful tonic.[16]

The same rationalistic mechanisms which explained recovery explained failure as well. One could not predict recovery in every case; even the most competent physician could only do that which the limited resources of medicine allowed—and the natural course of some ills was toward death. The treatment indicated for tuberculosis, as an ancient adage put it, was opium and lies. Cancer, too, was normally incurable; some states of disequilibrium could not be righted.

Early nineteenth-century American physicians unquestionably believed in the therapeutics they practiced. Physicians routinely prescribed severe cathartics and bleeding for themselves, and for their wives and children. A New England physician settling in Camden, South Carolina, for example, depended for health in this treacherous climate upon his accustomed cathartic pills. "Took two of the pills last night," he recorded in his diary; "they have kept me busy thro' the day and I now feel like getting clear of my headache."[17] Even when physicians felt some anxiety in particular cases, they could take assurance from the knowledge that they were following a mode of practice endorsed by rational understanding and centuries of clinical experience. A young New York City physician, in 1795, for example, felt such doubts after having bled and purged a critically ill patient:

> I began to fear that I had carried the debilitating plan too far. By degrees I became reassured; and when I reflected on his youth, constitution, his uniform temperance, on the one hand; and on the fidelity with which I had adhered to those modes of practice recommended by the most celebrated physicians, on the other, I felt a conviction that accident alone, could wrest him from me.[18]

Such conviction was a necessary element in medical practice; without belief, the system could hardly have functioned.

Individuals from almost every level in society accepted, in one fashion or another, the basic outlines of the world-view which we have described. Evidence of such belief among the less articulate is not abundant, but it does exist. Patients, for example, understood that a sudden interruption of perspiration might cause cold or even pneumonia, that such critical periods as teething, puberty, or menopause were particularly dangerous. The metabolic gyroscope which controlled the balance of forces within the body was delicate indeed, and might easily be thrown off balance. Thus it was natural for servants and laborers reporting the symptoms of their fevers to an almshouse physician to ascribe their illnesses to a sudden stoppage of the perspiration.[19] It was equally natural for young ladies complaining of amenorrhea to ascribe it to a sudden chill. The sudden interruption of any natural evacuation would presumably jeopardize the end implicit in that function; if the body did not need to perspire in certain circumstances, or discharge menstrual blood at intervals, it would not be doing so.[20] These were mechanisms through which the body maintained its health-defining equilibrium—and could thus be interrupted only at great peril.

Such considerations dictated modes of treatment, as well as views of disease causation. If, for example, the normal course of a disease to recovery involved the formation of a skin lesion, the physician must not intervene too aggressively and interrupt the process through which the body sought to rid itself of offending matter. Thus a student could record his professor's warning against the premature "exhibition" of tonics in a continued fever; such stimulants were "highly prejudicial they lock in the disease instead of liberating it from the system. After evacuations have been premised," the young man continued, "then the tonic medicine may be employed."[21] Yet physicians assumed that fevers normally accompanied by skin lesions could not "find resolution" without an appropriately bountiful crop of such blisters; and if they seemed dilatory in erupting, the physician might appropriately turn to blisters and counterirritation in an effort to encourage them. To "drive them inward," on the other hand, was to invite far graver illness. In such ailments it was the physician's task to prescribe mild cathartics, in an effort to aid the body in its efforts to expel the morbid material. Mercury, for example, might be desirable in small doses but perilous in "alterative" ones. In any case, however, it was the physician's primary responsibility to "regulate or restore" the normal secretions whenever they were interrupted; chronic constipation, or diarrhoea, or irregular menstruation similarly implied active steps on the physician's part. In constipation, mild cathartics were routine; in amenorrhea, drugs to restore the flow (emmenagogues) were indicated. (The use of emmenagogues could represent an ethical dilemma to physicians who feared being imposed upon by seemingly innocent young ladies who sought abortifacients under the guise of a desire to restore the normal menstrual cycle interrupted by some cause other than pregnancy.)[22]

The widespread faith in emetics, cathartics, diuretics, and bleeding is evidenced, as well, by their prominent place in folk medicine. Domestic and irregular practice, that is, like regular medicine, was shaped about the eliciting of predictable physiological responses; home remedies mirrored the heroic therapeutics practiced by regular physicians. In the fall of 1826, for example, when a Philadelphia tallow chandler fell ill, he complained of chills, pains in the head and back, weakness in the joints, and nausea. Then, before seeing a regular physician, he

> was bled till symptoms of fainting came on. Took an emetic, which operated well. For several days after, kept his bowels moved with Sulph. Soda, Senna tea etc. He then employed a Physician who prescribed another Emetic, which operated violently and whose action was kept up by drinking bitter tea.[23]

Only after two more days did he appear at the Alms-House Hospital. Physicians sceptical of traditional therapeutics complained repeatedly of lay expectations which worked against change; medical men might well be subject to criticism if they should, for example, fail to bleed in the early stages of pneumonia. Parents often demanded that physicians incise the inflammed gums of their teething infants so as to provoke a "resolution" of this developmental crisis. Laymen could, indeed, be even more importunate in their demands for an aggressive therapy than the physicians attending them thought appropriate. The indications for bleeding, for example, were carefully demarcated in formal medical thought, yet laymen often demanded it even when the state of the pulse and general condition of the patient contraindicated loss of blood. Some patients demanded, as well as expected, the administration of severe cathartics or emetics; they suspected peril in too languid a therapeutic regimen.

Botanic alternatives to regular medicine in the first third of the century were also predicated upon the routine use of severe cathartics and emetics, of vegetable origin. (In the practice of Thomsonian physicians, the most prominent organized botanic sect, such drugs were supplemented by sweat-baths designed, in theory, to adjust the body's internal heat through the eliciting of copious perspiration.)[24] Botanic physicians shared many of the social problems faced by their regular competitors; they dealt with the same emotional realities implicit in the doctor-patient relationship, and in doing so appealed to a similar framework of physiological assumption.

Nevertheless, there were differences of approach among physicians, and in the minds of a good many laymen who questioned both the routinism and the frequent severity of traditional therapeutics. (The criticisms which greeted the atypically severe bleeding and purging advocated by Benjamin Rush are familiar to any student of the period.) America, in 1800, was in many ways already a modern society, diverse in religion, in class, and in ethnic background. It would be naive to contend that the unity of vision which presumably, united most traditional non-Western cultures in their orientation toward particular medical systems could apply to this diverse and changing culture. Yet, as we have argued, there were surprisingly large areas of agreement. Even those Americans sceptical of therapeutic excess and inconsistency (and, in some cases, more generally of the physician's authority) did not question the fundamental structure of the body metaphor which I have described, however much they may have doubted the possible efficacy of medical intervention in sickness.[25]

In describing American medical therapeutics in the first quarter of the nineteenth century we have been examining a system already marked by signs of instability. Fundamental to this instability was rationalism itself. A key legitimating aspect of the traditional cognitive model was its rationalistic form (even if we regard that rationalism as egregiously speculative); yet by 1800, this structure of explanation was tied irrevocably to the institutions and findings of world science. And as this world changed, and provided data and procedures increasingly relevant to the world of clinical medicine, it gradually undercut that harmony between world-view and personal interaction which had characterized therapeutics at the opening of the century.

By the 1830s, criticism of traditional therapeutics had become a cliché in sophisticated medical circles; physicians of any pretension spoke of self-limited diseases, of scepticism in regard to the physician's ability to intervene and change the course of most diseases, of respect for the healing powers of nature. This point of view emphasized the self-limiting nature of most ailments, and the physician's duty simply to aid the process of natural recovery through appropriate, and minimally heroic means. "It would be better," as Oliver Wendell Holmes put it, in his usual acerbic fashion, "if the patient were allowed a certain discount from his bill for every dose he took, just as children are compensated by their parents for swallowing hideous medicinal mixtures."[26] Rest, a strengthening diet, or a mild cathartic were all the aid nature required in most ills. In those ailments whose natural tendency was toward death, the physician had to acknowledge his powerlessness and simply try to minimize pain and anxiety. This noninterventionist position was accompanied by increasing acceptance of the parallel view that most diseases could be seen as distinct clinical entities, each with a characteristic cause, course, and symptomatology.

These positions are accepted by most historians as reflecting the fundamental outline for the debate over therapeutics in the middle third of the nineteenth century. And, as a matter of fact, it does describe a significant aspect of change—the influence of high-culture ideas and of a small opinion-forming group in gradually modifying the world-view of a much larger group of practitioners and, ultimately, of laymen. But when we try to evaluate the impact of such therapeutic admonitions on the actual practice of physicians, realities become a good deal more complex. Medical practice was conducted at a number of levels—intellectual, economic, and regional—but demonstrated in each the extraordinary tenacity of traditional views.

American physicians were tied to the everyday requirements of the doctor-patient relationship and thus, even among the teaching elite, no mid-century American practitioner rejected conventional therapeutics with a ruthless consistency. The self-confident empiricism which denied the efficacy of any therapeutic measure not proven efficacious in clinical trials seemed an ideological excess suited to a handful of European academics, not to the realities of practice. It is no accident that the radically sceptical position was christened "therapeutic nihilism" by its critics. Nihilism, with its echoes of disbelief and destructive change, of "total rejection of current religious beliefs and morals" (to borrow a defining phrase from the *Oxford English Dictionary*) was not chosen as a term of casual abuse, but represented precisely the gravity of the challenge to a traditional world-view implied by a relentless empiricism, and by the materialism which seemed so often to accompany it.

There were enduring virtues in the old ways. "There is," as one leader in the profession explained, "a vantage ground between the two extremes, neither verging towards meddlesome interference on the one hand, nor imbecile neglect on the other."[27] The physician had to contend, moreover, with patient expectations: "the public," as another prominent clinician put it, "expect something more of physicians than the power of distinguishing diseases and of predicting their issue. They look to them for the relief of their sufferings, and the cure or removal of their complaints."[28]

The physician still had to create an emotionally, as well as intellectually meaningful therapeutic regimen; and throughout the middle third of the nineteenth century, this meant the administration of drugs capable of eliciting a perceptible physiological response. No mid-century physician doubted the efficacy of placebos (as little as he doubted that the effectiveness of a drug could depend on his own manner and attitude), but in a grave illness the physician's own awareness of their inertness made it impossible for him to rely on sugar or bread pills and the healing power of nature. One medical man, for example, after conceding the uselessness of every available therapeutic means in cholera, still contended that "a noble profession whose aims and purpose are the preservation of human life, should not be content with anything short of the adoption of remedial measures for so fatal a disease, which promise positive and beneficent results in every individual case."[29] Hospital case records indicate that even elite physicians maintained a more than lingering faith in cathartic drugs throughout the middle third of the century. (And in hospital practice, economic considerations could have played no role in the doctor's willingness to prescribe.)

Physicians shaped a number of intellectual compromises in order to maintain such continuity with traditional therapeutic practice. Despite the growing plausibility of views emphasizing disease specificity, for example, most physicians still maintained an emphasis on their traditional ability to modify symptoms. The older assumption that drugs acted in a way consistent with the body's innate pattern of recovery was easily shifted toward new emphases; the physician's responsibility now centered on recognizing the natural course of his patient's ailment and supporting the body in its progress to renewed health with an appropriate combination of drugs and regimen; even the course of a self-limited disease might be shortened, its painful symptoms mitigated. The secretions had still to be regulated, diet specified and modified, perhaps a plethora of blood lessened by cupping or leeching. Even in ills whose natural course was to death, the physician might still avail himself of therapeutic means to ease that grim journey. Finally, no one doubted, there were ailments in which the physician's intervention could make the difference between life and death; scurvy, for example, was often cited as a disease "that taints the whole system, [yet] yields to a mere change in diet."[30] The surgeon still had to set bones, remove foreign bodies, drain abscesses.

Second, even an explicit affirmation of the natural tendency to recovery, in most ills, did not obviate the place of traditional views of the body in explaining that recovery. Physicians, for example, spoke habitually of "vital power" and the need to support that vitality if the natural healing tendency were to manifest itself. The body could, that is, still be seen in traditional holistic terms, "vital power" constituting the sum of all its internal realities, and, by implication, a reflection of the body's necessary transactions with its environment. The use of the term *vital power* suggests, moreover, how deeply committed the medical profession still was to the communication of meaning through metaphor—in this case, a metaphor incorporating a shorthand version of the age-old view of the body which we have outlined, yet appearing in the necessary guise of scientific truth.

The decades between 1850 and 1870 did see an increased emphasis on diet and regimen among regular physicians, most strikingly a vogue for the use of alcoholic beverages as stimulants. It is hardly surprising that one reaction to the varied criticisms of traditional therapeutics was the acceptance of a "strengthening and stimulating" emphasis in practice; the new emphasis responded not only to criticisms by sectarian healers of "depleting" measures, such as bleeding and purging, but preserved an active role for the physician within the same framework of attitudes toward the body which had always helped order the doctor-patient relationship.

Practice changed a good deal less than the rhetoric surrounding it would suggest. "Nature," a South Carolina medical man explained to a patient troubled by a "derangement of the Abdominal organs," in 1850, "must restore their natural condition by gradually building them up anew, and time is necessary for the accomplishment of this." But, the physician continued, drug treatment was appropriate as well:

> The Medicinal treatment is to aid nature, by correcting irregularities and meeting untoward symptoms as they may occur. The Medicinal treatment consisted of an Alterative course of Tonics, chiefly Metallic, not Mercurial—

so combined with Laxatives as to regulate the Secretions of the Digestive organs.[31]

Less aggressive than it might have been a generation earlier, such a course of treatment still allowed the physician an active role.

The inertia of traditional practice was powerful indeed; older modes of therapeutics did not die, but, as we have suggested, were employed less routinely, and drugs were used in generally smaller doses. Dosage levels decreased markedly in the second third of the century, and bleeding, especially, sank into disuse. The resident physician at the Philadelphia Dispensary could, for example, report, in 1862, that of a total of 9,502 patients treated that year, "general blood-letting has been resorted to in one instance only, . . . cupping twelve times and leeching thrice."[32] Residents at Bellevue in New York and at Boston's Massachusetts General Hospital had reported the previous year that bloodletting was "almost obsolete."[33] Mercury, on the other hand, still figured in the practice of most physicians; even infants and small children endured the discomfort of mercury poisoning until well after the Civil War. Purges were still administered routinely in spring and fall to facilitate the body's adjustment to the changing seasons. The blisters and excoriated running sores so familiar to physicians and patients at the beginning of the century were gradually replaced by mustard plasters or turpentine applications, but the ancient concept of counterirritation still rationalized their use. Even bleeding still lingered, though increasingly in the practice of older men, and in less cosmopolitan areas. To divest themselves of such reliable means of regulating the body's internal equilibrium was, older physicians contended, to succumb to an intellectual fad with no compensation other than a morally irresponsible, if intellectually modish emphasis on the healing powers of nature. It seemed to many physicians almost criminal to ignore their responsibility to regulate the secretions, even in ailments whose natural course was toward either death or recovery. Hence the continued vogue of cathartics and diuretics (though emetics, like bleeding, faded in popularity as the century progressed).

The debate over therapeutics was characterized more by moderation than by a full-fledged commitment to either the old, or to the new and radically sceptical. Few physicians occupied either of these extreme positions. In the intellectual realm as well as in that of practice, clinicians sought, in a number of ways, to insure the greatest possible degree of continuity with older ideas. When smaller doses seemed as efficacious as those heroic prescriptions they had employed in their youth, it could be explained as a consequence of change in the prevailing pattern of disease incidence and perhaps even in the constitution of Americans.[34] More fundamentally, most physicians still found it difficult to accept the reductionist implications of the view that disease ordinarily manifests itself in the form of discrete clinical entities, with unique causes, courses, and pathologies. Physicians still spoke of epidemic influences, of diarrhoeas shifting into cholera, of minor fevers efflorescing into typhoid or yellow fever, if improperly managed.[35] The system was rich in confirmatory evidence; did not cases of "incipient" yellow fever and cholera recover, if treated in timely fashion? Traditionalists still found it natural to speak of general constitutional states—sthenic or asthenic—as underlying the symptomatology of particular ills or the response of the body to particular drugs. Drugs, on the other hand, were still assumed to reflect the influence of climate in their action. Man was still an organism reacting unceasingly, and at countless levels, with its environment.

Perhaps most significantly, even those who were most radical in their criticisms of traditional routinism and severity of dosage still emphasized that the physician's therapeutic effectiveness depended, to a good extent, on his familiarity with the patient's constitutional idiosyncrasies. "No two patients have the same constitutional or mental proclivities," the *Boston Medical and Surgical Journal* editorialized in 1883: "No two instances of typhoid fever or of any other disease, are precisely alike. No "rule of thumb," no recourse to a formula-book, will avail for the treatment even of the typical diseases."[36]

Indeed, it was not until the very end of the nineteenth century that an outspoken and thoroughgoing therapeutic scepticism came actually to be pronounced from some of America's most prestigious medical chairs. "In some future day," as one authority put it,

> it is certain that drugs and chemicals will form no part of a scientific therapy. This is sure to be the case, for truth is finally certain to prevail. . . . The principal influence or relation of materia medica to the cure of bodily disease lies in the fact that drugs supply material upon which to rest the mind while other agencies are at work in eliminating disease from the system, and to the drug is frequently given the credit. . . . Sugar of milk tablets of various colors and different flavors constitute a materia medica in practice that needs for temporary use only, morphin, codein, cocain, aconite and a laxative to make it complete.[37]

A dozen drugs, a Hopkins clinician argued, "suffice for the pharmacotherapeutic armamentarium of some of the most eminent physicians on this continent."[38] Not surprisingly, the sometimes aggressive depreciation of therapeutic routinism by such leaders in the profession as William Osler or Richard Cabot still provoked aggressive counterattack. "Expectant treatment," Abraham Jacobi contended bitterly, in 1908, "is too often a combination of indolence and ignorance. . . . Expectant treatment is no treatment. It is the sin of omission, which not infrequently rises to the dignity of a crime."[39] Not all medical men were willing or able to accept the newer kind of reassurance which characterized the world of scientific medicine.

Indeed, many nineteenth-century American physicians were keenly aware of a potential inconsistency between the demands of science and those of clinical practice—and, by implication, of humanity. This perceived conflict had a pedigree extending backward to at least the presidency of Andrew Jackson, while it is hardly a moot question today. The debate over therapeutics naturally reflected this conflict of values. "The French have departed too much from the method of Sydenham and Hippocrates to make themselves good practitioners," an indignant New York physician complained in 1836. "They are tearing down the temple of medicine to lay its foundations anew. . . . They lose more in Therapeutics than they gain by morbid anatomy—They are explaining how men die but not how to cure them."[40] To some American medical teachers, the newly critical demands of the Paris Clinical School and its emphasis on reevaluating traditional therapeutics in the light of "numerical" standards seemed almost antisocial, a reversion to a sterile and demeaning empiricism.

> The practice of medicine according to this view, is entirely empirical, it is shorn of all rational induction, and takes a position among the lower grades of experimental observations, and fragmentary facts.[41]

The polarization of values implied by such observations grew only more intense in the second half of the century, as traditionally oriented physicians expressed their resentment of a fashionable worship of things German, and what they felt to be a disdain for clinical acumen. The appeal of the laboratory and its transcendent claims seemed to many clinicians a dangerous will-o-the-wisp. Even S. Weir Mitchell, one-time experimental physiologist, could charge that "out of the false pride of the laboratory and the scorn with which the accurate man of science looks down upon medical indefiniteness, has arisen the worse evil of therapeutic nihilism."[42] The danger, as another prominent chairholder put it, was that young men, "allured by the glitter of scientific work, will neglect the important and really more difficult attainments of true professional studies."[43] To some extent, of course, this was a conflict between the elite and the less favored; but it was, as well, a clash of temperament and world-view within America's medical elite. Willingness to accept the emotional and epistemological transcendence of science, even at the expense of traditional clinical standards, provided an emotional fault line which marked the profession throughout the last two-thirds of the century and paralleled the kind of change and conflict implied by modernization in other areas of society.

In the second half of the twentieth century, the relationship between doctor and patient is much altered; its context has, in the great majority of cases, shifted from the home to some institutional setting. The healer is in many cases unknown, or known only casually, to the patient. Even the place of drug therapeutics has changed, changed not only in the sense that the efficacy of most drugs is beginning to be understood, but in the social ambience which surrounds their use. The patient still maintains a faith in the physician's prescription (often, indeed, demands such a prescription) but it is a rather different kind of faith than that which shaped the interaction of physician, patient, and therapeutics at the beginning of the nineteenth century.

Clearly the physician and the great majority of his patients no longer share a similar view of the body and the mechanisms which determine health and disease. Differing views of the body and the physician's ability to intervene in its mysterious opacity divide groups and individuals, rather than unifying, as the widely disseminated metaphorical view of body function had still done in 1800. Physician and patient are no longer bound together by the physiological activity of the drugs administered. In a sense, almost *all* drugs now act as placebos, for with the exception of certain classes of drugs, such as diuretics, the patient experiences no perceptible physiological effect. He does ordinarily have faith in the efficacy of a particular therapy, but it is a faith based not on a shared nexus of belief and participation in the kind of experience we have described, but rather on confidence in the physician and his imputed status, and, indirectly, in that of science itself. Obviously, one can draw facile parallels to many other areas in which an older community of world-view and personal relationship has been replaced by a more fragmented and status oriented reality. Such observations have become commonplace, as we try to ascertain the shape of a gradually emerging modernity in the nineteenth-century West.

It is less easy to evaluate the moral implications of such change, and its existential meaning for the participants in the healing ritual. Our generation is tempted by an easy romanticization of the loss of community; it would be tempting, that is, to bewail the destruction of a traditional medicine, of a nexus of shared belief and assured relationship. Clearly we have lost something; or, to be more accurate, something has changed. But it would be arrogant indeed to dismiss the objective virtues of modern medicine with the charge that it is somehow less meaningful emotionally than it was in 1800. For after all, if we have created new dimensions of misery through technology, we have allayed others. To the historian familiar with nineteenth-century medicine and conditions of life, it would be naive indeed to dismiss the compensatory virtues of twentieth-century medicine—its humane failings notwithstanding.

NOTES

This discussion is abstracted from a larger projected history of medical care in America between 1790 and 1910. I would like to acknowledge the support of the Rockefeller Foundation during the academic year 1976–77. I should also like to acknowledge the advice and encouragement given to me over many years by my teachers Erwin H. Ackerknecht and the late Ludwig Edelstein. My colleagues Drew Gilpin Faust, Saul Jarcho, Owsei Temkin, and Anthony F. C. Wallace read the manuscript carefully and made a number of important suggestions. A somewhat different version of this paper appeared in Perspectives in Biology and Medicine *20 (1977): 485–506.*

1. For examples of work which try to place traditional therapeutics in a more general framework, see Erwin H. Ackerknecht, "Aspects of the History of Therapeutics," *Bulletin of the History of Medicine* 36 (1962): 389–419 and his *Therapie von den Primitiven bis zum 20. Jahrhundert* (Stuttgart: Ferdinand Enke, 1970), and Owsei Temkin, "Therapeutic Trends and the Treatment of Syphilis before 1900," *Bulletin of the History of Medicine* 29 (1955): 309–16.

2. For an example of this position, see William Rothstein, *American Physicians in the Nineteenth Century. From Sects to Science* (Baltimore and London: The Johns Hopkins Press, 1972).

3. Within the meaning of the term *therapeutics,* I include any measures utilized by physicians or laymen in hopes of ameliorating or curing the felt symptoms of illness. In the great majority of instances this implied the administration of some drug, but might often include bleeding, and alterations in diet or other aspects of life style. This paper avoids the question of surgery and its place in the cognitive system which explained nonsurgical therapeutic practices.

4. For a more detailed discussion of one such cyclical crisis, see Carroll Smith-Rosenberg, "Puberty to Menopause: The Cycle of Femininity in Nineteenth-Century America," *Feminist Studies* 1 (1973): 58–72.

5. In some ways, it should be emphasized, constitutional ills fit more easily into this model than the acute infectious—and especially epidemic—ills. Cancer or tuberculosis, for example, could naturally be seen as resulting from long-term problems of assimilation. Acute and especially epidemic diseases seemed more sharply defined in time and, ordinarily, in their courses; nevertheless, the pathological mechanisms which caused the symptoms constituting the disease were still represented in terms similar to those we have described.

6. Digitalis was, similarly, categorized as a diuretic and prescribed in many cases in which the edema which indicated its employment was unrelated to a cardiac pathology.

7. The rapid fluid loss in severe bloodletting or purging might indeed lower temperature, while extremely copious bloodletting quieted agitation, as well!

8. The vogue of blisters, plasters and other purposeful excoriation or irritation of the skin was related, as well, to the prevailing physiological assumptions concerning the interdependence of all parts of the body, and the necessary balancing of forces which determined health or disease. Thus, for example, the popularity of "counterirritation," in the form of skin lesions induced by the physician through chemical or mechanical means, was based on the assumption that the excoriation of one area and consequent suppuration could "attract" the "morbid excitement" from another site to the newly excoriated one, while the exudate was significant in possibly allowing the body an opportunity to rid itself of morbid matter, and of righting the disease-producing internal imbalance. Such a path to healing could follow natural, as well as artificial lesions. "Every physician of experience," one contended as late as 1862, "can recall cases of internal affections, which, after the use of a great variety of medicines, have been unexpectedly relieved by an eruption on the skin: or of ailments of years' continuance, which have been permanently cured by the formation of a large abscess." John P. Spooner, *The Different Modes of Treating Disease: Or The Different Action of Medicines on the System in an Abnormal State* (Boston: David Clapp, 1862), p. 17.

9. Mary Ballard to Charles Brown, 12 May 1814, Charles Brown Papers, College of William and Mary, Williamsburg, Virginia.

10. E.B. Haskins, *Therapeutic Cultivation; Its Errors and its Reformation; An Address delivered to the Tennessee Medical Society, April 7, 1857* (Nashville, Tenn.: Cameron and Fall, 1857), p. 22.

11. Bleeding in a single large quantity was also seen as exerting such an alterative effect (and thus might be indicated where a number of smaller bleedings would have the opposite and undesirable effect). The term *alterative* was, in addition, most frequently associated with the treatment of long-standing constitutional ills, in the words of one physician, "subverting any vitiated habit of body or morbid diathesis existing." Samuel Hobson, *An Essay on The History; Preparation and Therapeutic Uses of Iodine* (Philadelphia: The Author, 1830), p. 22n.

12. Benjamin H. Coates, Practice Book, entry for 25 February 1836, Historical Society of Pennsylvania, Philadelphia, Pa.

13. For parallel discussion of medical explanation in relation to cosmology and symbolic form, see: Victor Turner, *The Forest of Symbols: Aspects of Ndembu Ritual* (Ithaca: Cornell University Press, 1967); Mary Douglas, *Purity and Danger. An Analysis of Concepts of Pollution and Taboo* (London: Routledge and Kegan Paul, 1966); Douglas, *Natural Symbols, Explorations in Cosmology* (New York: Pantheon, 1970).

14. Diary of Samuel W. Butler, 25 July 1852, Historical Collections, College of Physicians of Philadelphia.

15. As Benjamin Rush could explain to an English correspondent, for example: "The extremes of heat and cold, by producing greater extremes of violence in our fevers than in yours, call for more depletion, and from more outlets, than the fevers of Great Britain." Rush to John Coakley Lettsom, 13 May 1804, L.H. Butterfield, ed., *Letters of Benjamin Rush*, 2 vols. (Princeton, N.J.: American Philosophical Society, 1951), 2: 881.

16. Anonymous notebook, Materia Medica Lectures of John P. Emmett, University of Virginia, 1834–36, Perkins Library, Duke University, Durham, N.C.

17. The "busy" referred to the "operation" of the drug, not to the physician's schedule! Diary of William Blanding 4 July 1807, South Caroliniana Library, University of South Carolina, Columbia, S.C. As usual, Benjamin Rush was particularly enthusiastic. "Ten of my family have been confined with remitting fevers," he wrote to John Redman Coxe on 5 October 1795. "Twenty-four bleedings in one month have cured us all. I submitted to two of them in one day. Our infant of 6

weeks old was likewise bled twice, and thereby rescued from the grave." *Letters,* 2: 763.

18. Entry for 18 September 1795. *The Diary of Elihu Hubbard Smith (1771–1798)* (Philadelphia: American Philosophical Society, 1973), p. 59.

19. Such comments were made to examining physicians: for example, by laborer James McSherry, thirty-nine, and houseworker Sarah Mullin, nineteen, at the Philadelphia Alms-house, Hospital Casebook, 1824–27, Records of the Board of Guardians of the Poor, Philadelphia City Archives.

20. The logic of the system is usefully illustrated by the assumption that suppressed menstruation would cause a plethora, or superabundance of blood. During pregnancy, it was believed that the blood was utilized by the developing embryo, during lactation, by the body's need to produce milk for the nursling. If the mother became ill and the infant stopped nursing, a student in David Hosack's lectures noted during the winter of 1822–23, the lancet might be needed to "take off" the "plethora induced by the stoppage of the monthly discharge." J. Barratt, Medical Notebook, Lecture 49th, South Carolinian Library, University of South Carolina, Columbia, S.C. "A partial suppression of the menses," a housepupil at the Philadelphia Alms-House noted in 1825, "is sometimes the cause of Plethora. Give first an emetic of ipecac and then a laxative." Unpaged medical notebook in the Nathan Hatfield Papers, Historical Collections, College of Physicians of Philadelphia.

21. Abraham Bitner, "Notes taken from the Philadelphia Alms-House, Nvr. 1824," p. 3. Historical Collections, College of Physicians of Philadelphia.

22. Pious physicians sometimes found it difficult to balance their professional desire to restore a normal menstrual flow against a fear of being placed in the position of inducing abortion. For an example, see Diary of R. P. Little, 28 November 1842, Trent Collection, Duke University Medical Library, Durham, N.C.

23. Case of George Devert, 15 November 1826, Hospital Casebook, 1824–27, Philadelphia City Archives.

24. The most detailed account of the Thomsonian movement is still that by Alex Berman, "The Impact of the Nineteenth-century Botanico-Medical Movement in American Pharmacy and Medicine," (Ph.D. diss., University of Wisconsin, 1954); Berman, "The Thomsonian Movement and its Relation to American Pharmacy and Medicine," *Bulletin of the History of Medicine* 25 (1951): 405–28; 25 (1951): 519–38.

25. The absolute rejection of traditional therapeutics enunciated by mid-century hydropaths and other evangelically oriented critics of medicine did not involve a rejection of the central body metaphor, but rather an absolute rejection of "artificial" drugs and bleeding. They did not question, but, on the contrary, emphasized the traditional view of the body; it served, indeed, as the logical basis for their dismissal of conventional therapeutics. They emphasized instead the body's capacity to heal itself when aided by appropriate regimen alone. The physician's therapeutic intrusions into that system seemed literally blasphemous.

26. Holmes, *Valedictory Address, Delivered to the Medical Graduates of Harvard University, at the Annual Commencement, . . . March 10, 1858* (Boston: David Clapp, 1858), p. 5.

27. T. Gaillard Thomas, *Introductory Address Delivered at the College of Physicians and Surgeons, New York, October 17th, 1864* (New York: 1864), p. 31.

28. Jacob Bigelow, *Brief Expositions of Rational Medicine, to which is Prefixed the Paradise of Doctors . . .* (Boston: Phillips, Sampson and Co., 1858), p. iv.

29. A.P. Merrill, *Medical Record* 1 (1866): 275.

30. C. W. Parsons, *An Essay on the Question, Vis Medicatrix Naturae, How*

far is it to be relied on in the Treatment of Diseases? Fiske Fund Prize Dissertation No. 11 (Boston: Printed for the Rhode Island Medical Society, 1849), p. 7.

31. Edmund Ravenel to unknown correspondent, draft, [November 1850], Ford-Ravenel Collection, South Carolina Historical Society, Charleston.

32. Report of the Resident Physician, Philadelphia Dispensary, *Rules of . . . with the Annual Report for 1862* (Philadelphia: J. Crummill, 1863), pp. 12–13.

33. O.W. Holmes, *Medical Essays* (Boston and New York: Houghton Mifflin, 1911), p. 258. Cited from an essay published originally in 1861.

34. See, for example, Samuel Henry Dickson, "Therapeutics," *Richmond Medical Journal* 3 (1867): 12; Jared Kirtland, *An Introductory Lecture, on the Coinciding Tendencies of Medicines* (Cleveland, Ohio: M.C. Younglove, 1848), p. 7.

35. A New Orleans physician could, for example, write in 1849 that "we have some cases of *Yellow Fever*—that is, they are yellow fever at the death, though but few look like it at the *beginning.* It is the mildest type of Intermittent and Remittent fever, of which 99 in the 100 cases can be cured if taken in time and properly treated; but *neglected* or *maltreated* [they shift into classic yellow fever]." E.D. Fenner to James Y. Bassett, 18 September 1849, Bassett Papers, Southern Historical Collection, University of North Carolina, Chapel Hill.

36. "Routine Practice," 108 (11 January 1883): 43.

37. Elmer Lee, "How Far does a Scientific Therapy depend upon the Materia Medica in the Cure of Disease," *Journal of the American Medical Association* 31 (8 October 1898): 827.

38. Lewllys F. Barker, "On the Present Status of Therapy and its Future," *Johns Hopkins Hospital Bulletin* 11 (1900): 153. Critics of his sceptical position, the often acid William Osler put it, "did not appreciate the difference between the giving of medicines and the treatment of disease." *The Treatment of Disease. The Address in Medicine before the Ontario Medical Association, Toronto, June 3, 1909* (London: Oxford, 1909), p. 13.

39. Abraham Jacobi, "Nihilism and Drugs," *New York State Journal of Medicine* 8 (February 1908): 57–65.

40. Alexander H. Stevens to James Jackson, 14 April 1836, James Jackson Papers, Francis Countway Library of Medicine, Boston.

41. L.M. Lawson, *Western Lancet* 9 (1849): 196.

42. Mitchell, *The Annual Oration before the Medical and Chirurgical Faculty of Maryland, 1877* (Baltimore: Inness and Co., 1877), p. 5.

43. Roberts Bartholow, *The Present State of Therapeutics: A Lecture Introductory to the Fifty-sixth Annual Course in Jefferson Medical College . . . October 1, 1879* (Philadelphia: J.B. Lippincott, 1879), p. 21.

2 MEDICAL REFORM AND BIOMEDICAL SCIENCE: Biochemistry—a Case Study

ROBERT E. KOHLER

INTRODUCTION: MEDICAL SCHOOLS AND MEDICAL SCIENCE

The biomedical sciences are so integral a part of American medical schools and medical education that it is easy to see them as a natural necessity rather than a custom. How they became the basis of "scientific medicine" during the reform of medical schools between 1890 and 1920 has been the subject of many histories.[1] The role of the American Medical Association and of the Carnegie Foundation, which sponsored the Flexner Report in 1910, has been analyzed and celebrated.[2] It is only recently that historians have begun to look with a more sceptical eye at the sociopolitical role that the medical sciences played in addition to their role in improving clinical practice. A revisionist school has shown how "scientific medicine" provided a socially acceptable means of limiting access to the medical profession and regulating competition from poorly trained physicians and medical sects.[3]

In this view, everything is political, and the purist ideals of science seem a pious fraud. This seems to me to miss the point, which is that the political and technical are in actuality never separate categories. It is naive to believe that technical improvements could have been incorporated into medicine without being also politically advantageous to their possessors. It is equally naive to suppose that the medical sciences could have been adopted for purely political reasons, without there having been real technical benefits. The medical sciences must be seen as a vital and necessary part of a social system of medicine—not the only possible system, but one with real advantages to balance its equally real shortcomings.

There has recently been considerable discussion of the role of biomedical sciences in the medical curriculum, and the debate is certain to continue.[4] Where should the dividing line be drawn between premedical preparation in the biomedical sciences and professional training in the applied clinical sciences? Can society afford a uniform system of "high quality" (that is, highly scientific) medical training, when there is a need for less elaborate and less expensive kinds of professional services, to provide for health maintenance as well as curing; for cheap low-technology care as well as high-technology intervention; and for care adapted to the nonscientific mores of disadvantaged groups? Not surprisingly, it is proving difficult to create socially viable roles in which science does not play an important part. Ironically, we seem to be coming back to admiring certain features of the system of medical education and practice which preceded the medical reforms of the 1900s: open access, deregulation of supply, cheapness, and heterogeneity. The virtues of scientific medicine have become vices in their turn, just as those of the old system had before.

This essay does not focus on the biomedical sciences as a political or a technical aspect of medical practice. It is concerned rather with biochemistry as an example of a biomedical discipline developing in the context of the changing medical school. It also explores industrial and governmental settings within which biochemistry as a discipline took form. My main point is that histories of scientific disciplines are chapters in the history of scientific institutions, especially universities and professional schools. Disciplines are themselves institutions, built upon cultural or economic service roles, and their evolution must be understood as a part of larger historical processes. Biochemistry is a particularly interesting case: of all the biomedical disciplines, it is the one least directly involved in clinical practice. Moreover, its establishment as a separate discipline was an immediate result of the reforms in medical education in the 1900s. Its history illustrates how a science can lend symbolic or political significance to a medical reform movement, and how a scientific elite can make use of structural and ideological opportunities opened up by rapid changes in the social organization of medicine. This is a case study in the "ecology of knowledge."[5]

The process by which biochemistry became an independent discipline has two aspects: structural and strategic. These analytical concepts were developed by the business historian, Alfred Chandler, to explain institutional innovation in large corporations in the early twentieth century.[6] The basic idea is a simple one: the particular way that an institution has grown determines the organizational strategies employed by reformers, and these strategies, in turn, determine the structure of the new organization. Institutional forms—new disciplines, in this case—are shaped both by the historically evolving structure of university and professional school and also by the ideals and strategies of individuals.

In the case of biochemistry, the structural argument runs as follows: general or "medical chemistry" was a traditional part of the medical curriculum in the proprietary medical college. So long as the medical course was a collegiate, rather than a graduate-level degree course, there was no room in medical colleges for more specialized physiological or bio-chemistry (the terms came to be more or less synonymous). But when the medical course was reconstituted as a graduate professional school within universities, requiring one or two years of college study for admission, then basic chemistry was relegated to the premedical level, and a place was created in medical schools for courses devoted wholly to biochemistry. These roles required teachers with Ph.D.'s, trained in biochemistry, and proficient in specialized research—that is, they called forth the familiar apparatus and activities of an academic discipline. Intense competition for faculty and highly qualified students insured that the new specialty, introduced first by a few leading schools, became a necessity for all modern medical schools.

This continuity of institutional structure is only half the story, however. Why was biochemistry not relegated to the premedical level, along with general chemistry? Why did it not simply remain an advanced specialty, consisting of pathological and clinical chemistry, toxicology, and forensic medicine, as it had, to a degree, been before? Why, in short, did it become a biomedical discipline? The answer is that there were strategic reasons for establishing biochemistry as a full preclinical discipline. Precisely because it was closest in style to academic natural sciences, biochemistry had a symbolic value to reformers. A department of biochemistry exemplified the ideals of the medical reform movement. The proprietary college had been weakest in the biomedical sciences: a full roster of these intermediate, basic applied disciplines was central to the first and crucial phase of reform in the 1900s. Biochemists, physiologists, deans, and university presidents had a common interest in having biochemistry play a role no less important than medical chemistry had before.

Only in American medical schools was biochemistry routinely institutionalized as a separate department of knowledge. In most British universities it remained a subdepartment of physiology until the 1930s. So, too, in German universities, where biochemistry was divided between organic chemists and physiologists. The number of chairs in Germany actually declined between 1895 and 1925, from six to three.[7] Intellectually, biochemistry was no less deserving of recognition as a discipline in one nation than in another. The difference was a result of distinct institutional structures and the different "ecology" of the disciplines, and of variations in the timing and nature of the medical reform movement.

Ironically, the key to the institutional success of biochemistry in America was the archaic organization of medical colleges. The institutional weakness of the biomedical sciences, their existence more on the periphery of instruction rather than at the center, meant that physiologists and pathologists were not in a position to lay claim to biochemistry as a province of their own disciplines. Medical chemistry, however, was a strong department, with established service roles. The much lamented independence of medical colleges from universities also insulated medical chemists from university departments of chemistry. Physiological chemistry or biochemistry was regarded by university chemists as a medical school subject (and an academically inferior one). Even when they temporarily took over instruction in biochemistry for medical faculties, chemists made no effort to annex it as a chemical specialty. In the 1900s, only one in five universities taught biochemistry in a way that was satisfactory to medical schools.[8] As a result, there was virtually no opposition to the reorganization of medical chemistry as biochemistry, or any rival claims to the subject from other university faculties.[9] In short, American biochemistry was shaped by reform strategies acting upon the existing structure of the traditional medical college.

THE REORGANIZATION OF MEDICAL EDUCATION

The essential features of the transition of medical schools from proprietary medical colleges to university medical faculties are well known. First was the financial and administrative change from dependence on student fees to reliance on university endowment. Medical faculties relinquished their corporate authority over appointments and finance and became teaching faculties only. Appointments and policy became the responsibility of university administrations. Second, the role of the part-time physician-teacher was replaced by the role of the professor-researcher, first in the preclinical, and more gradually in the clinical disciplines. This new role entailed the acceptance of academic criteria for promotion: performance of research and advancement of the discipline, rather than performance as a physician or as a mentor to apprentice physicians. The ideal of scientific medicine, which reached new heights of prestige in the 1900s, was in part an ideological rationale for this new medical role. Third, and most important here, the location of medical schools in the educational system changed from college level to roughly the equivalent of graduate school, as entrance requirements were raised from a high school education, or less, to two years of college or more. In 1890, medical training was a vocational alternative to a liberal arts education; an M.D. from the better colleges was roughly equivalent to a B.A. By 1915, an M.D. from the better schools was more or less equivalent to a Ph.D. This relocation of the biomedical sciences to the graduate level enabled professors of anatomy, physiology, pathology, biochemistry, and pharmacology to make the ideals of scientific medicine an institutional reality. There was room in the curriculum for advanced courses; there was a student audience prepared to study specialized biomedical sciences in the university style. There were facilities, and time, for research.

The reform of medical education had been going on for a long time before the movement found its apotheosis in the Flexner Report of 1910.[10] By 1880, medical colleges having any pretensions at all had graded years. By 1890, terms had been lengthened, and the curriculum was extended to three years. In the 1890s, a fourth year became a regular feature of all the better schools. This expansion permitted the separation of clinical and preclinical years and made it possible to teach the preclinical subjects as experimental sciences, giving students extensive laboratory training. The increased income from tuition fees provided the capital to build and maintain the laboratories needed to teach these fields as experimental disciplines. Finally, some sort of official affiliation with universities was common by 1895, though even at the best medical colleges it seldom meant true organic union.

I would argue, however, that the addition of a fourth year, teaching laboratories, and a few full-time teachers in the preclinical sciences simply grafted onto the proprietary college some of the trappings of the German medical faculty, without changing the socioeconomic basis of the proprietary college in a fundamental way. It was German frosting on the traditional college cake. Though the role of professor-researcher was established in the leading medical schools (the University of Pennsylvania, Johns Hopkins, Harvard, Columbia, and Western Reserve) in the 1890s, facilities for research were generally poor, and research was not really expected. German training and qualification for research had a symbolic importance, especially in hiring, but reputations were made at this time for teaching, and for writing basic textbooks. These activities answered contemporary needs more than research. Edward T. Reichert, professor of physiology at the University of Pennsylvania, pursued a specialized (and sophisticated) line of research, in isolation. He showed no ambitions to establish disciplinary programs, and his circumstances certainly did not encourage a very large ambition for discipline-building. His colleages in chemistry and anatomy, John Marshall and George Piersol, were noted as authors and teachers. They and a few others constituted a marginal, somewhat enbattled clique in the medical faculty; the physicians who occupied the chairs of medicine and surgery called the tune.[11] In the 1900s, a more aggressive generation of reformers and scholars, such as Simon Flexner, saw the men of the 1890s as obstacles to scientific reform.

What really transformed the old medical college was raising the entrance requirement to two years of college; this occurred in the top twenty or so schools between 1895 and 1910. Unlike the earlier improvements, this reform stretched the financial resources of the proprietary school beyond the breaking point. Whereas the four-year course had increased the number of medical students in residence, higher entrance requirements disrupted the established market relation with high schools, diminished the pool of qualified applicants, and resulted in a drastic plunge in enrollment.[12] Medical schools henceforth could not survive on fees, and were forced to rely on large privately endowed or state-supported universities, which alone could afford the vastly increased costs of high quality medical training. Only university leaders had access to the private philanthropists who could provide endowment for medical schools and hospitals (and, increasingly, to the large foundations which were just being established). Medical schools relied on affiliated universities as sources of qualified students. Many instituted a six-year program combining the B.A. and the M.D. to entice more college students into medicine. This measure is indicative of the reformers' decision not to await passively the evolution of a market for quality medical training, but to actively create a market for it. In contrast to the prosperity of the mid-1890s, the 1900s were traumatic years, as organic relations with universities were established, and medical colleges became graduate professional schools.

As the medical reformers understood, the real issue behind the battle for higher entrance requirements was the division of labor between secondary, college, and graduate or professional education. The expansion of the system of public high schools in the 1890s made it possible for the first time to rationalize the system on a national scale. The unexpected flood of middle class sons to colleges in the 1900s, increasingly with preprofessional ambitions, made possible the symbiosis between college and medical schools. In the 1880s, Harvard's president Charles W. Eliot used all his influence to orient the high schools toward college preparation.[13] In the 1890s and early 1900s, he labored to ensure the college's role in preprofessional training.[14] Abraham Flexner's work with the Carnegie Foundation (1907–12) and with the Rockefeller-supported General Education Board, from 1913, was similarly inspired by a desire to establish a rational and uniform division of labor between college and professional schools,[15] as the General Education Board had previously tried to do for the high schools and colleges.[16] The reformer's insistence that medical schools require students to have college preparation coincided with the ambitions of professors in the preclinical sciences for more advanced and specialized roles.

Unlike the improvements of the 1890s, the reforms between 1900 and 1920 were not limited to the elite medical schools. They were planned and carried out on a national scale, initially by the Association of American Medical Colleges (AAMC), then by the American Medical Association (AMA) and the Carnegie, Rockefeller, and (later) the Commonwealth Foundations.[17] Owing to internal opposition from heads of proprietary colleges and from general practitioners antipathetic to medical specialization, the reformers within the AAMC and AMA were unable, in the 1890s, to mobilize their organizations for educational reform. This situation changed quite dramatically about 1900. Reorganization of the AMA, in 1901, brought state and county medical societies under national control. In 1901, the first educational issue of the AMA's *Journal* appeared, and AMA leaders joined state medical boards to press for uniform and higher standards of licensing.

The Council on Medical Education of the AMA was organized in 1904, and as a quasi-official regulatory body issued standards and prescriptions for entrance and degree requirements. In 1906, the council fixed a high school diploma as the minimum, and two years of college as the ideal preparation for medical school. The council's standards were a powerful stimulus for reform among the strong, as well as the weak schools. Public exposure in the Flexner Report and in the *Journal of the American Medical Association*, which unabashedly utilized the style of muckraking journalism, ensured that the ideals of scientific medicine, limited to a few schools in 1900, were the reality for all medical schools by 1920. State boards consolidated these reforms in licensing examinations.

Competition, as well as the ideals of scientific medicine, stimulated this educational reform. Up to about 1890, lowering the cost and quality of medical treatment had been an effective mode of competition for all but the elite physicians, and a serious threat to the minority of college-trained physicians. This style of competition was fostered by the open market of proprietary medical colleges, which likewise competed for students by keeping the cost and quality of medical training low. It took little capital to open a proprietary school, and the proliferation of new medical schools was greatest at precisely the time when the reform movement was getting under way: 33 new schools appeared in the 1880s, and another 33 by 1904, when there were no fewer than 166 in operation, teaching over 28,000 medical students.[18]

This pattern of unregulated competition and growth was typical of many social and economic activities in the Gilded Age (1880–1900). In many expanding industries the favored way to meet competition was to cut prices, lay down railway track, harvest more acres, or occupy markets, without worrying about long-range profitability. By the 1890s, this boom-and-bust style of competition was no longer effective or tolerable. Saturated markets, ruinous price wars, too many miles of unprofitable track, exhausted soil, and a similar phenomenon, too few patients per physician—made centralized regulation of competition and production under the aegis of government, trade association, or professional societies a more appealing arrangement. The rank and file of general practitioners in the AMA came around to supporting reform for the same reasons that the railroad tycoons led the movement for federal regulation: it was in their interest to do so.[19]

Longer and much more expensive medical training was acceptable because it meant both better medical practice and—because fewer physicians would be trained—predictable and adequate incomes. In a system dominated by competitive market rules, "scientific medicine" remained the ideal of a minority of urban, specialized physicians. As the purely intellectual program of a German-inspired elite, scientific medicine would have remained a small and isolated minority style within the profession. But in a market dominated by the new rules of regulated competition, "scientific medicine" was widely accepted as a means of improving physicians' economic and cultural status, and of promoting social progress at the same time. Thus after two decades of indifference to scientific medicine, the profession rapidly accepted it as the basis for a reorganized medical training. There is no better illustration that intellectual programmes have sociopolitical meanings, and that the history of science must be understood in the context of larger economic and cultural trends.

Scientific medicine was an appropriately neutral and plausible rationale for the new economic and social order of the Progressive Age. It was more consonant with contemporary democratic values than the establishment of a status hierarchy of physicians with different degrees and licenses to practice, as was the case in Britain and Eastern Europe.[20] Medical science was an effective therapeutic against the disease of sectarian rivalry, which had fulminated in the 1890s. It was an ideal criterion for regulating the medical market in an age which was unrestrained in its faith in experts and specialized expertise of all kinds.[21]

Though the reform movement was not primarily intended to promote the biomedical sciences as such (except, of course, by the biomedical scientists), these disciplines were the first beneficiaries of reform. The market for biomedical specialists expanded both horizontally (spreading into all eighty-seven of the medical schools which survived the AMA campaign and the Flexner Report) and vertically, as the leading universities, which supplied most holders of doctorates in these disciplines, expanded and diversified their biomedical science departments. In all of the biomedical disciplines the closer relation with universities and the infusion of scholar-teachers resulted in a new balance between clinical application and research on fundamental biological questions. There was a shift of interest from morphology to physiological process, from observation to experiment, from a strictly clinical to a comparative point of view. In some subjects this shift was very dramatic: materia medica was reborn as experimental pharmacology, and biochemistry emerged from medical chemistry. In these cases, reform created a demand for a kind of specialist who had not previously had a role in the medical college. In an institutional, if not an intellectual sense, reform virtually created new disciplines.

MEDICAL CHEMISTRY AND BIOCHEMISTRY

Although the new generation of biochemists regarded their predecessors as objects of scorn and derision, the medical chemists were by no means simply obstacles to scientific progress. Medical chemists created the roles and niches for biochemists to step into. The ungenerous rhetoric of a generation gap should not obscure the real continuity of succession.

So long as beginning medical students had little or no premedical scientific training, general chemistry was a necessary part of the medical curriculum, and teaching it was the major duty of medical chemists. "Medical chemistry" usually consisted of an introductory course in general chemistry, perhaps simplified for medical students, perhaps emphasizing applications to the analysis of blood and urine, to keep the students' interest. This course might conclude with a brief introduction to organic or physiological chemistry. Advanced courses generally consisted of physiological chemistry applied to clinical diagnosis, urinalysis, toxicology, and forensic medicine. Medical chemistry as a disciplinary package was thus a mixture of basic college chemistry and applied clinical chemistry. There was no room and no incentive in the structure of medical education to develop biochemistry as an intermediate preclinical discipline.

Courses in medical chemistry were often taught by chemical analysts or by physician-teachers who were waiting for chairs of medicine and surgery to fall vacant, or by physicians who were specialists in forensic medicine. Either as a variety of applied chemistry or as a medical specialty, teaching medical chemistry was a low-status role, performed by people whose training and career interests were not in biochemistry as such. Quality varied widely. Some medical chemists, such as Rudolph Witthaus, of Cornell Medical School, were distinguished medical jurists. Others, such as John Mandell, of New York University, were respected and productive biochemists. Others were chemists who were unable to succeed in academia or physicians moonlighting as chemical analysts; some were legal experts, or toxicologists for public health boards.

It was a marginal role, but also a transitional one, evolving even before it was overtaken by revolution. Because medical chemistry was on the frontier between university and medical school, professors of medical chemistry were often leaders in the movement for closer relations with universities. If they were chemists, they were often the first full-time, salaried professional teachers in the medical school. Professors of chemistry often served as medical deans, representing the interests of the medical schools in negotiations with university administrations. Some were active in the national movement to reform medical education. John Long, of Northwestern Medical School, was a mainstay of the AMA's Council on Education. Scientific medicine seemed to promise the medical chemists a more central, prestigious role in medical schools and upward mobility in the university pecking order. By 1900, the content of medical chemistry had changed. Courses in the better schools, such as Harvard or the University of Pennsylvania, consisted largely of physiological chemistry. It was not uncommon for medical chemists to spend summers studying biochemistry in Europe, in anticipation of inheriting more specialized departments and chairs, as general chemistry disappeared from the medical course. Some, such as Elbert Rockwood, at the University of Iowa, returned to school to get Ph.D.'s in biochemistry.[22] But, as is often the case with such transitional figures, their efforts at reform did not lead to the expected results.

The reorganization of the medical school did not provide upward mobility for most medical chemists. What had been a role for applied chemists or physician-chemists was redesigned as a specialized role for men with

Ph.D.'s in biochemistry. Toxicologists and medical chemists were rapidly replaced by professors of biochemistry. In 1907, for example, the professor of chemistry at the University of Texas Medical Branch, S. M. Morris, M.D. ("Old Test Tube"), foresaw the trend toward specialization. Realizing he had "neither the training nor liking for biochemistry," he relinquished his chair (and a profitable sideline as a chemical analyst) and eased into a new career in otorhinolaryngology.[23] Within a few years, a new department of biological chemistry was being organized by William C. Rose, a research-minded academic biochemist.[24]

Even some of the best of the medical chemists were rudely replaced by young biochemists with the right credentials and greater promise in specialized research. John Marshall, professor of chemistry at the University of Pennsylvania Medical School, had both an M.D. and a Ph.D. in physiological chemistry, and had had experience in physiological chemistry in Europe. As medical dean (from 1893), he pressed for closer relations with the university. By 1900, however, Marshall seemed cautious and old-fashioned. In 1902, Simon Flexner assessed the research activities of the preclinical sciences in dismal terms: "What outlook is there for a group of [research] workers? Chemistry can yield nothing, anatomy is doomed to sterility, and physiology is I fear, not very promising. When Wood retires, which must be soon, it is by no means a foregone conclusion that a trained man will be chosen to succeed him. Abbott alone of all the men in the Medical School is doing work."[25] In 1902, Provost Harrison ousted Marshall from the deanship, thinking him unsympathetic to reform. And in 1909, the scope of Marshall's chair was abruptly limited to the task of teaching chemistry to dental and veterinary students, to make way for a new chair of physiological chemistry created for Alonzo Taylor, a bright young research biochemist from Berkeley.[26] Many of those who began or ended their careers in the period from 1895 to 1910 had the experience of being the last of an old generation, or the first of a new.

The ideology of reform accentuated this discontinuity and facilitated the introduction of biochemists. Medical chemistry was easily tagged by the reformers as unprofessional and unscientific. The AMA's Council on Medical Education intoned: "It is inimical to good teaching and fatal to research to have [biochemistry and physiology] under the immediate control of men in active practice. . . . The old but still prevalent idea that almost any young practitioner with time on his hands would do as professor of physiology cannot be too forcibly condemned."[27] Given modern ideas of professionalism and academic quality, it was a far more politic course to replace medical chemists with outside experts than to encourage individuals or departments to upgrade themselves and evolve into new roles. In the context of medical reform, a biochemist represented the academically more prestigious science, and courses in biochemistry taught by specialists were a visible sign of progressive impulses in an institution. Biochemists with doctorates promised research performance along modern lines of work.

Behind the new faces and new voices, there was continuity between medical and biological chemistry. In most cases, biological chemistry did not arise out of physiology or chemistry, but developed out of departments of medical chemistry. That biochemistry belonged in the roster of preclinical disciplines was never disputed. Why was it not an issue? In the first place, as biochemistry occupied a growing place in medical·chemistry courses, specialized roles for biochemists were beginning to appear within medical chemistry. At the University of Pennsylvania, a "demonstrator" in physiological chemistry was appointed in 1903; at Harvard, Edward S. Wood had two assistants in physiological chemistry by 1904.[28] When chairs of medical chemistry fell vacant through deaths or resignations (many did in the 1900s), or when higher entrance requirements forced faculties to rethink roles and curricula, reform groups looked always to improvement, as they had for over a decade. They seized upon these occasions to press for more specialized biochemistry, more professional instructors, more modern research. There was no thought of dismantling existing departments in preclinical science. Reformers built upon the institutions and practices of the medical chemists, as reformers in Europe consolidated the practices of the chemical physiologists.

The existence of strong departments of medical chemistry also helped keep biochemistry from being attached to departments of physiology, within the medical schools. On this point there was discussion in the 1900s, and some variation in practice. American physiologists were no less keen than German physiologists in their belief that physiological chemistry was, intellectually, an integral part of physiology. In 1909, the subcommittee on organic chemistry, physiology, and physiological chemistry of the AMA Council on Education pronounced that efforts to separate physiology and biochemistry were misguided, and that the ideal was a dual department, with either a physical physiologist or a biochemist as head. In practice, however, such departments were exceptional: A survey by the AMA Council in 1909 showed that in the sixty schools offering courses in physiological chemistry, only four offered it as part of courses in physiology.[29] Independent departments of biochemistry were the rule by 1909.

Physiologists and pathologists were frequently the most active parties in efforts to replace medical chemists with biochemists. John G. Curtis and Mitchell Prudden played this role at Columbia when Charles Chandler retired in 1898.[30] Henry P. Bowditch and Walter B. Cannon played a similar role at Harvard in the struggle to prevent Wood from inheriting the new chair of biological chemistry in 1905.[31] Eugene Opie was largely responsible for the choice of a biochemist for the new chair at Washington University.[32] But seldom did physiologists try to annex biochemistry. Their aim was to have colleagues who were interested in the chemical aspects of physiology and pathology, rather than in toxicology and forensic medicine. Moreover, the tradition of independent departments of medical chemistry made it difficult to justify a radical change in departmental structures or in the allocation of funds. Where biochemistry did become attached (temporarily) to physiology, it was usually at places where medical chemistry was especially weak or physiology unusually strong. (At Chicago and California, for example, Jacques Loeb's presence and influence kept biochemistry within physiology.) In European universities, where there was no independent tradition of medical chemistry, biochemists had to make a special case for independence against physiologists who were already in possession of the subject. American biochemists simply stepped into the shoes of the old medical chemists.

Chemists likewise offered little competition to biochemists' claims. They had some occasion to do so: in the 1900s it was not uncommon for medical schools, as a first step in the reform of medical chemistry, to rely on university chemists for instruction in organic and physiological chemistry. This seldom led to a permanent role, however. The separation of colleges and medical schools made it more difficult for organic chemists to annex biochemistry than it was in the German universities, with their parallel faculties of science and medicine, and where organic chemists routinely gave the courses to medical students. Since, in American universities, organic chemistry became a required premedical course, university chemists gained a useful service role in premedical training, but had little incentive to acquire biochemistry, which was accepted as a preclinical discipline, in close connection with physiology, pathology, and clinical medicine.[33]

The independent status of biochemistry as a preclinical department was a real advantage to American biochemists in discipline-building. The important role of college chemistry in premedical study provided recruits who had been exposed to laboratory work. Independence permitted biochemists to develop their own lines of work, rather than serving the aims of other disciplines. The connection with clinical disciplines provided important problems for research and vital service roles. These advantages were observed by Wilmot Herringham and Walter Fletcher during their official tour of American Medical Schools for the University Grants Committee (U.K.) in 1921. They reported that the American system of elaborate and prolonged premedical training was a great stimulus to research in the biomedical fields, though it made an American M.D. twice as expensive as a European one. Although physiology suffered, they felt, in an exclusively clinical context, they noted the high state of development of biochemistry and pharmacology as independent disciplines.[34]

Once the pattern of independent departments of biochemistry was set by the leading schools (Johns Hopkins, Harvard, Columbia) it spread through the system with remarkable speed. In 1909, the AMA Curriculum Committee found that sixty of the ninety-seven surviving medical schools reported courses in physiological or bio-chemistry. With a few exceptions (Fordham, Louisville, Tulane, Buffalo, Jefferson, and Marquette), the thirty-seven schools which reported no courses in biochemistry were small proprietary schools, many of which sank in the waves created by the Flexner Report. The others instituted programs in biochemistry within a few years. In 1911, the University of Pennsylvania medical faculty surveyed fifty-eight leading schools and concluded that twenty-three gave courses in biochemistry equal in quality to that given by Alonzo Taylor—a very high standard indeed.[35] Introduction of collegiate entrance requirements were routinely followed by reorganization of the departments of medical chemistry.

Courses entitled "physiological chemistry" differed greatly in quality, of course; some were surely little more than the old medical chemistry, with an alias. The American Society of Biological Chemists (ASBC) grumbled, in 1919, that some courses, even in the better schools, were still being taught by persons who did not have the credentials or accomplishments which would make them eligible for membership in the society.[36] But the point is that by 1919, virtually every medical school had a separate course in biochemistry, which included laboratory work. In each there was a potential niche for a professional biochemist, and increasing pressures of prestige—indeed of survival—to acquire a trained specialist. More indicative than the complaints of the ASBC was the fact that it deliberately did not set forth an "official" standard course: most departments were in the hands of professional biochemists, who did not want or need to be told what to teach.[37]

The establishment of departments of biochemistry in medical schools closed out other options for establishing it as a department in science faculties. Duplicating programs taught in the medical school in other parts of the university was economically and politically difficult. The few exceptions to the rule were universities in which strong programs in biochemistry already existed in other professional schools: at Wisconsin, in the Agricultural College; at Yale, in the Sheffield Scientific School; at Illinois (Urbana), in the College of Science and Letters. In some instances, competition between departments made the reorganization of the medical school more difficult. Medical biochemistry at Wisconsin remained overshadowed by the large and aggressive agricultural department.[38] Russell Chittenden's department in the Sheffield School, the oldest and most prestigious department of biochemistry in the United States, was not transferred to the Yale Medical School until 1921, and even then maintained, de facto, an independent course.[39] At the University of Illinois, biochemistry shared (in a modest way) in the prestige and influence of the dominant school of chemistry in America, while in the University's Medical Department, in Chicago, biochemists remained a small group, primarily teachers, within physiology.[40] But the vast majority of departments of biochemistry, including most of the largest and most influential, were independent departments in medical schools.

By 1915 or 1920, the standard best department of biochemistry consisted of a staff of four (professor, associate or assistant professors, and instructors), with an annual budget of about $14,000.[41] In size and share of resources it was on a par with the departments of physiology and (except for the expensive autopsy and dissection budgets) with those of anatomy and pathology. The faculty had diverse roles. Otto Folin's staff, at Harvard Medical School, were exemplary: in addition to teaching between 70 and 120 medical students, they guided between 5 and 7 Ph.D. candidates, several foreign researchers and advanced medical students, and a dozen or so physicians, on month-long research projects. Laboratories in local hospitals provided material for research, as well as employment and experience for Folin's graduate students.[42]

Courses, too, had achieved a more or less standard form by 1920.[43] There were many good laboratory manuals, and a new generation of textbooks of biochemistry had begun to replace the older medical chemistry texts. Older biochemists complained that they were unable to keep up with the demand for biochemists with Ph.D.'s, and marvelled at the sudden and unexpected popularity of their profession. Young biochemists made the most of a seller's market.[44]

A professional infrastructure was also created to consolidate the various groups interested in biochemistry. In 1904, the *Journal of Biological Chemistry* was organized by Christian Herter and John J. Abel.[45] By 1915, it had doubled its rate of publication to over 200 articles a year, 90 per cent from American institutions. In 1906, Abel and William J. Gies, professor of biological chemistry at Columbia, organized the American Society of Biological Chemists.[46] With 80 founding members, its membership had grown to over 500 by 1940 (figure 1).

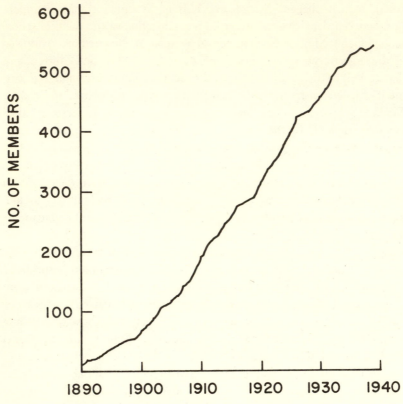

Figure 1. Number of individuals elected to the ASBC from 1906 to 1942 who were professionally employed between 1890 and 1940.

THE ECOLOGY OF A DISCIPLINE, 1890–1940

Medical schools were the major, but by no means the only place in which biochemists were finding professional employment. The medical reform movement was only one part of a general reorganization of American institutions in the Progressive period. Institutions of all sorts were restructuring occupational roles and creating a demand for trained experts. Larger and more complex institutions could afford departments for research and development. The growing regulatory roles and interventionist style of government agencies were hospitable to university-trained professional scientists. The new corporate style of economic competition (depending upon planned technical improvement achieved through research and development) likewise resulted in new professional roles for scientific specialists, including biochemists.

At the same time that biochemists were filling more diverse service roles, their disciplinary identity was becoming more sharply and narrowly defined. Precisely because biochemists had never been able to develop specialized institutions, outside of the medical schools their field had been cultivated by an unusual variety of other kinds of specialists: chemists, biologists, physiologists, pathologists, pharmacologists, plant physiologists, bacteriologists, and clinicians. Long after chemistry, botany, or physiology were monopolized by chemists, botanists, and physiologists, professional biochemists were still only one group in a loose network of specialty groups primarily located in other disciplines. All laid claim to parts of what biochemists increasingly saw as their domain. Harvard's Lawrence J. Henderson was one of the many who was distressed by the absence of specifically *biochemical* methods, problems, and a sense of professional identity, even in the outstanding department of physiological chemistry at Strassburg.[47]

These groups of amateurs, part-time biochemists, and well-wishers were instrumental in the creation of specialized institutions for biochemistry. In medical schools the replacement of medical chemists by biological chemists was frequently carried through by physiologists, pathologists, or clinicians. Both the *Journal of Biological Chemistry* and the American Society for Biological Chemists were initiated and supported in their early years by users, more than by producers, of biochemical knowledge, notably the pharmacologist John J. Abel, and pathologist Christian Herter. The popularity of the multidisciplinary terms "biochemistry" or "biological chemistry," in the early 1900s, reflected the need to appeal not just to a disciplinary group, but to all of the diverse constituencies interested in biochemistry.[48]

This pattern changed rapidly, however. The development of a professional infrastructure encouraged the trend toward professional self-consciousness and a more exacting division of occupational space. Just as medical schools insisted that positions in biochemistry be filled by biochemists, so, too, did other institutions. The ill-defined boundaries with other disciplines became more definite as the core of skills, methods, problems, and ideals coalesced. Physiologists who had themselves done biochemistry increasingly turned to biochemists to play specialized roles in departments, laboratories, or research teams.

These two trends—consolidation of the core discipline and diversification of constituencies—are common themes in the history of most disciplines,[49] but especially so in the history of biochemistry.

The membership of the American Society of Biological Chemists (ASBC) is an ideal population in which to take the measure of these trends. The group constitutes what Daniel Kevles has called a productive elite.[50] Unlike most professional societies, the ASBC nominated and elected members on the basis of research achievement.[51] Most of the biochemical professoriate from the top dozen medical schools were members. But a systematic effort was apparently made to include representatives of other institutions—hospitals, government agencies, industrial laboratories, agricultural stations—and of small subspecialties within the field, such as nutrition, home economics, and clinical and agricultural biochemistry. Important people in other disciplines who promoted or performed biochemical research were also enlisted, especially in the early years.[52] The ASBC membership is thus an almost ideal sample of the discipline, a group self-selected according to the prime index of status in academic disciplines, but inclusive of a variety of nonacademic constituencies.[53] The successive editions of *American Men of Science* provide career information on 92 percent of the 721 individuals elected from 1906 to 1942, and with the aid of a computer, this information can be made to yield trends showing where, and how, society members (or members-to-be) were trained and employed, in each year from 1890 to about 1935.[54]

A rough measure of the trend toward consolidation of the discipline is the declining proportion of ASBC members employed in disciplines other than biochemistry. Only 29 percent of individuals active in 1900 who were later elected to the ASBC were employed as biochemists. In 1935, the figure was 55 percent. The number of individuals affiliated with biology and the other biomedical sciences declined from 30 percent to 12 percent in the same period,[55] and the proportion employed as chemists declined from 35 percent to 12 percent (figures 2 and 3). In contrast, the proportion of biochemists in the applied branches of the discipline—in clinical medicine, agriculture, and nutrition—increased from 3 percent to nearly 20 percent. Consolidation at the center and expansion of constituencies—that was the pattern.

These figures must be interpreted with care. The decline in the biomedical class reflects the fact that the number of individuals elected from these disciplines dropped precipitously after the early years. Three-fourths of all of the members admitted (up until 1942) from clinical and other biomedical sciences had been elected by 1920, compared with one-fourth of those in biochemistry as such. Fully one-third of the biomedical members had been founders. There was no massive shift of individuals from biomedical disciplines to biochemistry. Rather, individuals doing the kind of research that qualified them for membership were increasingly professional biochemists. Physiologists, pharmacologists, and clinicians increasingly left biochemical research to the biochemists, as they were leaving teaching to the newly independent departments of biochemistry in medical schools.

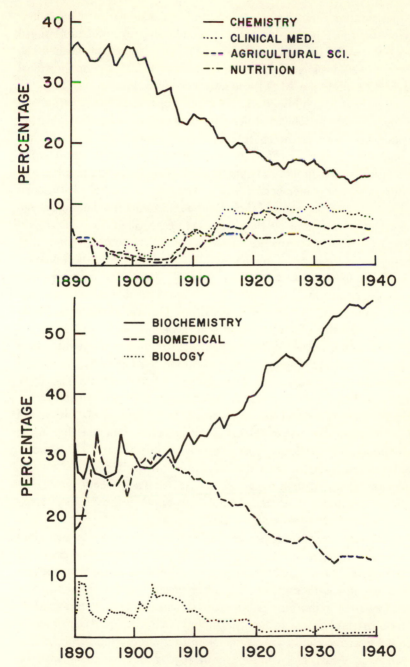

Figures 2 and 3. Proportions of professionally employed ASBC members affiliated with various disciplines (shown as percentage of those with known affiliation).

Specialization entailed a narrowing of professional interests. One indicator of this trend is the decline of comembership in other professional societies (besides the ASBC) in successive "generations" of biochemists, where generations are defined as Ph.D. cohorts.[56] The later an individual received his Ph.D. (or M.D.), the less likely he was to join certain other societies (figure 4). While comembership in the Society for Experimental Biology, a multi-disciplinary society, declined only slightly, comembership in disciplinary societies, notably other biomedical societies, dropped sharply for individuals acquiring a Ph.D. or M.D. after 1900. Comembership in the American Physiological Society plummeted from 56 percent to 6 percent. A high degree of comembership in the American Society of Pharmacologists was characteristic only of the 1895–99 Ph.D. cohort, who came of age when biochemistry and pharmacology were especially close. Comembership in the Society of American Bacteriologists, always low, dwindled to almost zero in the 1920s; comembership in the American Medical Association dropped from 28 percent to 3 percent.[57] Thus at the same time that biochemistry was institutionalized as a biomedical discipline in medical schools, fewer biochemists were involved in a professional way in neighboring preclinical disciplines and in clinical medicine.

As horizontal linkages between biochemistry and its sister disciplines atrophied, vertical linkages between chemistry, biochemistry, and applied biochemistry (especially clinical biochemistry) grew stronger and more numerous. These vertical linkages were no longer mediated by hybrid roles, however, but by channels for recruitment, in the case of chemistry, and employment, in the case of clinical medicine. Thus comembership in the American Chemical Society rose dramatically in younger Ph.D. cohorts. And employment in the applied areas of biochemistry in clinical medicine, agriculture, and nutrition remained modest but steady (see figure 3). Recruitment became routinized and employment options became more diversified.

The importance of these new professional roles is revealed by analysis of the varied kinds of institutions in which biochemists were employed (figures 5, 6). Since membership in the ASBC was based on research achievement, it is not surprising that a large majority of the productive elite were employed in universities and medical schools—a steady two-thirds to three-quarters of all society members professionally employed were academics. Between 1900 and 1920, academic institutions created some 200 new positions for ASBC biochemists, and by 1930, nearly 200 more. In 1915, biochemists at academic institutions accounted for 55 percent of the 206 articles published in the *Journal of Biological Chemistry;* that proportion increased to 72 percent by 1948 (see table 1). The number of academic

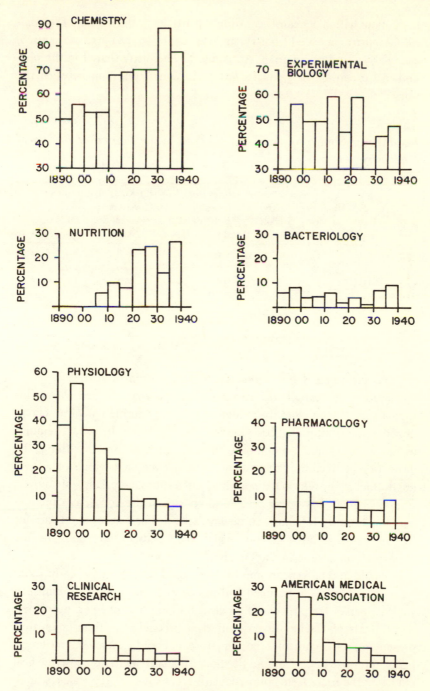

Figure 4. Comembership of ASBC members in other disciplinary and professional societies (shown as percentage of Ph.D. or M.D. cohorts).

institutions with biochemists contributing articles to the *Journal of Biological Chemistry* increased from 15, in 1907–08, to 19, in 1915, 32, in 1926, 40, in 1937, and 51, in 1948. Academic biochemistry shared in the phenomenal expansion of graduate and professional education between the wars.[58]

Table 1
Institutional Sources of Articles Published in the *Journal of Biological Chemistry*

Year	Total Num.	University & Med. Schools	Agric. Schools & Stations	Medical Research Institutes	Hosps.	Government (Federal & State)	Industry	Private
1907–8	106	61	5.7	5.7	2.8	3.8	—	21.0
1915	206	55	9.7	20.0	8.8	4.9	2.9	—
1926	236	63	6.7	17.0	6.4	4.2	1.7	0.8
1937	338	69	3.8	19.0	5.3	2.1	1.2	—
1948	553	71	3.0	10.0	4.3	7.2	3.8	—
1959	599	73	1.8	8.5	1.8	13.0	1.2	—

Percentage of Articles from Different Kinds of Institutions[1]

1 Percentage of total articles in the journal, from all American institutions.

More surprising is the decline in the proportion of ASBC members employed in medical schools between 1895 and 1920. At first glance this trend seems to contradict the argument that the reformed medical schools provided the institutional basis for the new discipline. In fact, it reminds us not to oversimplify a complex historical process. For one thing, the distinction between the categories of university and medical school became less distinct in the reform period. Many universities, especially state universities, inaugurated two-year preclinical courses in the 1900s, as a preliminary step toward a full four-year medical school. These account, in part, for the rise in the number of "university" biochemists after 1900, and the corresponding decline in the "medical" category.[59]

It should also be kept in mind that medical schools in the early 1900s were often financially troubled and insecure. Because of the diminished student market for postcollege medical training, the opening up of new departments of biochemistry occurred at precisely the time of greatest pressure for retrenchment. Departments could not be expanded until prosperity returned in the 1920s. Positions in many, perhaps most medical schools in the 1900s were not particularly conducive to large-scale research. Research funds were scarce, and in all but the top schools teaching remained the chief duty of biochemists, as it had been for the medical chemists.

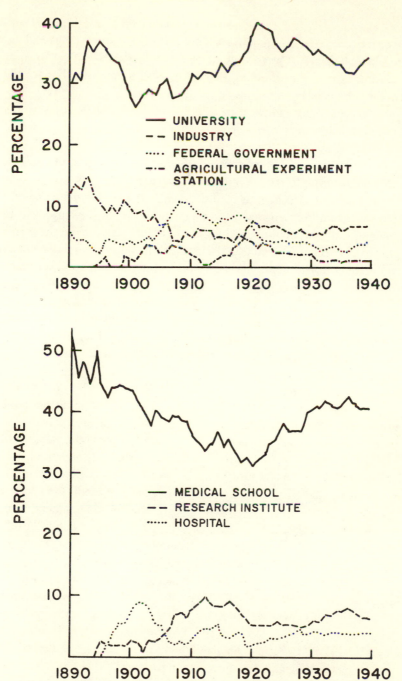

Figures 5 and 6. Proportions of ASBC members employed in various types of institutions (shown as percantage of the total professionally employed).

In the better schools, the reform period was one of political turmoil, and frequently, of bitter confrontations between preclinical reformers and entrenched clinicians. It was a time to create departments, not yet to enjoy the fruits of settled institutions. It was, in short, a promising but volatile market. The exhilaration of new opportunities was inseparable from conflict, risk, and uncertainty as to whether medical schools really would succeed in becoming places where academic research and graduate teaching could be done on a large scale.

Shortages of trained biochemists also hindered expansion of the new departments. Prior to 1900, Chittenden's department at Yale was virtually the only source of biochemists with doctorates. It took about a decade for a supply system to be created. Moreover, the success of the movement to promote academic clinical teaching and clinical research in the 1910s resulted in a decline in recruits to the biomedical sciences. Clinical research paid better and had more prestige. World War I and the postwar boom in industrial chemistry compounded the shortage of biochemists in the universities, as they opted to work in industry. Philip Shaffer, at Washington University, Folin, at Harvard, and William Gies, at Columbia, were left almost single-handed, with only student assistants to keep their departments going. Complaints of a "crisis in the preclinical sciences" were widespread in the early 1920s.[60]

In short, the structural opportunities for growth created in the new departments between 1900 and 1914 were not fully realized until the 1920s, when student enrollments increased, and a balance between biomedical and clinical departments was attained. The postwar generation of biochemists reaped the rewards of the labors of the institution-builders.

The most important cause of the relative decline of ASBC members employed in medical schools, however, lay outside of medical schools: it was the appearance of professional opportunities in nonacademic institutions. State and federal bureaus of agriculture and of public health, hospitals, medical research institutes, and industry were beginning to offer attractive careers in biomedical research. Employment with these institutions offered real advantages over academic jobs. The medical research institutions, of which there were some two dozen by 1910, provided their researchers with personal freedom, economic security, and insulation from routine teaching and administration. John D. Rockefeller and Andrew Carnegie deliberately established separate institutes, instead of grant programs for university researchers.[61] As for industries, they offered salaries, research facilities, and budgets far beyond what medical school departments could afford.

It was not really clear that medical school departments were ideal places for biomedical research on a large scale until the 1920s, when the unprecedented prosperity of universities, and large-scale patronage of academic biomedical science by state legislatures and foundations erased all doubt about the central role of medical schools in biomedical research. Moreover, the expansion of nonacademic roles for basic research in biochemistry was limited: in research institutes, by fixed endowments; in hospitals and industries, by practical institutional goals that allowed only a limited margin for basic research. Other institutions, such as teaching hospitals and agricultural experiment stations, were, in effect, absorbed by universities, and became parts of diversified educational institutions.

The earliest of these institutions were the state agricultural experiment stations, in which a generation of "scientist-entrepreneurs" combined a modest amount of basic research with substantial service roles in fertilizer and soil analysis.[62] In the 1890s, these stations employed 15 percent of future ASBC members, but this figure rapidly dwindled to less than 2 percent by 1930 (see figure 5). In part, this trend reflects administrative changes: as experiment stations became laboratories for graduate training, biochemists who worked there saw their primary role in the agricultural college, rather than in the station as such. This trend is reflected in the increase in the number of ASBC members affiliated with agricultural sciences from 2 percent to 9 percent, between 1910 and 1915.

Agricultural colleges never provided the kind of support system for biochemistry that medical schools did. Enrollment in agricultural colleges soared in the 1900s, while medical enrollments plummetted, and many new agricultural disciplines were established.[63] But agricultural chemistry remained an omnibus discipline, including biochemistry as one of its parts; in most schools, agricultural biochemistry did not become a separate discipline, as biochemistry did in medical schools. The most important reason was that agricultural colleges remained professional undergraduate colleges, much like the early medical colleges. Thus there was less room for specialized biochemistry in the curriculum and less demand for teachers with Ph.D.'s in agricultural biochemistry, and for advanced specialized research. Graduates of agricultural colleges went mainly into management and agribusiness, and science played a less important role in their professional practice than it did in medicine. Science did not regulate professional competition in agriculture as it did in medicine. A few very large and successful departments of biochemistry developed in agricultural colleges, notably at the University of Wisconsin (which had a professorial staff of eight by 1930, and an international reputation for its work on vitamins). The University of Minnesota, Iowa State, and a few others had separate departments of agricultural biochemistry, but these few saturated the field. By and large, in schools of agriculture, biochemistry remained a part of agricultural chemistry.

Hospitals were the second class of research institutions to expand research roles for biochemists. The representation of ASBC biochemists in hospitals grew rapidly in the late 1890s, peaked in 1902–3, and declined in relative importance from 1907. The early 1900s were marked by optimistic statements about the promise of hospitals, then being constructed at an unprecedented rate, as contexts for basic biomedical research.[64] Pathology laboratories, which had previously performed routine blood and urine analyses for clinicians, were transformed from dark and evil-smelling basement rooms to modern laboratories. Staffs of professional biochemists used the service role in clinical testing and diagnosis to get material for basic research on metabolism. At some of the larger hospitals—Roosevelt in New York, Massachusetts General and its McLean Asylum, Philadelphia General, and the Johns Hopkins Hospital—this Cinderella story was true.[65] The vast majority of civic hospitals, of course, did not support basic research, and the rapid growth of hospital roles for ASBC biochemists slowed to rather less than the growth of the discipline as a whole.

The hospitals that most regularly supported basic research were the teaching hospitals associated with medical schools. As hospitals became operating divisions of universities, research laboratories were increasingly staffed by biochemists whose primary appointment was on medical school faculties. Hospital laboratories, like the agricultural experiment stations, became, in effect, research extensions of university departments for employment, support, and training of graduate students. Biochemists were eager to have hospital connections.[66] It assured them of a supply of clinical material for research; hospital laboratories were, prior to the development of *in vitro* techniques, the best places for research on metabolism.

The third type of research institution to show a spurt of growth were agencies of the federal government, notably the Public Health Service and the Department of Agriculture.[67] The proportion of ASBC members in federal laboratories rose sharply from about 1905, peaked in 1908–9 at over 10 percent, then declined steadily for the next thirty years, relative to the proportion employed in medical schools. This rapid increase in government jobs in the 1900s coincides with the great expansion of the regulatory roles of the Department of Agriculture, and the increased acceptance of a federal role in the food-processing industries, as well as in research and development directed to the efficient utilization of agricultural by-products.[68] The Food and Drug Administration, under Harvey Wiley's aggressive leadership in the Bureau of Chemistry, provided jobs for hundreds of chemical analysts and a smaller number of research biochemists. The rapidly expanding Bureaus of Plant and Animal Industry employed the largest proportion of ASBC biochemists in government jobs.

Civil service codes and competition from universities resulted in improving working conditions for government biochemists. Government posts had been considered second rate, and scientists coming from academia had expected to be less well paid and to stick it out for only a few years. When Carl Alsberg left Harvard Medical School, in 1907, to accept a post in the Bureau of Animal Industry, he noted that things had changed in the Department of Agriculture. Alsberg wrote his own ticket; he was assured of autonomy, and expected to stay.[69] (In 1912 he succeeded Wiley as the chief of the Bureau of Chemistry.) Facilities for research were excellent, and in the 1900s it became a common practice for young biochemists with doctorates to acquire research experience for a few years in the Department of Agriculture before going on to an academic post.

In contrast to the medical schools, however, the basic mission of government bureaus was practical and bureaucratic, and the funding for basic research was limited. As medical schools improved their facilities for research, the proportion of ASBC members in government declined.

The private medical research institutes that began to proliferate after the opening of the Rockefeller Institute in 1904 also offered attractive alternatives to academic jobs. The proportion of society members in these institutes grew most rapidly between 1905 and 1912, declined relative to the other institutions in the 1920s, and increased again during the Depression, as academic jobs grew scarce. These institutes reflected the new significance that was attached to the idea of research in the Progressive period: research as a profession, as service, as producer of new kinds of goods and services. Following the model of the Pasteur Institutes in Europe, the new philanthropists put their money into special institutions devoted solely to the production of fundamental and useful medical discoveries.[70] The ideal was neatly expressed in a letter from Rockefeller counsel Starr J. Murphey to John D. Rockefeller, Jr.:

My own feeling . . . is that the Institute will eventually form the crown of medical research in this country. A great deal of research is being done in the hospitals, but this is necessarily limited in its character by the purposes for which hospitals are created. . . . The managers of hospitals should be limited to such work as is a direct aid in the treatment of the sick patients in the wards. The medical schools extend the scope of their research work considerably beyond that of the hospitals. Their primary function is that of teaching, and they, therefore, are at liberty to engage in research covering general problems of much broader scope than that which is proper in the hospitals, and yet . . . they are limited . . . to the work which has a bearing upon medical instruction. And finally, above them all, should come the work of your Institute for Medical Research which would take up the problems where the medical schools leave them, and treat them in their broadest aspects, and thus the hospitals and the medical schools . . . will lead up to and be feeders for the Institute, which will be the crown of the system.[71]

Philanthropists' preference for separate institutes created anxieties among university scientists that they might lose their role in large-scale research. These fears evaporated in the 1920s, with the growth of support for academic research, and the initiation of fellowship and grant programs by the large foundations, most notably the Rockefeller Foundation. (Biochemistry became a central part of the Foundation program in "molecular biology" in the 1930s.)[72]

For biochemists, the Rockefeller Institute was far and away the most important research institute. Peter Levene's and Donald D. Van Slyke's laboratories at the Institute and the Hospital produced five to ten times more papers for the *Journal of Biological Chemistry* than all the other institutes combined until after 1945. The Institute became a favorite place for postdoctoral research by young biochemists in the 1930s. For biochemists such as A. Baird Hastings, appointment to research institutes attached to departments of medicine was a step up the academic ladder.[73] E. C. Kendall, later to win a Nobel Prize, found a supportive context for a research career in the Mayo Foundation after moving successively through university, hospital, and industrial laboratories.[74]

But as figure 6 suggests, there were definite limits to the ability of independent research institutes to expand. Private endowment was a more limited basis for increasingly expensive research than the service roles in government, industry, or medical schools. Medical school departments also offered biochemists the promise of greater influence in the discipline through teaching on a graduate faculty. William Mansfield Clark was enticed away from his research team at the Public Health Service to the chair of biochemistry at Johns Hopkins in 1927; Hans T. Clarke left Eastman Kodak to succeed Gies, at Columbia, in 1928; Baird Hastings gave up research to succeed Folin, at Harvard, in 1937. The research institutes remained not the "crown," but a minor partner in a system dominated by the medical schools.

The last new market for biochemists was in industrial research. Opportunities increased sharply from 1915 to 1921, and kept pace with the expansion of universities through the 1920s and 1930s (see figure 5). The expansion of industrial roles for biochemists was part of the general boom in the chemical industry during and after World War I. The seizure of German chemical patents, and government-supported research and development in chemical warfare provided impetus for growth. The food processing and pharmaceutical industries developed rapidly to exploit the commercial opportunities resulting from the discoveries of new vitamins and hormones. Essential amino acids, the A, B, and D vitamins, insulin and the steroid hormones, and sulfa drugs, in turn, provided opportunities for the immediate application of basic biochemical research. And, as in other industries, increasing reliance on strategies of patent monoply and long-term market development through research and development created a favorable context for basic biochemical research in industry.[75]

Financial constraints limited the overhead of basic research in industry. Contributions to the discipline of biochemistry remained incidental to industrial goals. The most important role of biochemical industry for the discipline was in providing employment for the many biochemists with M.A.s and Ph.D.'s who were never elected to the ASBC, but whose training supported graduate programs and research in universities and medical schools.

Between 1900 and 1920, these new professional roles for biochemists were both stimulus and competition to hard-pressed medical schools. Industry, hospitals, bureaus, and research institutes were challenging the university monopoly in biochemical research at the same time that universities were reorganizing to meet the demand from these institutions for trained experts. The reestablishment of the medical school as the major context for biochemical research reflects the implicit division of labor which emerged in the 1920s, with medical schools carrying out general research in the basic applied sciences and providing research institutions with experts to carry out the more specialized research relevant to their institutional missions.

In the 1890s, biochemists were a small group of specialists working primarily in medical schools, with very limited opportunities for institutional expansion, and dependent on the goals and professional infrastructures of neighboring disciplines such as physiology, pathology, and clinical medicine. Between 1900 and 1920, the discipline was institutionalized as a regular department of the reformed medical schools, training physicians, but also training professionals for roles in other institutions. The recognition of biochemistry as a formal discipline resulted in fewer linkages with other biomedical disciplines, but in more diversified roles in applied biochemistry, notably in clinical medicine. Horizontal compartmentalization and vertical integration developed hand in hand. A social organization suited to the scattered and dependent structure of the emergent community in the 1890s gave way to an organization characteristic of modern academic disciplines and professions. This structure was complete by 1920, and for the next twenty years, biochemists exploited the opportunities for growth which were built into the system.

INSTITUTIONAL STRUCTURES AND INTELLECTUAL STYLES

In this account of the creation (or re-creation) of a discipline, I have deliberately emphasized the role of social structures and service roles over intellectual achievement. Obviously, a degree of intellectual accomplishment is necessary for claims to disciplinary status to be plausible. Physiologists, pathologists, and clinicians, in the 1890s and 1900s, exhorted university leaders that biochemistry was vital to their own disciplines. Biochemists argued that their subject was the foundation of all the biological disciplines. Some chemists were impressed by the promise of biochemical discovery. Those who made these assertions obviously had some reason to do so. The 1890s and 1900s were unusually rich in grand chemical theories of life processes: theories that all diseases were caused by the chemical action of bacterial toxins; Paul Ehrlich's side-chain theory of the immune response; the enzyme theory of cell function; Jacque Loeb's chemical theory of fertilization, development, and behavior.[76] There was widespread scepticism as to the details of such global theories, but widespread agreement that biochemistry would be indispensable to future progress in the biological and medical sciences. One can also spot some less sensational but more specific discoveries that seem to have played a special role in claims for biochemistry. The emerging understanding of the role of acidosis in causing the symptoms of diabetes is one such discovery.

My point is that there were almost always a sufficient number of such paradigms and theories to justify claims to disciplinary status for biochemistry. Acceleration in the pace of biochemical discovery between 1870 and 1920 was not great enough to have been the primary cause of its sudden recognition in the 1900s. It is most unlikely that specific discoveries of the sort that interest intellectual historians had any direct role in the establishment of biochemistry as a discipline. One small but suggestive example: Charles W. Eliot's brief for appointing Otto Folin to the Harvard Medical Faculty in 1907 did not mention Folin's two 1905 papers on the theory of protein metabolism, which were already famous. Eliot cited Folin's work on improved methods of urinalysis, and the relevance of his metabolic studies to clinical medicine.[77]

If we want to see the actual linkage between intellectual achievement and institutional rewards, we must look at the accumulation of technical knowledge, especially in applied biochemistry. The first generation of bio-chemists were not hired by other biochemists; they were hired by users of biochemical knowledge. The dramatic improvement in the rewards and incentives offered to biochemists has less to do with changes internal to biochemistry than with changes in the perceptions and programs of groups using biochemistry for their own purposes. These changes, in turn, reflect the new ideals of scientific medicine and the new service roles for biochem-ists in medical instruction.

Once established, of course, a discipline does gain a large degree of internal control over appointments and priorities, and its evolution will reflect the pace and nature of discovery. But the relationship between intellectual inquiry and social structure is a symbiotic one. The social organization of a discipline profoundly influences the kinds of problems that are addressed and the kinds of answers that are given. American biochemistry was shaped by the fact that it evolved out of medical chemis-try, rather than physiology, and that its primary service role was in turning out clinicians, rather than chemists or biologists. One can distinguish national styles, and these reflect differences in origins and institutional support systems.

I would argue, for example, that the rapid transition from medical chem-istry to biochemistry closed as many intellectual options as it opened. Biochemistry crystallized as a discipline in a single generation, in a way that put a premium on technical specialization and clinical application, rather than on investigating the intellectual connections between biochemistry and the other biomedical disciplines. American biochemists were not forced to think programmatically or to cultivate linkages with biology, whereas in Europe the social situation of biochemists encouraged these intellectual connections. Chittenden's programmatic statements describ-ing biochemistry as a broadly biological discipline ran afoul of Yale presi-dent Arthur Hadley's plans for a complete medical school.[78] Gies's cultiva-tion of linkages with Columbia biologists led to no institutionalized relations, and Gies drifted away from biochemistry into dental reform.[79] L. J. Henderson, who envisioned biochemistry as general physiology, lost out to Folin, who flourished on the connection to clinical medicine.[80] Loeb fled from the constraints of medical schools to the Rockefeller Institute, leaving his program for a discipline of chemical biology unrealized.[81]

Biochemistry is customarily regarded as a "hybrid" of chemistry and physiology, or as a filial branch of physiology. In Europe, biochemistry did evolve out of physiology, and the style of at least some departments re-flected this evolution. German biochemists, were (by necessity) trained in physiology and medicine and had few opportunities for specialized roles;

they dealt more easily with larger, more biological themes. Similarly, the close connection with organic chemistry led to a rich development in bio-organic chemistry. In England, a broadly biological program for bio-chemistry flourished in F. G. Hopkins's department at Cambridge University, which evolved out of physiology, and enjoyed almost complete independence from medicine.[82] Incomplete institutionalization in Germany and England kept intellectual options open to the few who managed to become professional biochemists. In the 1930s, American biochemists were going to Europe to learn a broader kind of "general biochemistry" from Hopkins, Otto Warburg, Otto Meyerhof, Adolf Butenandt, and others.

In America, however, biochemistry was not an offshoot of physiology but of medical chemistry, and its style reflected its historical evolution. The physiologists on the AMA Curriculum Committee took the standard view that intellectual affinity should be reflected in institutional structure: "Chemistry and physiology cannot be entirely separated in the organic world. Still less can they be separated in studying living things. . . . Physiologic or biochemistry should be considered a part of physiology rather than of chemistry. . . . It is probably expedient and even desirable that the two branches of physiology be included under one department of instruction."[83] But in practice, American biochemistry was shaped by its institutions and the structure of careers. American biochemists were trained in independent departments for careers in medical schools, generally in clinical biochemistry. Only a handful of ASBC members employed as biochemists had Ph.D.s in physiology; few biochemists shifted into or out of other biomedical diciplines. By 1925, there was a dramatic decline in the proportion of papers in the *Journal of Biological Chemistry* from departments of physiology and pathology, and an increasing proportion from departments of biochemistry, (table 2). Systematic influence from biology through recruitment or propinquity dwindled.

In contrast, chemistry and clinical medicine both exerted a continuing influence on biochemistry: the one through recruitment, the other through employment. Many biochemists were professionally trained as chemists. Of the 519 ASBC members with Ph.D.'s, 31 percent had degrees in chemistry, and 48 percent in biochemistry.[84] Comembership in the American Chemical Society jumped from 50 percent to 70 percent among those who got their Ph.D.'s after 1920, and reached a peak of 87 percent for the cohort of 1930–34. The appointment of pure chemists, such as W. M. Clark, Hans T. Clarke, and Vincent duVigneaud to major chairs at Johns Hopkins, Columbia, and Cornell, in the 1920s and 1930s, is indicative of the growing prestige of physical and organic chemists. Roger Adams and James B. Conant, The leading American organic chemists, received frequent offers of biochemical chairs. Chemists saw biochemistry become a prestigious field for professional careers. Conant urged Clarke to take the Columbia chair on the grounds that it would greatly advance the cause of organic chemistry in America.[85] Established patterns of recruitment meant that biochemistry in America was constantly infused with the disciplinary ideals, first, of medical and analytical chemistry, and later, of physical and organic chemistry. One would exaggerate only somewhat to say that American biochemistry remained a chemical specialty within a medical context.

The influence of the clinical connection came not through recruitment or choice of research tools but through employment and choice of research problems. It is evident in the steady, but modest, proportion of ASBC members affiliated with clinical medicine (figure 2). Medical research institutes were second only to universities in contributions to the *Journal of Biological Chemistry* (see table 1). Departments of medicine were the source of an increasing share of the papers from academic institutions (see table 2). Many of the most distinguished American biochemists made their reputations in clinical biochemistry: for improved analytical methods, or studies of pathological metabolism, electrolyte balance, and the physiology of urine secretion. Otto Folin, Donald Van Slyke, Stanley Benedict, and a host of lesser-known but influential department heads reflected this style of biochemistry. A survey of the twenty-four or so most productive departments of biochemistry shows that half were led by individuals who were involved in work of this sort, many of whom were students of Folin or Van Slyke.

This American style of biochemistry reflects the ecology of biochem-

Table 2

Disciplinary Sources of Articles Published in the *Journal of Biological Chemistry*

Year	Total Num.	Percent. of total articles	Percentage of Articles from Academic Departments					
			Bio-chemistry	Medical Sciences	Physiology	Pathology	Chemistry	Others
1907–8	65	61	35	—	23	11.0	17.0	7.7
1915	113	55	37	6.2	19	7.1	8.9	18.0
1926	148	63	47	14.0	7	4.0	18.0	10.0
1937	233	69	41	22.0	5	0.4	13.0	14.0
1948	394	71	59	6.9	8	1.8	11.0	10.0
1959	440	73	61	14.0	4	0.5	5.9	12.0

[1] Percentage of all articles from American universities and professional schools.

istry as an independent department in medical schools, with its main service role in training clinicians, and its links to hospital laboratories. It also reflects the historical process by which these departments and roles were taken over from medical chemists. It is striking how many of the first generation of American biochemists resembled their predecessors, the medical chemists, in their interest in analytical techniques and clinical applications. There were new faces, but old service roles, programmes, and intellectual preferences. The difference between medical chemistry and biochemistry is more a difference of generations than of species—moreso than the young Turks would have cared to admit. And the legacy of the medical chemists helps to explain why, thirty years later in the 1950s, a "molecular biology" developed by physicists, physiologists, geneticists, and microbiologists took another generation of biochemists by surprise. But that is another story.

CONCLUSION

The history of the modern biomedical sciences is an extremely rich and seriously underdeveloped field of research. Each of these disciplines was as profoundly affected as biochemistry by the reform of medical practice and training. Anatomy, pathology, pharmacology, and microbiology, to say nothing of the clinical fields, offer equal promise to historians of science and medicine. Interesting differences in the evolution of different fields are to be expected: the evolution of pharmacology out of pharmaceutical chemistry and materia medica was strikingly similar to that of biochemistry, for example, while anatomy presents a different picture of an established discipline torn apart by the conflicting ideals, service roles, and research interests of gross anatomists and cytologists, and with its dominance in the medical curriculum under attack from all sides. Physiology was threatened in a different way, losing provinces as separate disciplines or research specialties. The transition from pathological anatomy to physiological pathology was intimately involved with the changing ideals of scientific medicine and the changing ecology of medical disciplines. Bacteriology may prove to have the most complex and interesting set of social relations, for it had connections with pathology, hygiene and public health, agriculture, and general microbiology. I hope that this study may provide a model for comparative exploration of these disciplines in the common context of the medical reform movement, the strategies of "scientific medicine," and the structure of the new medical institutions.

NOTES

This paper was prepared with the support of the National Institutes of Health (grant no. LM–02630). I am greatly indebted to P. Thomas Carroll for his help in developing a program for the analysis of the American Society of Biological Chemists data, and for initiating me into the mysteries of computers.

1. John Field, "Medical Education in the United States: Late 19th and 20th Centuries," in Charles D. O'Malley, ed., *The History of Medical Education* (Berkeley: University of California Press, 1970), pp. 501–30; Richard Shryock, *The Unique Influence of the Johns Hopkins University on American Medicine* (Copenhagen: Munksgaard, 1953).

2. Morris Fishbein, *A History of the American Medical Association: 1847–1947* (Philadelphia: W. B. Saunders, 1947); V. Johnson and A. G. Weiskotten, *A History of the Council on Medical Education and Hospitals of the AMA, 1904–1957* (Chicago: American Medical Association, 1960); Robert P. Hudson, "Abraham Flexner in Perspective: American Medical Education, 1865–1910," *Bulletin of the History of Medicine* 46 (1972): 545–61; James G. Burrow, *Organized Medicine in the Progressive Era* (Baltimore: Johns Hopkins University Press, 1977); Rosemary Stevens, *American Medicine and the Public Interest* (New Haven: Yale University Press, 1971).

3. Stephen Kunitz, "Professionalism and Social Control in the Progressive Era: the Case of the Flexner Report," *Social Problems Journal* 22 (1974–75): 16–27; H.D. Banta, "Medical Education: Abraham Flexner, A Larger Perspective on the Flexner Report," *International Journal of Health Services* 5 (1975): 573–92; G. E. Markowitz and K. D. Rosner, "Doctors in Crisis: A Study of the Use of Medical Education Reform to Establish Modern Professional Elitism in Medicine," *American Quarterly* 25 (1973): 83–107; E. Richard Brown, *Rockefeller Medicine Men: Medicine and Capitalism in America* (Berkeley: University of California Press, 1979).

4. G. E. Berry, "Medical Education in Transition," *Journal of Medical Education* 28 (1953): 17–42; M.H. Littlemeyer, "Annotated Bibliography on Current Changes in Medical Education," idem, 43 (1968): 14–28; O. Cope and J. Zaccharias, *Medical Education Reconsidered* (Philadelphia: J. B. Lippincott, 1966).

5. Charles E. Rosenberg, "Toward an Ecology of Knowledge: on Discipline, Context and History," in Alexandra Oleson and John Voss, eds., *The Organization of Knowledge in Modern America, 1860–1920* (Baltimore: Johns Hopkins University Press, 1979).

6. Alfred D. Chandler, Jr., *Strategy and Structure: Chapters in the History of the American Industrial Enterprise* (Boston: MIT Press, 1962), chap. 1.

7. Hans-Heinz Eulner, *Die Entwicklung der medizinischen Spezialfächer an den Universitäten des deutschen Sprachgebietes* (Stuttgart: Ferdinand Enke Verlag, 1970).

8. See Frederick C. Waite, "What Medical Subjects Can be Taught Efficiently in the College of Liberal Arts?", *Proceedings of the American Association of Medical Colleges* 16 (1906): 25–33. See also other contributions and discussion in this volume.

9. It is significant that medical chemistry was established in independent institutes in Austrian medical faculties, which, like the American medical colleges, were much less developed academically than German medical faculties. See Eulner, *Die Entwicklung.*

10. Abraham Flexner, *Medical Education in the United States and Canada* (New York: Carnegie Foundation, 1910).

11. George Corner, *Two Centuries of Medicine: A History of the School of Medicine, University of Pennsylvania* (Philadelphia: Lippincott, 1965).

12. For data on enrollment, see *Journal of the American Medical Association* 87 (21 August 1926): 565–73.

13. Edward A. Krug, *The Shaping of the American High School, 1880–1920* (Madison: University of Wisconsin Press, 1969), chap. 3; Hugh Hawkins, *Between Harvard and America* (New York: Oxford University Press, 1972).

14. Thomas F. Harrington, *The Harvard Medical School: A History, Narrative and Documentary* (New York: Lewis, 1905); correspondence between Henry Christian and Jerome Greene (1908–10), C. W. Eliot Papers, box 207, Harvard University Archives, Cambridge, Mass.

15. Raymond B. Fosdick, *Adventure in Giving: the Story of the General Education Board* (New York: Harper and Row, 1962); General Education Board, *Annual Reports*, 1903–10.

16. See Abraham Flexner, *Medical Education, A Comparative Study* (New York: Macmillan, 1925), chap. 3, for the most explicit statement of Flexner's policies.

17. See n. 2.

18. See n. 12.

19. See Gabriel Kolko, *Railroads and Regulation, 1877–1916* (Princeton: University Press, 1965). Revisionist historians see the reform in medical education as an elitist conspiracy to create a professional monopoly. It is more accurate, I think, to see it as a response by many interest groups to a new social and economic context. For a more subtle interpretation of interest politics, see Samuel P. Hays, "New Possibilities for American Political History; the Social Analysis of Political Life," in S. M. Lipset and R. Hofstadter, eds., *Sociology and History: Methods* (New York: Basic Books, 1968), esp. p. 201, and Richard Hofstadter, *The Progressive Historians* (New York: Knopf, 1969), pp. 244–45.

20. Stevens, *American Medicine*, chap. 2. See also her *Medical Practice in Modern England: The Impact of Specialization and State Medicine* (New Haven: Yale University Press, 1966).

21. See Robert H. Wiebe, *The Search for Order, 1877–1920* (New York: Hill and Wang, 1967); Richard Hofstader, *Anti-intellectualism in American Life* (New York: Knopf, 1963).

22. John A. Mandel to William Welch, 15 April 1894, J. J. Abel Papers Johns Hopkins Medical School, Baltimore, Md.; John H. Long, "The Relation of Modern Chemistry to Modern Medicine," *Science* 20 (1904): 1–14. On Rockwood: Henry Mattill to P. A. Shaffer, 24 August 1936, Shaffer Papers, box 8, folder 81, Medical Archives, Washington University, St. Louis, Mo. Harvard University, *Catalogue* [s], 1895–99. John Marshall's budget for general and physiological chemistry, in 1908, was $550 and $1350, respectively: University of Pennsylvania Medical Council Minutes, 1907–8, University of Pennsylvania Archives, Philadelphia, Pa.

23. Various authors, *The University of Texas Medical Branch-Galveston* (Galveston: University of Texas Press, 1967), pp. 41–42.

24. Ibid., p. 83.

25. Corner, *Two Centuries of Medicine*, pp. 205–7. Horatio C. Wood was professor of pharmacology, nervous diseases, and materia medica; Alexander Abbott, professor of bacteriology; Flexner had just accepted the directorship of the Rockefeller Institute.

26. Ibid., pp. 210, 223–24.

27. "A Model Medical Curriculum, Report of the Committee of 100—Council on Medical Education of the AMA," *American Medical Association Bulletin* 5 (1909): 48–62 (also issued separately); quotation, pp. 54–55.

28. Harvard University, *Catalogue,* 1904–5; University of Pennsylvania, *Catalogue,* 1903–4; Philip Hawk to Howard B. Lewis, 24 May 1952, H. B. Lewis Papers, Bentley Historical Library, University of Michigan, Ann Arbor, Mich.

29. "Model Medical Curriculum," pp. 50–51.

30. Correspondence between John G. Curtis and Seth Low, 1897–99, folder "Curtis," Columbia University Central Files, Low Library, Columbia University, New York.

31. Henry P. Bowditch to C. W. Eliot, 13 August 1902, 6 December 1905; Walter B. Cannon to C. W. Eliot, 28 October 1904, C. W. Eliot Papers, boxes 203, 205.

32. Correspondence between Eugene Opie, John Howland, George Dock, and Joseph Erlanger, 1910. Eugene Opie Papers, American Philosophical Society, Philadelphia, Pa.

33. The arguments presented to the AAMC for and against allowing credit toward an M.D. for courses taken in liberal arts colleges are very revealing of these attitudes. *Proceedings of the Association of American Medical Colleges* 16 (1906).

34. Herringham and Fletcher, "Memorandum Presented to the University Grants Committee" (London: H. M. Stationery Office, May 1921). Fletcher deplored the fact that pharmacology, as it became independent, took away vital parts of physiology.

35. University of Pennsylvania Medical Council Minutes, 13 February 1911, vol. 1, pp. 361–63. The twenty-three medical schools were: Harvard, Columbia, Johns Hopkins, Wisconsin, Michigan, Chicago-Rush, Minnesota, Western Reserve, Cornell, Yale, Washington University, California, Stanford, Syracuse, Virginia, Missouri, North and South Dakota, Utah, Northwestern, Toronto, McGill, Southern California, and Indiana.

36. Untitled MS, "Folin Mins," undated (circa 1920), P. A. Shaffer Papers, box 6, folder 60; Otto Folin, "Teaching of Biological Chemistry," in "Reports of Committee on Medical Education to the AAMC and AMA Council, Chicago 1–3 March 1920," *Journal of the American Medical Association* 74 (1920): 823–26.

37. Ibid.

38. Paul F. Clark, *The University of Wisconsin Medical School: A Chronicle, 1848–1948* (Madison: University of Wisconsin Press, 1967), pp. 112–18; Merle Curti, *The University of Wisconsin,* 2 vols., (Madison: University of Wisconsin Press, 1949), vol. 2, pp. 485 ff. See also Harold C. Bradley to Joseph Erlanger, 5 September 1906, and other correspondence in the Joseph Erlanger Papers, Washington University Medical School, St. Louis, Mo.

39. Russell Chittenden, *History of the Sheffield Scientific School of Yale University, 1846–1922* (New Haven: Yale University Press, 1928), chaps. 15, 19; various authors, *Past, Present and Future of Yale University School of Medicine* (New Haven: Yale University Press, 1922). See also Charles H. Warren to James R. Angell, 3 April 1936; Warren to Stanhope Bayne-Jones, 24 March 1936, and other correspondence in the Yale Medical Deans' Files, box 21, folder, "Dept. Physiological Sciences," Yale University Archives, New Haven, Conn.

40. University of Illinois, "Special Circular by the Department of Chemistry, 1916–1927" (Urbana: The University of Illinois, 1927); see also University of Illinois *Catalogues.*

41. Philip A. Shaffer to Abraham Flexner, 16 March 1920; Alonzo Taylor to Flexner, 1 June 1920; Otto Folin to Flexner, 9 March 1920; Simon Flexner to Abraham Flexner, 5 March 1920, General Education Board Archives, series B19, file "Columbia P and S," Rockefeller Archives Center, North Tarrytown, N.Y. Shaffer to A. Flexner, 16 March 1921, Shaffer Papers, box 6, folder 57.

42. Otto Folin to Abraham Flexner, 9 March and 18 March 1920, Shaffer Papers, box 6, folder 57.

43. See "Folin Mins.," pp. 5–6, 9.

44. For example: William J. Gies to N. M. Butler, 17 October and 15 June 1905, Columbia Central Files. Otto Folin to J. J. Abel, n.d. (circa 1909), Abel Papers.

45. See correspondence between Abel and Herter, 1904–5, in the Abel Papers.

46. R. H. Chittenden, *The First Twenty Five Years of the American Society of Biological Chemists,* (New Haven: for the Society, 1945). See extensive correspondence between William J. Gies and J. J. Abel in the Columbia Central Files (folder W. J. Gies), and the Abel Papers.

47. Lawrence J. Henderson, "Memories," undated MS (circa 1939), pp. 86 ff., 121 ff., L. J. Henderson Papers, Harvard University Archives, Cambridge, Mass.

48. See Robert E. Kohler, "The Enzyme Theory and the Origins of Biochemistry," *Isis* 64 (1973): 181–96.

49. See Daniel J. Kevles, *The Physicists* (New York: Knopf, 1978); D. J. Kevles, "The Physics, Mathematics and Chemistry Communities: a Comparative Analysis," in Oleson and Voss, *The Organization of Knowledge in Modern America,* pp. 139–72.

50. Kevles, "Physics, Mathematics and Chemistry."

51. Stanley Benedict to P. A. Shaffer, 26 January 1915, Shaffer Papers, box 4, folder 29. Benedict was complaining that some professors got their students elected before they had demonstrated their research ability. In fact, a good number of ASBC members elected with fresh Ph.D.'s had undistinguished careers.

52. Membership lists up to 1940 are given by Chittenden, *First Twenty-Five Years;* for subsequent years, membership lists were obtained from the society.

53. The ASBC sample underrepresents the larger "profession," i.e., biochemists whose rewards were for the effective use of knowledge, not for the publication of research. The "discipline" is a special subgroup within the "profession."

54. The population considered in any year consisted of all individuals who were then, or subsequently, members of the ASBC. As a result, employment patterns are given for some years before the society was founded. Medical practice, schoolteaching, and chemical consulting were not scored as "professional employment," and individuals (when so employed) were dropped from the sample. A special category of eighteen "clinical members" elected between 1922 and 1925 were not included.

55. Discipline affiliation was inferred, for more than 85 percent of the sample, from job title, department, title of Ph.D. dissertation, self-identification, and research interests. Disciplinary affiliation was not necessarily the same for each job. Disciplinary affiliation is, of course, conventional and means different things in different contexts, especially outside of academia. "Other biomedical sciences" include anatomy, physiology, pathology, bacteriology, and pharmacology.

56. The sample for fig. 4 is 618, since 37 of the total of 655 did not have a Ph.D. or M.D. Note that each set of bar graphs does not indicate changes in the comembership of the entire population, but only of successively "younger" Ph.D. or M.D. cohorts.

57. Adjunct members of the AMA (non-M.D.'s) were not scored as comembers.

58. R. F. Bud, P. T. Carroll, J. L. Sturchio, and A. W. Thackray, *Chemistry in America, 1876–1976: An Historical Application of Science Indicators: Report to the National Science Foundation* (Philadelphia: University of Pennsylvania, 1978); National Research Council, Board on Human-Resource Data and Analysis, *A Century of Doctorates: Data-Analyses of Growth and Change* (Washington D.C.: National Academy of Science, 1978).

59. This bias toward the university category is magnified by the fact that uncertain cases were arbitrarily assigned to "university." The proportions of medical school biochemists are minimum figures. However, a subsequent survey of individual medical schools revealed that all but a handful depended almost entirely on their role in medical education, even those in university preclinical departments.

60. K. P. Bunnell, "Liberal Education and American Medicine," *Journal of Medical Education* 33 (1958): 319–40 (see pp. 328–34); C. P. Emerson, "The Danger of the Stereotyped Curriculum," *Journal of the American Medical Association* 80 (1923): 1009–11; P. A. Shaffer to A. Flexner, 16 March 1920, Shaffer Papers, box 6; Otto Folin to A. Flexner, 10 March 1920, General Education Board Archives, series B19, file "Columbia P and S."

61. George W. Corner, *The Rockefeller Institute, 1901–1953* (New York: Rockefeller Institute Press, 1964); Howard S. Miller, *Dollars for Research* (Seattle: University of Washington Press, 1970), chap. 9. See also the series of articles on the Carnegie Institution by Henry Pritchett, J. C. Branner, James McKeen Cattell *et al.* in *Science* 16 (1902).

62. Charles E. Rosenberg, "Science, Technology, and Economic Growth: the Case of the Agricultural Experiment Station Scientist, 1875–1914," in *No Other Gods* (Baltimore: Johns Hopkins University Press, 1976).

63. Margaret Rossiter, "The Agricultural Sciences in the U.S., 1860–1920," in Oleson and Voss, *The Organization of Knowledge in Modern America*.

64. For example, Otto Folin, "Chemical Problems in Hospital Practice," *Harvey Lectures* 3 (1909): 187–98. Folin was at McLean Hospital, which had an unusually strong research department as early as the 1880s; see *Annual Report of the Massachusetts General Hospital* 87 (1900): 161–62; 88 (1901): 170–72; 89 (1902): 205–7.

65. Frederic A. Washburn, *The Massachusetts General Hospital. Its Development 1920–1935* (Boston: Houghton Mifflin, 1939); Nathaniel W. Faxon, *The Massachusetts General Hospital 1935–1955* (Cambridge: Harvard University Press, 1959); Albert R. Lamb, *The Presbyterian Hospital and the Columbia-Presbyterian Medical Center 1868–1943* (New York: Columbia University Press, 1955); Alan M. Chesney, *The Johns Hopkins Hospital and the Johns Hopkins University School of Medicine: A Chronicle,* 3 vols. (Baltimore: Johns Hopkins University Press, 1943, 1958, 1963); Samuel Bookman, "Twenty-five Years of Physiological Chemistry at Mt. Sinai Hospital, 1902–1927, *"Journal of Mt. Sinai Hospital* 12 (1940): 87–90; various authors, *The Roosevelt Hospital, 1871–1957* (New York: Roosevelt Hospital, 1954).

66. William J. Gies to Dean Hallock, 9 June 1906; Gies to Dean Lambert, 28 September 1911, Columbia Central Files, folder "Gies"; H. Gideon Wells to James B. Angell, 16 January 1912, University of Chicago Presidents Papers, box 58, folder 5, University of Chicago Archives, Chicago, Ill.; F. S. Hollis to J. J. Abel, 14 June 1911, Abel Papers; Rufus Cole to Frank Underhill, 27 May 1910, F. Underhill Papers, Yale University Archives, New Haven, Conn.; Philip Shaffer, untitled address to the ASBC Anniversary, 18 March 1956, Shaffer Papers, box 2, folder 18; Philip Shaffer to Dean Allison, 14 February 1922, Washington University Medical Deans' Files, box 6, folder "Biological Chem.," Medical Archives, Washington University, St. Louis, Mo.; and documents in n. 41.

67. The Public Health Service employed far fewer ASBC biochemists prior to World War II than the Department of Agriculture. The military services and the Bureau of Standards employed almost none.

68. A. Hunter Dupree, *Science in the Federal Government* (Cambridge: Harvard University Press, 1959), chaps. 8, 13.

69. Carl Alsberg to C. W. Eliot, 27 August 1908, Eliot Papers, box 213; Joseph S. Davis, *Carl Alsberg, Scientist at Large* (Stanford: University Press, 1948).

70. See n. 61.

71. S. J. Murphy to J. D. Rockefeller, Jr., 19 December 1901, in "Papers Concerning the Proposed New Buildings and Endowment for the Medical School," Eliot Papers, box 104, folder 47. See also Harrington, *Harvard Medical School*.

72. Nathan Reingold, "The Case of the Disappearing Laboratory," *American Quarterly* 29 (1977): 79–101; Stanley Coben, "Foundation Officers and Fellowships: Innovation in the Patronage of Science," *Minerva* 14 (1976): 225–40; Robert E. Kohler, "The Management of Science: the Experience of Warren Weaver and the Rockefeller Foundation Programme in Molecular Biology," *Minerva* 14 (1976): 279–306, and "The Patronage of Scientific Research: Reorganization in the Rockefeller Foundation, 1922–1929," *Minerva* (in press).

73. Maurice Visscher to A. Baird Hastings, 2 May 1928, Hastings Papers Countway Medical Library, Boston, Mass.

74. Edward C. Kendall, *Cortisone* (New York: Scribners, 1971).

75. David Nobel, *America by Design* (New York: Knopf, 1978); Bud, Carroll, Sturchio and Thackray, *Chemistry in America*.

76. See Robert E. Kohler, "The History of Biochemistry: A Survey," *Journal of the History of Biology* 8 (1975): 275–318. A case for the importance of such paradigmatic ideas is made in my article, "The Enzyme Theory and the Origins of Biochemistry," *Isis* 64 (1974): 181–96.

77. Memo in Eliot's hand, 27 May 1907, Eliot Papers, box 222, folder "C. L. Jackson."

78. *Report of the President of Yale University, 1905*, pp. 116–18; idem, *1906*, pp. 9–13; R. H. Chittenden to Arthur T. Hadley, 7 December 1909, Hadley Papers, box 17, folder 322 Yale University Archives, New Haven, Conn.; Chittenden, *Sheffield Scientific School*.

79. W. J. Gies to Dean Hallock, 9 June 1906, and other correspondence with N. M. Butler, Columbia Central Files; Benjamin Harrow, unpublished biographical sketch of Gies (circa 1956) in the Hans T. Clarke Papers, American Philosophical Society, Philadelphia, Pa.

80. Henderson, "Memories," Henderson Papers, Harvard Archives, Cambridge, Mass.; Walter Bloor to P. A. Shaffer, 6 June 1949, Shaffer Papers, box 6, folder 60; David Edsall to A. Lawrence Lowell, 29 January 1920, David Edsall Papers, Countway Medical Library, Boston, Mass.

81. W. J. V. Osterhout, "Jacques Loeb," National Academy of Sciences *Biographical Memoirs*, 13 (1930): 318–400; see Loeb to Simon Flexner, pp. 326–28.

82. "Walter Fletcher, F. G. Hopkins, and the Dunn Institute of Biochemistry: A Case Study in the Patronage of Science," *Isis* 69 (1978): 331–55.

83. "Model Medical Curriculum."

84. The degree fields of 21 percent of the sample could not be determined from information in *American Men of Science*. This vital datum was given first in the 1949 edition.

85. James B. Conant to Hans T. Clarke, 23 May 1928, Clarke Papers, American Philosophical Society, Philadelphia, Pa. See Julius Stieglitz, *Chemistry and Recent Progress in Medicine* (Baltimore: Williams and Wilkins, 1926).

When you enter my wards your first duty is to forget all your physiology. Physiology is an experimental science—and a very good thing no doubt in its proper place. Medicine is not a science, but an empirical art.

Samuel Gee (1888)[1]

3 DIVIDED WE STAND: Physiologists and Clinicians in the American Context

GERALD L. GEISON

INTRODUCTION

By the mid-nineteenth century, European physiologists had largely won their campaign to secure the independence of their subject from medical anatomy. They had achieved this emancipation by self-consciously adopting an experimental approach toward the study of vital processes. They exploited for their own purposes recent advances in physics and chemistry, and they especially emphasized the value of vivisection experiments in the investigation of animal function. Henceforth they could claim to belong to a separate discipline no longer to be regarded as a mere "handmaiden" of medicine.[2]

A generation later, English and American physiologists had begun to enjoy a similar sense of independence. Yet the prospects of the new discipline remained closely bound up with the destinies of medicine and medical education. If physiology found its most receptive home in universities (occasionally even in philosophical faculties rather than medical schools), its audience nonetheless consisted overwhelmingly of intending physicians. Without those premedical and medical students, and without the resources that came to it by virtue of its association with medicine, the newly "independent" discipline would have withered on the vine. However distasteful it may have been for some research physiologists to admit it, they remained essentially parasitic on the larger medical enterprise from which they had emerged.

But perhaps medicine was itself becoming dependent upon its new disciplinary offspring. Perhaps, to modify my earlier metaphor, it was less the case that physiology remained parasitic on medicine than that the two had entered into a symbiotic relationship. Many physiologists certainly believed (or hoped) so. The benefits that medicine derived from this symbiosis have traditionally been described (by physiologists and medical historians alike) in terms of the presumed utility of physiological theories, techniques, and instruments for the medical problems faced by practicing doctors. The word "presumed" is used advisedly, for these traditional allusions to the medical utility of physiology are disappointingly brief and vague.[3] They tend to take for granted the point at issue. No one, to my knowledge, has yet made a sustained effort to identify the specific ways in which experimental physiology has contributed to the healing task.

Some readers may feel that the contributions of the discipline to medical practice were (and are) so obvious as to require neither detailed elaboration nor systematic defense. Yet repeated assertions as to the medical value of experimental physiology have failed to still a remarkably persistent stream of skepticism toward the discipline on the part of practicing doctors. The evidence for this skepticism is admittedly somewhat fragmentary, and must usually be surmised from the remarks of physiologists themselves. But since medical history, like other history, reflects the views of academic elites, one may wonder whether there have not been thousands of fellow travelers in spirit for every busy doctor whose skepticism has found its way into print. Moreover, it is the persistence of this attitude, rather than its extent, that is perhaps more striking and more in need of explanation.

Although this essay focuses on the division between physiologists and clinicians in the American context, it is important to recognize that there was nothing uniquely American about the situation. We do not have to do here with some trivial manifestation of the alleged pragmatism of American society. As the discipline of physiology took root in Europe, so, too, did the skepticism of clinicians toward it. When the great French physiologist Claude Bernard began to lecture on the medical significance of experimental physiology, he lamented the number of physicians who believed that "physiology can be of no practical use in medicine," that it was "but a science *de luxe* which could well be dispensed with."[4] It was presumably in an effort to change this attitude that Bernard wrote his famous *Introduction to the Study of Experimental Medicine* (1865). He offered there his vision of a new "scientific" medicine as the way out of the therapeutic uncertainty and nihilism of that era. Obviously irritated by the "false opinion" that medicine was not a science but a mysterious art, Bernard went on to dispute the long-standing claim that the best physiologists are the worst doctors, the "most awkward when action is necessary at the patient's bedside." To Bernard it seemed obvious that "solid instruction in physiology . . . , the most scientific part of medicine," was precisely the one thing that physicians most needed.[5]

Skeptical doctors may have been bemused to compare Bernard's prescription with that of his contemporary, the Prussian pathologist Rudolf Virchow. For Virchow, writing in the 1840s and 1850s, the royal road to medical certainty lay not through ordinary physiology ("a 'respectable' science but thus far a very incomplete one"), but rather through Virchow's own specialty of "pathological physiology." Unlike ordinary physiology, pathological physiology recognized that even a complete knowledge of drug action under normal conditions would be inadequate for understanding the therapeutic effects of drugs under pathological conditions. Moreover, pathological physiology "does not stand before the gates of medicine but lives in its mansion":

> [It] receives its questions in part from pathological anatomy, in part from practical medicine; it derives its answers partly from observation by the sickbed, to this extent being a division of the clinic, and partly from animal experiment.[6]

For all of that, however, the similarity between Bernard's campaign and Virchow's was more striking than their differences in matters of detail. Both would have medicine built upon basic science, and for both (as Virchow put it in 1847) "experiment is the final and highest court."[7] From Virchow himself, we gain some sense of the reception his program got from medical men. A surgeon named Schuh, whom Virchow had accused of failing to grasp the real significance of the new scientific knowledge and techniques, responded by saying that he was no more competent than anyone else to undertake the task Virchow had in view. As Virchow reported it, Schuh said that "he gladly left to others the saccharine practice of dreaming and the enjoyment of infallibility; meanwhile he, as a practical surgeon, stood on the same field of observation as his forebears had for centuries."[8]

One can, of course, look upon such reactions as merely inevitable in an era when the new or emerging disciplines of experimental biology had yet to establish their relevance and value for medical practice. For physiology, as I have suggested elsewhere, the yoke of utility was especially burdensome. At least as late as the 1870s, even the most aggressive spokesmen for the discipline found it difficult to think of any physiological discovery that had made a significant, direct impact on the art of healing. In his *Introduction*, Bernard could only point rather weakly toward the experimental eradication of the "itch" (scabies). In 1874, Michael Foster, founder of what was to become the great Cambridge School of Physiology, tried to justify vivisection by claiming that it had already played an important role in the advance of the healing task. But he could offer only two specific examples, both of them dubious: allegedly experimental advances in methods of ligature had improved the treatment of aneurysms, and Claude Bernard's work on the glycogenic function of the liver provided the only available source of illumination into the problem of diabetes, which unfortunately remained outside the therapeutic pale.[9]

What Bernard and Foster really sought to convey was the medical promise of experimental physiology, but their efforts won only guarded and partial acceptance from medical men. Before the 1870s, precisely because its therapeutic value was considered dubious, experimental physiology (and laboratory science in general) found no place in the English medical curriculum, which was shaped predominantly by the pragmatic demands of the London hospital schools. Foster's colleague and compatriot, John Scott Burdon Sanderson, faced the problem candidly and directly in 1872, when he told the British Association for the Advancement of Science that the revival of English physiology depended above all on overcoming "that practical tendency of the national mind which leads us Englishmen to underrate or depreciate any kind of knowledge which does not minister directly to personal comfort or advantage."[10]

Burdon Sanderson's address came on the eve of the exciting work of Koch and Pasteur in bacteriology and immunology. Obviously encouraged by these dramatic developments in neighboring fields, some physiologists (and "pathological physiologists") now found it easier to speak confidently about the medical utility of their research. As early as 1877, in fact, Virchow could write as follows:

> It is no longer necessary today to write that scientific medicine is also the best foundation for medical practice. It is sufficient to point out how completely even the external character of medical practice has changed in the last thirty years. Scientific methods have been introduced everywhere into practice. The diagnosis and prognosis of the physician are based on the expe-

rience of the pathological anatomist and the physiologist. Therapeutic doctrine has become biological and thereby experimental science. Concepts of healing processes are no longer separated from those of physiological regulatory processes. Even surgical practice has been altered to its foundations, not by the empiricism of war, but in a much more radical manner by means of a completely theoretically constructed therapy.[11]

Nonetheless, there is evidence to suggest that many clinicians continued long afterward to doubt the utility of all this newfangled science. The epigraph with which this essay begins reminds us that as late as 1888 an academic clinician could advise his ward clerks that their "first duty" was to "forget all [their] physiology."[12] Especially now, when the scientific basis of modern medicine is taken so much for granted, the long-standing split between doctors and research physiologists seems worthy of more systematic attention than it has hitherto received.

In what follows, the persistence of this division after 1870 is explored with specific reference to the American context. The latter half of the paper very briefly surveys several factors that may help to explain the phenomenon, including the possibility that the skeptical physicians may actually have had some justification for their doubts about the medical utility of laboratory physiology.

But two cautionary and qualifying remarks should be recorded now. First, this is an exploratory effort, not yet buttressed by the sort of extensive evidence we shall surely need to do full justice to the issues it raises. Second, while every effort has been made to focus on the attitudes of practicing doctors toward physiology per se, these attitudes almost invariably reflect a very similar posture toward experimental science in general. Indeed, a much longer essay (or book) might well be written on the persistent skepticism of many ordinary doctors toward experimental science from its beginnings to the present day.

THE PERSISTENCE OF THE DIVISION IN THE UNITED STATES AFTER 1870

Like his colleagues in Europe, Henry Newall Martin, first professor of biology at the new Johns Hopkins University (from 1876 to 1893), insisted that physiology "should be cultivated as a pure science absolutely independent of any so-called practical affiliation." Yet he could scarcely ignore the fact that his discipline's raison d'etre "in the mind of even the educated public rested on its relation to medical instruction." Martin therefore worked hard to establish rapport with the medical profession, at one point inviting local physicians to his course of physiological demonstrations.[13]

But in Baltimore, as elsewhere, experimental physiology must have seemed very far removed from the immediate problems of practicing doctors. There was as yet, in the 1870s and 1880s, precious little evidence of its pragmatic value, and no obvious reason to suspect that the situation might soon change. In a sense, American doctors probably agreed with Martin that experimental physiology, if it were to be pursued at all, must indeed be pursued independently of pragmatic medical concerns.

That assessment was clearly shared by those most directly responsible for medical education. For while many medical students might want or need some exposure to human physiology, few indeed would perceive any special need for the sort of experimental training emphasized by the emerging band of professional investigators in the discipline. Insofar as these students did represent a natural (or even captive) audience for physiology, their primary need was for oral (rather than laboratory) instruction in the settled points of functional human anatomy. Thus, even as medical schools did begin increasingly to employ professional, laboratory-trained physiologists, they did not really expect their students to repeat the most salient features of the training those physiologists had themselves received.

Even at Harvard Medical School, which had established an assistant professorship in physiology as early as 1870 and had provided a laboratory for the first incumbent (H. P. Bowditch), two decades passed before students were required to take a course in laboratory physiology. By then, laboratory courses had been established at two other major medical schools (the University of Michigan, in 1887, and Columbia University, in 1891), but both courses were elective, rather than required. The course at Columbia did not become required of medical students until 1902.[14] Partly, no doubt, because it was so expensive to provide, laboratory physiology found precious little place in the American medical curriculum before 1900. The process by which it finally did become a regular part of medical education has gone virtually unexplored, though it seems likely that laboratory physiology was one of the chief beneficiaries of that more general reform movement in medical education associated with the activities of the American Medical Association's Council on Medical Education (established in 1904) and with the famous Flexner Report of 1910.[15]

Even then, the AMA's classification of the discipline suggests some continued uncertainty about its precise relationship to medicine. From 1901 until at least the 1930s, physiology was placed in the AMA's section on "Pathology and Physiology," having previously been relegated to sections on "Medical Jurisprudence, Hygiene and Physiology" (1847–73),

"Practical Medicine, Materia Medica and Physiology" (1874–91), and "Physiology and Dietetics" (1892–1900).[16] Professional physiologists doubtless preferred their new union with the pathologists to those earlier sectional associations, but they may also have wondered whether their own research interests would now be subordinated to the interests of pathologists, "pathological physiologists," or bacteriologists. Perhaps that concern helped to motivate the provision, adopted at the outset, that a physiologist would serve as chairman of the new section every third year.[17]

Implicit, at any rate, in the curricular neglect of laboratory physiology was the assumption that practicing doctors had little or no need of it. Occasionally, that assumption found explicit verbal expression as well. In the 1890s, when the American Physiological Society almost collapsed from lack of interest, even some spokesmen for "scientific medicine" were heard to say that "physiology had done all it could for medicine".[18] In the 1902 edition of his spectacularly popular *Book on the Physician Himself, and Things that Concern His Reputation and Success,* D. W. Cathell claimed that the new scientific knowledge might actually be damaging to his primary readership, ordinary general practitioners. He warned his readers not to be "biased too quickly or too strongly in favor of new theories based on physiological, microscopical, chemical or other experiments, especially when offered by the unbalanced to establish their abstract conclusions or preconceived notions." To submit too readily to the appeal of theoretical science "may impair your practical tendency, give your mind a wrong bias and almost surely make your usefulness as a practicing physician diminish." Scientific curiosity was all well and good for those "scholars and scientists" who did not depend upon practice for their "bread and butter." But the "first question for you, as a practitioner, seeking additional and better tools, to ask yourself in everything of this kind is 'What is its use to me?' "[19] Very different in tone, but not remarkably different in its conclusions about the direct utility of experimental physiology, was the complaint of clinician S. J. Meltzer, in 1904, that internal medicine had received little benefit from physiology "because this science is keeping aloof from medicine and its problems."[20]

As laboratory physiology became an established part of the medical curriculum, the number of skeptics perhaps declined, but they certainly did not disappear. From Meltzer through Rufus Cole and Alfred Cohn, in the 1920s and 1930s, to Frank McLean, in the 1960s, one can trace the theme that physiology—if it had once been useful for clinical medicine—was becoming less so every day. That, at any rate, was part of the justification these men offered for their efforts to establish and extend a new independent discipline of experimental clinical medicine. They hoped that this new discipline would reduce some of the obvious distance between the laboratory and the ward.[21]

In a way, the frequency with which physiologists and academic clinicians continued to insist upon the need for closer interaction between the two fields is itself a striking indication of the persistence of their separation. Physiologist W.H. Sewall might insist, in 1923, that "today . . . every physician recognizes that he is likely to understand his sick man in proportion as he apprehends 'clinical physiology',"[22] but that same year, one such "clinical physiologist," A.B. Luckhardt, lamented the continuing split between the clinician and the laboratory worker. "Although both groups are intensely interested in the progress of medicine," he wrote, "each group, curiously enough, views the work of the other either with a silent disregard or more often with disdain or openly expressed contempt."[23] Five years later, physiologist C. J. Wiggers thought he detected a few encouraging signs of increased cooperation between clinicians and physiologists, but he could still only hope that they would soon be "walking arm in arm," rather than "making mere gestures of shaking hands across the street."[24]

As a matter of fact, most such appeals for greater cooperation between the clinician and the laboratory worker probably understated the extent and depth of the split. The problem went beyond the mere indifference or skepticism of clinicians toward laboratory science. Some clinicians, including a few of the most celebrated, continued to echo D. W. Cathell's concern that laboratory training might actually *damage* the practitioner's ability to treat patients effectively. Although my first two examples of this sentiment will be drawn from statements by great English clinicians, there is no doubt that American counterparts could be found. Sir Archibald Garrod, renowned for his work on the "inborn errors of metabolism," wrote in 1911 of his belief that "laboratory findings are little less fallible than clinical inferences, and . . . in some cases they actually mislead."[25] In 1919, the eminent cardiologist Sir James Mackenzie expressed the same reservation far more harshly in his book, *The Future of Medicine.* "Laboratory training," he wrote, *"unfits* a man for his work as a physician, for the reason that, not only does the laboratory man fail to educate his senses, but he puts so much trust in his mechanical methods that he never recognizes their limitations and he fails to see that there are other methods which are essential to the interpretation of disease."[26] A decade later the American clinician, Alfred Cohn, who generally adopted a more nuanced and less hostile tone, did nonetheless insist that "the history of medicine since the Renaissance has shown plentifully that whenever the approach to an understanding of disease is made by scholars trained primarily in other pursuits of knowledge [including physiology] . . . the result, so far as understanding disease is concerned, is disappointing and sometimes grotesque."[27] As recently as 1967, in his book *Clinical Judgment,* American cardiologist Alvan Feinstein produced a perceptive and sometimes eloquent statement of the position that reliance upon "scientific" medicine—simplistic animal experiments, elegant physiological theories, and elaborate diagnostic instruments—can actually distort the clinician's judgment when he encounters disease, in all its complexity, in real human beings. For Feinstein, not so incidentally, the persistence of the split between experimental biology and clinical medicine is reflected in the continued division of medical journals and conferences into separate scientific and clinical sections, which seem to have little to do with each other.[28]

To be sure, the major aim of Feinstein's book is to lay the foundations for his own version of a truly scientific clinical medicine. But the "science" upon which he would have clinicians build is mathematical logic. More specifically, he advocates the use of Boolean algebra and Venn diagrams as the basis of a new and subtler form of disease "taxonomy." Whatever its merits, Feinstein's version of scientific medicine is clearly a world apart from Bernard's (or Virchow's) experimental "determinism," and it is the skepticism of clinicians toward that experimental vision of medicine that we shall now seek to explain.

THE ROLE OF ECONOMIC AND TEMPERAMENTAL FACTORS IN THE DIVISION

We cannot begin to understand the persistence of the division between doctors and research physiologists unless we emphatically reject one of Virchow's more exasperated admonitions. "Whether someone is or is not a practitioner *ex professo* has little to do with the matter," he insisted. "If only people would finally stop finding points of disagreement in the personal characteristics and external circumstances of investigators."[29] What Virchow would have us do is to ignore an important part of reality—as if unanimity of opinion or convergence of interest could be expected from individuals and groups with deeply different "personal characteristics" and "external circumstances."

In the case at hand, differences in "personal characteristics" were decidedly reinforced by wide differences in "external circumstances"—both in the nature of the tasks performed and in the structure of the respective reward systems. It is one thing to publish papers; it is quite another to treat patients. And surely no reader of this volume need be told that eminent American doctors (and, increasingly since the 1930s, ordinary doctors too) have always enjoyed higher social status and higher incomes than eminent research scientists. Even in the first decade of this century, the difference was already obvious. In 1909, when S. J. Meltzer sought to entice a group of graduating physicians into his proposed new discipline of experimental clinical medicine, he felt the need to appeal to the example of the German university system. There, he claimed, scientific research was more highly valued than medical practice, and the character of youth was not formed by "sport and the habits of millionaires' sons." There, unlike the United States, "the worth of the individual is not measured exclusively by a gold standard." Should anyone in his audience remain unclear, Meltzer warned them that medical practice was "a bewitching graveyard in which many a brain has been buried alive with no other compensation than a gilded tombstone."[30]

Meltzer's ally, that ubiquitous layman Abraham Flexner, also had good reason to respect the power of the "gold standard." Throughout the 1910s and 1920s, his efforts to create "full-time" salaried clinical chairs ran into serious difficulties, initially even at John Hopkins—perhaps partly because American physicians rather oddly found the very concept of a salary in some way unprofessional, but surely also because the proposed amount of the salary (initially, $10,000) was so much less than the income to which leading clinicians had become accustomed from their practices.[31]

From the mid-1940s on, the income differential between research physiologists and practicing doctors became so striking that the American Physiological Society considered it a serious obstacle to the recruitment of high quality personnel. According to the data collected in the society's remarkable self-survey of the 1950s, the average net income of physicians in 1940 was $4400, compared to $3700 for physiologists. A mere five years later this modest gap had widened to $11,000 for physicians and $4625 for physiologists, while by 1952 it was $14,080 for physicians and $6360 for physiologists. The absolute differential is surely much larger now—with physicians earning a tremendous range of incomes, with a median of perhaps $65,000, while the salaries of employed physiologists cluster within a much narrower range, around $30,000.[32] Already in the 1950s, the American Physiological Society was more concerned about the loss of "brainy people" to medical practice than Meltzer had once been about the "loss to clinical medicine of the brainy men who now devote their energies to the pure sciences."[33] In the academic market of the 1970s, a cynical (or honest) physiologist might warn potential aspirants to the field that "research is a bewitching graveyard in which many a body has been buried alive with no other compensation than an occasional published paper."

Yet throughout the period of widening income differentials, an apprecia-

ble (if declining) number of students proved willing to make economic
sacrifices for the sake of physiological research. And as late as the 1950s,
at least, most physiologists expressed general satisfaction with their chosen
career.[34] Once captured by research, few physiologists with M.D.s (from
Claude Bernard on) forsook it for the medical practice they could have
entered. For most of them, the obvious and growing financial appeal of a
medical career could not divert them from their personal inclination; for
them, an unfavorable difference in "external circumstances" could not
overwhelm a more profound difference in "personal characteristics." It did,
however, help to increase the distance separating them from practicing
doctors.

By now the available sociological and psychological data seem sufficient
to establish the existence of significant differences in background, personality, and values between those intending to be physicians and other members of their age cohort, including those who undertake careers in scientific
research.[35] Indeed, the so-called "Two Cultures" gap between humanists
and scientists may be as nothing compared to that which separates pragmatic, action-oriented, client-dependent professionals (including physicians) from those with essentially scholarly sensibilities (including research
physiologists).[36]

Long before any data were systematically compiled, experimental scientists and practicing physicians were aware of deep differences between
them. Such major nineteenth-century physiologists as Claude Bernard,
Carl Ludwig, and Emil du Bois Reymond, although sometimes at odds over
issues within science itself, were united in that mixture of disdain and
grudging envy with which they regarded practicing doctors. Vallery-Radot,
in his *Life of Pasteur*, captures some of this ambivalence in a presumably
apocryphal, but nonetheless revealing exchange said to have been initiated
by Bernard, who, unlike Pasteur, did at least possess an M.D. degree.
Vallery-Radot has Claude Bernard ask Pasteur, "with a smile under which
many feelings were hidden, 'Have you ever noticed that when a doctor
enters a room, he always looks as if he was going to say, "I have just been
saving a fellow man"?' "[37]

The physiologists of more recent times have continued to feel, and
occasionally to express, that sense of ambivalence. In 1945, for example,
the Harvard physiologist Walter Cannon wrote as follows:

My father's wish that I might become a physician was . . . never realized. Instead
of engaging in practice I engaged in teaching medical students. This was what
my predecessor, Dr. [H. P.] Bowditch had done. He told the tale of a conversation between one of his children and a little companion. The companion asked,

"Has your father many patients?" and the answer was, "He has no patients."
"What! A doctor and no patients?" Thereupon the apologetic answer, "Oh, no,
he is one of those doctors who don't know anything!" Possibly the children of
other physiologists suffer from the same sense of inferiority. One of my daughters, on being informed proudly by a little friend that *her* father was a doctor,
remarked somewhat sadly, *"My* father is only a father."[38]

If that is a joke, it is a deeply symbolic one, and we may wonder whether
Cannon (like Bowditch before him) is not indulging the familiar parental
habit of speaking through their children.

That is not to say that Cannon himself actually felt an outright "sense
of inferiority" vis-à-vis doctors; the rest of his autobiography suggests otherwise. Rather, it is as if he felt the need to call attention to the high (but
ephemeral) social status of individual doctors in order to distinguish the
very different and basically intellectual motivations that lay behind his
calling. That self-identification with intellectual goals, which also perme-
ates most other autobiographical accounts by research physiologists, helps
us to understand the existence and persistence of the split between them
and practicing doctors. If physicians have often looked upon research
physiologists as remote "dreamers," or worse, the physiologists have tended
to regard doctors as mere "technicians" who cannot or will not appreciate
the value of basic scientific research or of scholarship in general. The result,
quite obviously, has been to increase whatever distance between them
might have been accounted for by any actual disjunction between physiological knowledge and medical practice.

In the following section, these psychological (or temperamental) differences between physiologists and physicians are invoked to help us understand the response of physiologists to the fragmentation of physiology as
a discipline. Because of this fragmentation, physiologists faced the charge
that their discipline had become both intellectually sterile and progressively
less relevant to medical science. The physiologists, it seems, found the
former charge more worrisome than the latter.

THE FRAGMENTATION OF PHYSIOLOGY: THE PRIORITY OF THE INTELLECTUAL CHALLENGE

Quite steadily, from about 1900 onward, physiology lost its privileged
place in the world of experimental biology. Just as physiology had once
declared its independence from medicine and medical anatomy, so new
fields and specialties now seemed to declare their own independence from

physiology. Actually, we know very little as yet about the emergence of these new disciplines. It is certainly premature, and probably misleading, to claim that the new disciplines evolved directly and simply out of physiology. But that was the way many physiologists saw it. For them, a sense of fragmentation resulted from the creation of independent societies by specialists who had begun to feel some dissatisfaction with the American Physiological Society, founded in 1887. In the early years of the twentieth century, there appeared in rapid order the Society for Experimental Biology and Medicine (1903), the American Society for Biological Chemists (1906), the American Society for Pharmacology and Experimental Therapeutics (1908), and the American Society of Experimental Pathology (1913).[39] As early as 1911, the increasing fragmentation of what had once seemed to be physiology inspired the following remark from physiologist Henry Sewall. Ever ready to deploy (or mix) metaphors, Sewall voiced his impression that:

> the course of evolution has ordered it that whereas physiology was then [in the 1870s] the dependent runt of the medical family, it is today the eldest son in a stable system of primogeniture. As with a noble jewel, whose beauty depends upon the cutting, we may name one facet Pathology, another Pharmacology, another Bio-chemistry, another Psychology, and so on, the jewel remains and ever will be Physiology.[40]

Other physiologists, then and later, expressed similar sentiments with remarkable frequency, and their common use of biological metaphors in which physiology remains the "trunk" or "mother-stem" of the vigorous new disciplinary branches does not entirely mask an underlying concern. Along with a growing sense of estrangement from the increasingly intricate methods, techniques, and instruments of modern experimental biology or "biophysics," some "classical" medical physiologists began to wonder whether physiology any longer existed as a discrete intellectual entity at all. The conceptual doubt was reinforced by recruiting difficulties, for the number of new Ph.D.s in physiology actually declined in the 1940s—not only absolutely, but also (and more importantly) in proportion to new Ph.D.s in other biological disciplines.[41]

Certainly, by then, if not before, the situation had provoked something of an internal crisis in the field. In the early 1950s, the American Physiological Society, funded by the new National Science Foundation, undertook a remarkably complete and revealing survey of the discipline. The survey addressed itself in part to the question of how physiology could be defined, and in one striking aside, survey director R. W. Gerard carried Sewall's evolutionary metaphor to one of its possible conclusions. For if Sewall, in 1932, could still see physiology as the "eldest son in a stable system of primogeniture," Gerard raised the possibility that its new disciplinary off-shoots might be better adapted to the age, while physiology itself faced the prospect of extinction, of becoming "a fossil on musty library shelves."[42]

The threat of extinction came from at least two directions simultaneously. For the new disciplinary subspecies not only included fields which seemed intellectually more exciting than physiology—biochemistry, cytology, genetics, cellular physiology, and biophysics—but also others which seemed (at least on the surface) of more immediate utility to medicine—notably bacteriology or microbiology, pharmacology, nutrition, immunology, and endocrinology. And so, as the fragmentation became increasingly obvious, physiologists had to decide which of these two developments they considered more threatening.

On the whole, despite the once aggressively utilitarian rhetoric of spokesmen like Bernard, physiologists apparently found the charge of intellectual sterility more immediately damaging that that of medical irrelevance. They certainly noticed both aspects of the challenge, but they responded to the latter with rather considerable restraint. Often enough, they referred to the value that physiology might derive from a closer interaction with clinical medicine (rather than the other way around), and they rarely exaggerated the direct medical utility of their work—even on so profoundly practical a problem as wound shock, which occupied a truly staggering proportion of American physiologists and their *Journal* after the nation entered World War I.[43]

Insofar as physiologists did confront the clinical challenge, they seemed most concerned about such "academic" clinicians as Meltzer, Cole, Cohn, and McLean. The challenge these critics posed was at once intellectual and institutional. For Meltzer and his three spiritual descendants, all of whom had significant ties to Abraham Flexner and the Rockefeller Foundation, took the almost paradoxical position that the best solution to the medical remoteness of physiology was to create yet another entirely new independent discipline, "experimental clinical medicine." In the more or less typical language of biomedical reformers, Meltzer claimed that this new discipline would keep more firmly in touch with medical problems. Yet he also insisted that it absolutely required independence from actual medical practice—more so, even, than such "ancillary" sciences as physiology.[44]

Physiologists, already concerned about the fragmentation of their subject into new academic fields, began to wonder aloud what would be left of the discipline if it now faced a frontal assault from the proposed new discipline of "experimental medicine." When physiologist C. A. Lovatt Evans expressed open concern about these "Meltzerian" proposals, in 1928, Alfred Cohn probably did little to reduce that concern when he responded as follows:

> Although physiology has made itself independent, Professor Evans still harbors fears. He fears to cut the guiding strings of the alma mater [medicine], lest physiology lack nourishment. And like many . . . children, he fears lest the ancient mother be too feeble intellectually and too powerless, having reared and weaned her children, to be able to continue to order and to develop her own house. But the situation is just this: having learned as it were and indicated to her many offspring how they might best set up houses of their own, medicine is at length free to cultivate her own garden.[45]

At this point, it seems to me, the rank-and-file practitioner might have been excused for casting a smile at the medico-academic elite. So the long campaign of research physiologists to achieve independence from medicine was to end, after all, in nothing more than an opposing effort by "academic" clinicians to reclaim part of the lost territory! To the ordinary doctor, the situation was doubtless reminiscent of other comical but irrelevant disputes among academics. In addressing themselves above all to the challenge posed by fellow academics, the physiologists were responding to the intellectual inclinations that had attracted them to research in the first place. But ordinary doctors can only have felt still further estrangement from such physiologists as Nobel Laureate Otto Loewi, who actually suggested in 1954 that the discipline might never have entered its "crisis" if only its practitioners had pursued problems of even more "remote usefulness for medicine."[46]

AN HERETICAL SUGGESTION: COULD THE SKEPTICAL CLINICIANS HAVE A POINT?

Medical historians have not entirely ignored the skepticism of practicing doctors toward experimental physiology (or experimental science in general), and doubtless most would agree that economic and temperamental factors contributed importantly to it. But perhaps the most common "explanation" for the phenomenon—essentially an echo of Claude Bernard's position—is that one could not expect "short-sighted" clinicians to appreciate the benefits that medicine would "soon" reap from the triumph of experimental science. On this view, older clinicians, who had not been trained in the new scientific methods, would be especially unwilling to acknowledge their dependence on experimental science and especially likely to persist in the delusion that medicine was essentially an art. These older clinicians were also most likely to feel vulnerable to any economic threat posed by the rising breed of "scientific" and presumably more effective physicians. And so, out of ignorance and self-interest, they would naturally dispute the medical utility of laboratory science.[47]

At some point, however, this sort of explanation can no longer suffice. Surely by about 1920, when most doctors would have been exposed to laboratory science, its value should have been so obvious as to overwhelm their skepticism, except perhaps for a few quacks and cranks. From the evidence already presented, it should be clear that skeptics nonetheless remained, including at least a few leading clinicians. If such an eminent clinician as Feinstein can continue even today to express reservations about the medical value of laboratory science, medical historians ought to be willing at least to reconsider the matter. Insofar as the skeptics have focused on physiology per se, there is perhaps particular reason not to dismiss their views out of hand.

Twenty years ago, the Downstate Medical Center of the State University of New York sponsored an ambitious symposium on "the historical development of physiological thought," resulting in a book of that title. The book contains sixteen essays, many of which remain valuable studies, but only one directly confronts the relationship between physiology and medical practice. That essay, by Owsei Temkin, begins as follows: "If we were to awaken a man from sleep by shouting into his ear: 'medicine depends upon basic scientific thought,' he might unthinkingly say 'amen!' " With typical perspicacity, Temkin goes on to show how thoroughly complicated the issue looks when the immediate response is replaced by a thoughtful one. Indeed, the thoughtful response soon threatens to dissolve into utter confusion because of the difficulty of even defining such terms as "physiology," "science," "medicine," or "health." In the end, Temkin seems to suggest, medicine does indeed depend partly upon basic scientific thought, but often of a sort that research physiologists might fail to recognize as "scientific" at all.[48] At the same conference (though his paper was published separately), Paul Cranefield briefly pondered the far more specific question of whether the preceding half-century of "infinitely delicate and beautiful studies of microscopic physiology" had influenced medical practice. His rather rueful answer: no, "by and large they have not."[49]

In other cases, too, in which it has seemed obvious that experimental physiology must have made vital contributions to medical practice, it may prove instructive and sometimes surprising to examine the situation critically. Consider, for much too brief a moment, the clinical field in which the pragmatic value of physiology might seem to be most obvious—cardiology. This is, moreover, a field of direct concern to the average office-based practitioner, and one in which physiological research has been accorded a quite immediate and specific role. As C. J. Wiggers put it in 1951, referring to the "clinical applications" of modern circulatory physiology:

> The physiological interpretations of graphic recordings of the pulse enabled [Sir James] Mackenzie to give physiological interpretations to many of the common [cardiological] irregularities. Additional experiments by [Joseph] Erlanger and [Arthur] Cushny elucidated the phenomena of heart block and atrial fibrillation, and their discoveries soon proved valuable in clinical diagnoses. The foremost step in the decade was the invention in 1903 of the string galvanometer by Einthoven and his prompt application of this tool to the study of physiological and clinical problems . . . while the discerning mind of Thomas Lewis immediately envisaged the great strides that could be made in the field of clinical cardiology through correlation of electrographic phenomena in patients and experimental animals.[50]

Upon closer inspection, however, the situation begins to look rather more problematic than Wiggers's summary suggests. To be sure, electrocardiography did emerge from an important tradition in purely "academic" electrophysiology. But can one trace any major innovations in therapeutic cardiology to this new physiological knowledge? At the turn of the century, physiological experiments on dogs led Arthur Cushny to the diagnosis of auricular fibrillation for the clinical condition previously known as *delerium cordis*. In the course of this research, Cushny complained bitterly that clinicians had failed to keep abreast of the recent avalanche of knowledge in the physiology of the mammalian heart. Yet his own further research, and that of others, produced no dramatic departures in therapy, but mainly provided a new rationale for the use of the digitalis compounds that had already been introduced "empirically" for the treatment of such cases.[51]

Astonishingly, some leading clinicians even disputed the diagnostic value of the new electrophysiology and electrocardiography. Among them was Sir James Mackenzie himself, who figured prominently in the clinical developments to which Wiggers refers, not only through his own contributions, but also as sometime collaborator with Arthur Cushny and as mentor of Sir Thomas Lewis. It was Mackenzie, we should recall, who warned in 1919 that laboratory training could actually distort the clinician's judgment and "unfit" him for his work as a physician. Mackenzie, moreover, practiced what he preached, eventually abandoning even the primitive polygraph he had used in his early cardiological studies for the more direct and more traditional methods of clinical observation.[52] Recall, too, that Feinstein, who to some degree shares Mackenzie's skepticism toward laboratory science, is also a cardiologist.

Thus, even in the apparently straightforward case of cardiology, the medical utility of physiological research is open to some qualification, at the least. Surgery represents a second major clinical field in which experimental physiology has seemed to play an important and immediate role. Quite obviously, future surgeons can enhance their surgical skills by performing animal experiments, even if the immediate object is physiological. Moreover, some leading surgical mentors, notably Owen Wangensteen of the University of Minnesota, certainly did, and do, stress the value to surgeons of a thorough training in physiology. Indeed, one branch of modern "total surgery" even bears the name "physiologic surgery." In the 1964 edition of a leading American surgical textbook, this branch of surgery is said to have as its aim the alteration of "normal" but deleterious bodily function for the general good of the patient and to have its theoretical roots in Walter Cannon's concept of homeostasis.[53] Cannon himself was considerably more restrained about the medical utility of his physiological work: "It is said," he wrote in 1945, "that our researches on the bodily effects of emotions have been helpful because they give the doctor pertinent information in explaining to his nervous patients the reasons for their functional disorders."[54] Perhaps Cannon was being excessively modest here, and perhaps his work has had an immense impact on medical and surgical practice. Yet it is not immediately obvious exactly how and in what sense his physiological insights should have led to any significant reorientation of medical or surgical practice.

But let us not carry our own skepticism too far. Let it be clear that it would require infinitely more research to examine the wealth of possible contributions experimental physiology may in fact have made to clinical medicine or to health. At least on the surface, it seems obvious that experimental physiology must have made important contributions to the so-called "replacement therapies," of which insulin for diabetes, thyroid extract for myxodema, and liver extract for pernicious anemia serve as classic examples. It also seems clear that experimental physiologists must have contributed importantly to our understanding of such medically significant aspects of blood chemistry as pH levels, electrolyte balance, and incompatible blood types.[55] The existing literature provides a host of other possible examples, thus far mostly in the form of schematic lists, which clearly deserve more extensive inquiry.[56]

In the course of this more extensive research, a number of distinctions should be kept very firmly in mind. Different sorts of medical practitioners would doubtless come to very different sorts of conclusions about the utility of particular investigations in experimental physiology. What is useful to hospital-based specialists, for example, is liable to be very different from what is useful to office-based pediatricians, internists, and general practitioners. It is also vital to distinguish between the therapeutic, diagnostic, and preventive aspects of medicine with respect to the possible utility of experimental physiology. And whatever conclusions one may reach about the direct medical utility of laboratory physiology, one may well wish to consider separately its cultural value and its proper role in medical education. Let me conclude with some preliminary conclusions growing out of this last distinction.

REFLECTIONS ON THE GENERAL ROLE OF LABORATORY SCIENCE IN MEDICAL EDUCATION

Throughout much of this paper, I have insisted upon the persistent skepticism of practicing doctors toward the medical utility of experimental physiology. In the section immediately above, I have raised the question whether that skepticism may not have had some justification for at least some sorts of physicians. Yet Abraham Flexner, in his famous report of 1910 on American medical education, called physiology "the central discipline of the medical school."[57] It has retained an importance place in the American medical curriculum ever since. For some readers, that will surely serve as prima facie evidence of its value to medical practice. Unless laboratory physiology is medically useful, why did it acquire and why does it retain such an important role in medical training?

To address this question, which might seem to dismiss out of hand any need to reexamine the relationship between experimental physiology and medical practice, we must give at least passing attention here to the more general role of laboratory science in medical education. What especially needs to be recognized is that doctors have gained at least one important benefit from the study of experimental science, quite apart from whatever direct medical utility it has, and quite apart from any indirect contribution it may make to medically effective modes of thinking.[58] For the experimental sciences, like Latin in an earlier era, have given medicine a new and now culturally compelling basis for consolidating its status as an autonomous "learned profession," with all of the corporate and material advantages that such status implies.

It was Flexner, once again, who asserted that the "possession of certain portions of many sciences arranged and organized with a distinct practical

purpose in view . . . makes [medicine] a 'profession'."[59] Underwritten by
the Carnegie Foundation for the Advancement of Teaching, supported in
crucial ways by the AMA's Council on Medical Education, and dependent
for much of its influence on Flexner's skillful use of Rockefeller money, the
Flexner Report accelerated the process by which the supply of American
doctors was greatly reduced, as the expense, duration, and quality of their
education was greatly increased.[60] The eventual result was to elevate the
American medical profession to the remarkable position it enjoys today.
Along the way, the basic sciences came to occupy a newly central role in
the medical curriculum. And in a society that reveres (even as it fears)
science, doctors clearly owe some of their status to the Flexnerian perception that they are in some sense "scientists."

This is not to claim that the medical profession, either in its "prescien-
tific" or "scientific" phases, has consciously and cynically exploited the
available cultural resources (whether polite Latin learning or experimental
science) for its own self-serving ends. Even if the medical profession, like
other professions, has sometimes acted in a patently self-interested way,
there is no *necessary* conflict between professional self-interest, responsible
medical care, and the humanitarian ideals traditionally espoused by physicians. And even if proper examination should reveal that our "scientific"
medicine has contributed only marginally, if at all, to any measurable
improvement in health, it does not automatically follow (as Ivan Illich
assumes) that our medical system is misconceived or unduly expensive.[61]
Perhaps the most striking feature of the recent wave of controversy over
the cost and quality of American medicine is the tendency of both critics
and apologists (but especially "academic" critics) to forget that sick people
do not think in statistical terms and that medicine serves vital functions
not yet captured in "vital statistics"—among them, prevention or relief of
pain and morbidity, preservation or restoration of physical or social function, making sense of illness, and the dispensing of peace of mind and
general human support.[62]

But if we do not yet really know the extent to which physicians influence
ordinary vital statistics, we have even less sense of whether or how much
their scientific training enhances their ability to perform their less dramatic
"supportive" functions. The slim available evidence does suggest—contrary
to a segment of popular opinion—that scientific orientation and training
are not inimical to the humanitarian aspects of the physician's role.[63] But
it remains to be established that physicians so trained perform *more* effectively in their supportive tasks, and there is perhaps particular reason to
wonder whether such primary-care physicians as pediatricians and internists are being appropriately trained to handle the medical problems that

they actually face.[64] Especially in view of the high cost of training "scientific" doctors, we deserve rather better evidence that the expense is justified.

For Flexner, who had graduated from Johns Hopkins during its golden early years as the American embodiment of "Germanic" research ideals, it was a self-evident proposition that an expansion of laboratory training in the medical curriculum would result in improved health for Americans. Thus he noted in passing—as if establishing a causal connection between two parallel phenomena—that "the century which has developed medical laboratories [roughly, 1810–1910] has seen the death-rate reduced by one-half and the average expectation of life increased by ten or twelve years."[65] It is precisely this alleged connection between laboratory training and health that requires critical scrutiny. And surely it will not do for medical historians to assume in advance the health benefits of experimental science or to ignore entirely the other functions that laboratory training plays in medical education.

NOTES

This is a considerably revised version of the paper I delivered at the conference, "Two Hundred Years of American Medicine," in Philadelphia, 2–4 December 1976. As originally presented, the essay included a section that argued for the existence of an "Anglo-American" style of physiology. I now expect to develop that theme in a separate publication. Moreover, since giving my paper, I have profited from the criticisms of James Secord, Robert Bernstein, and an anonymous referee for the University of Pennsylvania Press, and (especially bibliographically) from reading an as yet unpublished essay on the "social and intellectual location of physiology in America" by David Bearman. In the footnotes that follow, I have tried to indicate my more specific debts to Mr. Bearman.

1. Quoted by K.D. Keele, *The Evolution of Clinical Methods in Medicine* (London: Pitman Med. Pub., 1963), p. 105.

2. On the emergence of physiology as an independent discipline, see Joseph Schiller, "Physiology's Struggle for Independence in the First Half of the Nineteenth Century," *History of Science* 7 (1968): 64–89; and John E. Lesch, "The Origins of Experimental Physiology and Pharmacology in France, 1790–1820: Bichat and Magendie," (Ph.D. diss., Princeton University, 1977).

3. A perhaps typical, if not classic, example of the genre is Carl J. Wiggers, "The Interrelations of Physiology and Internal Medicine," *Journal of the American Medical Association* 91 (1928): 270–74, where a long but utterly schematic list is given of the "physiologic researches . . . of immediate interest to the clinician."

4. Rene Vallery-Radot, *The Life of Pasteur,* trans. Mrs. R.L. Devonshire (N.Y.: Garden City Publ. Co., n.d.), p. 226.

5. Claude Bernard, *An Introduction to the Study of Experimental Medicine,* trans. H.C. Greene (N.Y.: Dover, 1957), pp. 203–5.

6. Rudolf Virchow, *Disease, Life and Man,* trans. L.J. Rather (N.Y.: Collier, 1962), pp. 50, 66, 76; indented quotation on p. 50.

7. Ibid., p. 50.

8. Ibid., p. 91. This was almost certainly Franz Schuh, one of the most "scientific" surgeons in Europe. See Erna Lesky, *The Vienna Medical School of the 19th Century,* trans. L. Williams and I.S. Levij (Baltimore: Johns Hopkins University Press, 1976), pp. 168–73. If so, one can only imagine the response of less academic surgeons.

9. See G.L. Geison, "Social and Institutional Factors in the Stagnancy of English Physiology, 1840–1870," *Bulletin of the History of Medicine* 46 (1972): 30–58, esp. 41–42.

10. Ibid., p. 55.

11. Virchow, *Disease,* p. 163.

12. See Keele, *Evolution,* p. 105.

13. See Henry Sewall, "The Beginnings of Physiological Research in America," *Science* 58 (1923): 187–95, esp. 194–95.

14. Walter J. Meek, "The Beginnings of American Physiology," *Annals of Medical History* 10 (1928): 111–25, esp. 122–24.

15. See text below, section 6, and the sources cited in n. 60.

16. Arthur H. Sanford, "The Role of the Clinical Pathologist," *Journal of the American Medical Association* 95 (1930): 1465–67.

17. Ibid., p. 1466.

18. See Frederick W. Ellis, "Henry Pickering Bowditch and the Development of the Harvard Laboratory of Physiology," *New England Journal of Medicine* 219 (1938): 819. I owe this reference to David Bearman.

19. As quoted by William G. Rothstein, *American Physicians in the Nineteenth Century: From Sects to Science* (Baltimore: Johns Hopkins University Press 1972), pp. 265–66.

20. S.J. Meltzer, "The Science of Clinical Medicine: What It Ought to Be and the Men to Uphold It," *Journal of the American Medical Association* 53 (1909): 508–12, quotation on 510.

21. See Franklin C. McLean, "Physiology and Medicine: A Transition Period," [1960], in *The Excitement and Fascination of Science* (Palo Alto, Calif.: Annual Reviews, Inc., 1965), pp. 317–32, esp. 317–19.

22. Sewall, "Beginnings," p. 190.

23. Arno B. Luckhardt, "The Progress of Medicine: A Plea for the Concerted Efforts of the Clinician and the Laboratory Worker," *Journal of the American Medical Association* 81 (1923): 347–49.

24. Wiggers, "Interrelations," p. 274.

25. A.E. Garrod, "The Laboratory and the Ward," in *Contributions to Medical and Biological Research: Dedicated to Sir William Osler* (N.Y.: P.B. Hoeber, 1919), pp. 59–69, quotation on 63. I owe this reference to David Bearman.

26. Quoted by Keele, *Evolution,* p. 105.

27. Alfred E. Cohn, "Medicine and Science," *Journal of Philosophy* 25 (1928): 403–16, quotation on 409.

28. Alvan R. Feinstein, *Clinical Judgment* (Baltimore: Johns Hopkins University Press, 1967), esp. introduction.

29. Virchow, *Disease,* p. 163.

30. Meltzer, "Science," pp. 511–12.

31. See Donald Cousar, "The Establishment of Full-Time Clinical Chairs at Johns Hopkins," unpublished essay for Junior Independent Work, Princeton University, 1975. Cf. Abraham Flexner, *Universities: American, English, German* (London: Oxford, 1930), pp. 85–96.

32. For the 1940 to 1952 data, see R.W. Gerard, *Mirror to Physiology: A Self-Survey of Physiological Science* (Washington, D.C.: American Physiological Society, 1958), p. 66. I owe the estimate of current physician income to my colleague, medical economist Uwe Reinhardt. The estimate for current physiologists' salaries is merely a rough guess based on the salary of chairmen of physiology departments at medical schools ($35,000–$40,000).

33. Meltzer, "Science," p. 511; and Gerard, *Mirror,* passim.

34. See Gerard, *Mirror,* chap. 6.

35. See, *inter alia,* Rashi Fein and Gerald I. Weber, *Financing Medical Education* (N.Y.: McGraw Hill, 1971); James A. Knight, *Medical Student: Doctor in the Making* (N.Y.: Appleton-Century-Crofts, 1973); and the flood of papers on the topic in virtually any issue of the *Journal of Medical Education.*

36. Perhaps useful in this connection is Eliot Freidson's distinction between consulting and other professions. See Freidson, *Profession of Medicine* (N.Y.: Dodd, Mead, 1970). Cf. also Norman W. Storer, *The Social System of Science* (N.Y.: Holt, Rinehart, 1966), esp. pp. 91–97.

37. See Vallery-Radot, *Life of Pasteur,* pp. 225–26.

38. Walter B. Cannon, *The Way of an Investigator* (N.Y.: Norton, 1945), p. 21.

39. See Sewall, "Beginnings," p. 190.

40. Henry Sewall, "Henry Newell Martin . . . ," *Johns Hopkins Hospital Bulletin* 22 (1911): 327–33, quotation on 328.

41. See Gerard, *Mirror,* esp. p. 39.

42. Ibid., p. 249.

43. See, e.g., Carl J. Wiggers, "Physiology from 1900–1920: Incidents, Accidents, and Advances," [1951], in *Excitement and Fascination of Science,* pp. 547–66, who says (on p. 558) that his haemodynamic studies "tended to confuse rather than clarify" the problems of shock. More generally, see the other essays in *Excitement.*

44. Meltzer, "Science," p. 508.

45. Quoted by McLean, "Physiology," p. 319.

46. Otto Loewi, "Reflections on the Study of Physiology," [1954], in *Excitement,* pp. 269–78, quotation on 276.

47. This attitude is at least implicit in Rothstein, *American Physicians,* and perhaps also in R.H. Shryock's classic, *The Development of Modern Medicine* (New York: Knopf, 1947).

48. Owsei Temkin, "The Dependence of Medicine upon Basic Scientific Thought," in *The Historical Development of Physiological Thought,* ed. Chandler McC. Brooks and Paul Cranefield (N.Y.: Hafner, 1959), pp. 5–21.

49. Paul F. Cranefield, "Microscopic Physiology Since 1908," *Bulletin of the History of Medicine* 33 (1959): 263–75, quotation on 274.

50. Wiggers, "Physiology," 553–54.

51. See G.L. Geison, "Arthur Cushny," *Dictionary of Scientific Biography,* (N.Y.: Scribner's, 1978), vol. 15, pp. 99–104, esp. the primary sources cited on p. 104.

52. See Thomas M. Durant, *The Days of Our Years: A Short History of Medicine and the American College of Physicians* (brochure, American College of Physicians, Chicago, 1965), p. 14.

53. Loyal Davis, ed., *Christopher's Textbook of Surgery,* 8th ed. (Philadelphia: W.B. Saunders Co., 1964), pp. 1–3, 19–20.

54. Cannon, *Way,* pp. 213–14.

55. I am indebted to Robert Bernstein for emphasizing to me the examples from studies of blood chemistry. It may well be significant that Rufus Cole, who

was otherwise somewhat skeptical about the utilitarian claims of physiologists, did concede the medical value of their research in these areas. See Rufus Cole, "Progress of Medicine During the Past Twenty-Five Years as Exemplified by the Harvey Society Lectures," *Science* 71 (1930): 617–27.

56. Cole, ibid., offers a few other examples that may be all the more deserving of investigation since they come from a clinician and moderate critic of physiologists' claims for medical utility. For an expansive list of such claims, I refer the reader again to Wiggers, "Interrelations."

57. Abraham Flexner, *Medical Education in the United States and Canada* (New York: Carnegie Foundation, 1910), p. 63.

58. I mean to suggest here, though none of my sources develops the idea, that laboratory training may encourage a receptivity to novelty. That claim is sometimes made on behalf of liberal studies in general.

59. Flexner, *Medical Education*, p. 58.

60. See Robert Hudson, "Abraham Flexner in Perspective: American Medical Education, 1865–1910," *Bulletin of the History of Medicine* 46 (1972): 545–61; and the remarkable series of annual reports by the AMA Council on Medical Education that began to appear in the *Journal of the American Medical Association* from 1904.

61. Ivan Illich, *Medical Nemesis* (London: Marion Boyars, 1975).

62. Cf. Walsh McDermott, "Evaluating the Physician and His Technology," in "Doing Better and Feeling Worse: Health in the United States," ed. John Knowles, *Daedalus*, 106 (1977): 135–57.

63. See Earl R. Babbie, *Science and Morality in Medicine* (Berkeley: University of California, 1970).

64. Cf. Kerr L. White *et al.*, "The Ecology of Medical Care," *New England Journal of Medicine* 265 (1961): 885–92.

65. Flexner, *Medical Education*, p. 62.

4 *"PHYSICIAN VERSUS BACTERIOLOGIST": The Ideology of Science in Clinical Medicine*

RUSSELL C. MAULITZ

INTRODUCTION

Of what came to be known as the "basic sciences" (those domains of natural knowledge "basic" to medicine) in America's second century, none had as precipitous or as great an impact on clinical medicine as bacteriology. In the critical decades following the Centennial rites of 1876, hospitals, government agencies, medical schools, and laboratories were linked in an intricate web of relationships. In the United States, as in Europe, the emerging pattern of institutions reflected in part an equally complex set of relations between overlapping disciplines in the biomedical sciences. Some disciplines, such as physiological chemistry and bacteriology itself, grew out of parent subjects: physiology and pathology. Others, especially those which were older and better established, such as hygiene and pathology, strove to transform themselves, after the mid-1880s, by incorporating the stream of new insights emanating from bacteriological laboratories.[1]

In the United States and in Germany (from which many American physicians derived the ideology as well as the substance of medical science, around the turn of the twentieth century), and probably elsewhere in Europe, the set of mind among many medical men was changing, in response to the study of the bacterial pathogenesis of disease.[2] Bacteriology, as an array of etiologic notions and instrumental imperatives, both diagnostic and therapeutic, was beginning to change the face of medicine. That bacteriology helped to bring about the convergence of science and medicine could be demonstrated convincingly in terms of the texture and substance of bacteriology itself. One could illumine its impact by showing how physicians came to embrace a constellation of concepts and techniques associated with bacteriology, from Listerian antisepsis in the 1870s, through pathogenic specificity in the 1880s, to the new serum and chemotherapeutic regimens of the 1890s and 1900s.[3]

It was not only the substance of bacteriology, but its role as a vehicle for the infusion of the ideology of science into medicine which made it pivotal in the history of scientific medicine. More than any other laboratory domain, bacteriology spoke to the clinician. It did so in a manner at once authoritative and paradoxical. It did not merely promise to change the way the practitioner thought about the patient's illness and sought to ameliorate it. While it offered clinicians these new tools, it also threatened them by suggesting that scientific values, so promising of enhanced efficacy and legitimacy, might remove them from the bedside to the bench. An inherent irony lay in this state of affairs, a contradiction between spheres of action.

The contradiction could generate tensions at several levels. Ultimately, clinicians would resent the diversion of governmental and institutional funds from clinic to laboratory. And ultimately, perhaps, some clinicians might even come to envy the unequivocal success of their pure-science cousins in the bacteriology laboratories at the dawn of the antibiotic era. Yet long before any economic threat or therapeutic success had insured the influence of laboratory medicine, the tension between physician and bacteriologist, between bedside and laboratory, began to develop and to lay down a global, and uniquely modern pattern of fault lines on the surface of medicine.[4] Well in advance of any full understanding of carrier states, host resistance factors, or antimicrobial compounds, these fault lines had come to characterize medical men's efforts to answer a central, critical question: What was the proper path by which science might be assimilated into medicine?

LIMITS OF THE DISCUSSION

I shall maintain, then, that the early decades of medicine in America's second century were characterized by a debate over the appropriate locus of scientific medicine. Often, though by no means always, the ideas of the bacteriologist served as the fulcrum of the debate. In the pages which follow, I shall identify some of the principal actors. A few caveats and qualifications apply. First, the quarrel was to some extent one-sided, especially in the United States. This was partly because bacteriology was as yet (circa 1900) not a fully separate discipline. It was, in fact, still largely a subdomain of pathology. The debate's one-sidedness also owed something to the fact that it was primarily the clinicians who felt the creative ambivalence which lies at the core of my argument. They were therefore most vocal in expressing an ambivalence toward the ideology of scientific medicine, as they encountered it in the new science of bacteriology. Second, I shall be discussing almost exclusively a group of physicians who belonged to some subset of the German or American medical mandarinate. The most vocal among those responding to the germ theory and bacteriologic technique were the opinion leaders and academic elite of medicine. They were, however, by no means identical in social, institutional, or economic location.[5]

Third, an implicit subtheme regarding the international transfer of ideas should be made explicit and then qualified. It is clear that strains between the instrumental imperatives of laboratory and bedside were present in Germany by 1880 and may be discerned in American medicine a few years later. I shall provide examples of both, noting especially the limiting case of Ottomar Rosenbach in Germany. Clearly, there is a parallel between the two countries with respect to the fault lines separating the possibilities of the bacteriological laboratory and those of the sickbed. I do not propose either to endorse or to refute the standard, causal formulation relating to the two countries. I shall, rather, present certain case studies in sequence, leaving to future research a more finely-grained analysis of the specific lines of influence.

Fourth, in the context of the argument presented here, I regard technique as being of perhaps even greater importance than any purely notional implications of bacteriology.[6] Hence bacteriologic technique looms larger in the discussion than anything so nebulous as "germ theory." To the physician, whether he was laboratory or bedside-oriented, it was the appeal of technique, the routine and habitual stuff of his workaday existence, which determined where he fell on the spectrum between those two orientations.[7] Nowhere were the tensions dictated by these instrumental possibilities better captured than in the fictionalized account of the career of Martin Arrowsmith, presented to a receptive post-Flexnerian American public by Sinclair Lewis in 1924.[8] In Arrowsmith and his colleagues we find alternative attempts to resolve the tension between the importance of laboratory medicine to the clinician and his need to distance himself from it.

THE NINETEENTH CENTURY

Among members of the American medical community, the need to measure carefully one's intellectual and social distance from the pure culture of science was little in evidence in 1876. In that year of the Centennial, Joseph Lister visited the United States, proselytizing for his new application of the germ theory to surgical disorders. It is becoming rather clear that the 1870s, and even the 1880s, represent too early a period to look for intellectual or institutional meaning in American bacteriology. Lister's incursion into the United States met an exceedingly ambiguous response, in fact, and might better be conceived in terms of the transfer of a clinical technique, a matter of praxis, rather than of a body of knowledge rooted in scientific theory.[9]

It is not surprising, then, to discover that in 1876, the noted American practitioner Edward Clarke, in his Centennial retrospect on "Practical Medicine", gave barely a nod to laboratory investigation. Dismissing in less than two pages the contributions of the laboratory, Clarke devoted seventy-odd pages to bedside achievements at home and abroad.[10] The "indifference to basic science" reflected in Clarke's essay was not so much a matter of explicit conviction as it was an expression of the lack of any interface between clinic and laboratory.[11]

By contrast, German clinicians were already acutely aware of the liabilities, as well as of the institutional potentials of the new disciplines of laboratory medicine. In the waning days of the decade, the Berliners Friedrich von Frerichs and Ernst von Leyden combined their efforts to create a new journal which might convey the values of medical science, yet lay primary stress upon clinical diagnosis and treatment. In 1880, Frerichs and Leyden published the first volume of the *Zeitschrift für klinische Medizin*. A veritable manifesto of clinical science, the journal proclaimed the autonomy of clinical medicine as a discipline which might, in its own right, participate in the ethos of science.[12]

Throughout the 1880s and 1890s, while a new generation of bacteriologists, led by Robert Koch, went from achievement to achievement in their laboratories, the self-styled German "scientific clinical" school attempted to remain close to the patient. The clinicians pursued their goal by means of a variety of tactics. There were two chief tactics, one essentially negative and one positive. Frerichs and Leyden, along with Adolf Kussmaul, Bernard Naunyn, and a number of their clinical colleagues, rejected those sciences which tended to remove the physician's sphere of activity from bedisde to bench.[13] Hence they also proposed to deemphasize laboratory physiology and the sort of experimental pathology which had appeared so promising in the hands of men such as Julius Cohnheim.[14]

In the place of laboratory research, the clinicians proposed a set of techniques of clinical investigation that promised to be every bit as rigorously "scientific," but which returned their practitioners to the bedside. Now, instead of discerning the morphologic lesion or the isolated strain of pathogenic microbe, they sought to investigate those functional parameters in the human body which, in health or disease, were uniquely susceptible to study on the hospital wards. Physiological derangements, often lacking recognizable morphologic hallmarks, were to be scrutinized. Words like *insufficiency* and *failure* of the body's organ systems entered clinical parlance.

In order to achieve a positive program of clinical science, German physicians seized on two basic tools. The first was borrowed from an earlier tradition, that of nosography, the classification and description of disease in the older, natural-historical mode. Within this framework, one was to resist identifying tuberculosis, for example, with the acid-fast bacillus, hence conceiving of it as a unified disease process. One should rather study the various natural histories of tuberculosis, a disease process which assumed a protean range of manifestations.

A positive, and equally important response to the new laboratory techniques was the clinicians' own technologic innovations. Methods for the investigation of fever, gastric acidity, and muscle tone were brought to bear at the bedside. A variety of methods were devised to permit observation of previously unexplored body orifices. Early internists sought to monitor functional parameters such as cardiac reserve. The gastric tube took the place of the microscope, the thermometer that of the agar plate. The clinical case description was to supercede, as it had preceded, the controlled laboratory experiment.[15]

By the mid-1880s, a group of elite American clinicians had arrived at a posture, which, though it was both less clearly defined and more optimistic about the place of the scientific laboratory in clinical medicine than its German counterpart, began to reflect a keen awareness of the interface between the two settings. The Association of American Physicians (AAP) was formed in 1885 by a group of seven doctors led by the prominent clinician William Osler.[16] Of the list of founders, six were academicians, six were European-trained, and all seven were consulting specialists.[17] Most were socially prominent, and all were graduates of elite medical schools.[18]

A precipitating factor in the founding of the AAP was the anticipation of the International Medical Congress of 1886, the first such to be held in the United States. In 1885, a group of physicians coalesced around the felt need to find a new voice, to put forward a new face of American medical science. But that new scientific sensibility was but the thinnest end of the entering wedge, borne still by a minority voice. The AAP and the American Medical Association (AMA) leadership broke rather bitterly; the rupture never fully healed, and the congress was held in Washington, with the American medical profession reaching no consensus.

The particular issues involved in the polarization between the AMA and the AAP are here secondary in importance to both the timing of the split and the very fact that it occurred. The fact of it underscores the notion that at least a quarter century before Abraham Flexner's Bulletin Number Four, an ideology of science can be seen emerging within the profession. The timing of the affair draws our attention to the first successful and widely publicized bacteriologic identifications of specific pathogens. Americans, in 1885, were well aware of the successful unmasking, in Robert Koch's laboratory, of the causative agents of anthrax, tuberculosis, and cholera.

The impact of the laboratory techniques of the 1880s, emphasizing etiology and diagnosis, was great. It was but a foreshadowing of the response in the early 1890s to the techniques of serology, techniques which brought the bacteriological laboratory directly to bear on the clinician's therapeutic armamentarium. The account of Emil Behring's curative administration of antidiphtheritic serum to a dying Berlin child at Christmas, 1891, for example, has taken on an almost mythic quality: it was a turning point, a watershed. Americans rushed to exploit the German's serum-production techniques. In the following year, Herman Biggs and William Park in New York mounted an effort similar to Behring's, which in turn led to a public, and highly publicized, antidiphtheria campaign in 1894.[19] Their success initiated a process which, by the end of the decade, had helped to redefine the roles of hygiene as a discipline, the public health specialist as a professional, and the laboratory as an institutional form.

THE EARLY TWENTIETH CENTURY: THE PREWAR YEARS

The promise of bacteriology in 1896, and the role of the laboratory dictated by that promise, eclipsed what had gone twenty or even ten years before. Clinicians in both countries were now faced with the prospect of dramatic changes in their sphere of action. Some, like Theodor Billroth in Germany, selected problems for investigation which allowed them to discount or ignore the deepening fissure. Others struck polar stances, and took sides.

In Germany, such an extreme posture was maintained by a neglected, but central figure, Ottomar Rosenbach.[20] An important opinion leader in the German clinic, a prolific writer, an articulate if splenetic spokesman for the ideology of science qua clinical investigation, Rosenbach was a key proponent of the physiologically-oriented clinical medicine championed earlier by Traube and Frerichs. Bacteriology, by contrast, was virtually anathema.

In 1903, Rosenbach published a polemical volume, *Arzt contra Bakteriologe,* which effectively made him the limiting case in any analysis of a newly emerging sensibility characterized by a mistrust of the fruits of the bacteriological laboratory. Of his laboratory-based brethren he wrote:

> Now that an unquestionable change of viewpoints, and hence of the scientific points at issue, has taken place, I once more present for unbiased consideration those evidences which are characteristic of the various stages of the controversy. . . . More particularly have I fought against bacteriologists operating *in absentia,* a court council of war, as it were, who, remote from the raging battle, consider themselves capable of giving directions to the real fighters in the battle against disease. On the other hand, bacteriology as a biological science, concerning itself with qualities of smallest organisms, can not be too much promoted. . . . I do not hesitate, even to-day when the heat of battle has passed, to state the opinion that nothing has so injured the standing of the practitioner and of the medical profession as the eagerness of bacteriologists to transfer decisions from the bedside to the laboratory, and to regulate etiology, diagnosis and therapy . . . according to an artificial scheme, instead of making full allowance for the requirements of actual conditions which can only be judged by those who are present at the bedside and who are familiar with local conditions.
>
> The course of events [in the investigation of cholera] has shown that the destiny of patients must not be decided in the laboratory, . . . *still the claim of bacteriology to control the sole determining vote in diagnosis* will continue to prevail for some time to come. . . . For what do we need physicians if the diagnosis of cholera can be made, not from the clinical picture of the disease . . . but solely in the laboratory, without . . . examination of the patient?[21]

Rosenbach's work was soon translated into English for American consumption. His translator, the New York physician Achilles Rose, depicted Rosenbach, in 1904, as one who was "well aware" of the value of bacteriology. But the German clinician was nevertheless willing to "raise his voice against the unjustified, the unwarranted claims of the bacteriologists . . . diagnosticians *in absentia* with their disinfectants and measures based on unsupported theory."[22]

It is difficult to gauge how much influence Rosenbach's book had in America. Some medical journalists welcomed it as a useful corrective to the excesses of simplistic diagnostic logic and therapeutic zeal anticipated from the bacteriology laboratories.[23] What is clear, though, is that the cognitive and social tensions which Rosenbach had, for himself, so resoundingly resolved in favor of science at the bedside were present to stay in America. In the first decade of the twentieth century, the critical years before the Flexner Report, many American medical professionals were gripped by this tension, and, when they failed to resolve it as Rosenbach had done, by the ambivalence it engendered—and that ambivalence in itself became a motive force in working out the boundaries of what American "scientific medicine" could and should mean.

THE INTERURBAN CLINICAL CLUB

Three men who, between 1904 and the First World War, attempted to delineate those boundaries of medical science in the United States were William Osler, Rufus Cole, and Samuel J. Meltzer. Each dealt with the bedside-bench ambivalence differently, and each thereby took a different tack in his respective career. Osler, glimpsed through the veils of many years of hagiography, stands as the paradigmatic ideologue of clinical science. Already having served as a guiding light of the AAP, Osler saw the need for a newer, more manageable organizational entity. In 1905, he convened the first meeting of the Interurban Clinical Club. Patterned on a surgical club which, in addition to surgery, would also be devoted to scientific medicine, geared in part to expand the hegemony of the now ascendant Johns Hopkins, and avowedly elitist, the Interurban would pursue several objectives. It would stimulate the growth of scientific internal medicine. It would improve methods of teaching and research. It would promote the scientific investigation of disease. And it would serve as a forum for the interchange of information about work in the clinics of the four cities represented.[24]

Osler's agenda for the Interurban hardly stopped with the articulation of lofty sentiments. Meeting twice each year in one of the four cities (in rotation) the group's members shared a range of sensibilities learned in most cases in the polyclinics of Germany. The minutes of the meetings make it clear that, paradoxically, they valued laboratory science and yet were alienated from it. Repeatedly, they spoke of the value of the clinic as the primary locus of scientific medicine.

There is, of course, something of a self-serving quality to the pronouncements of Osler and the other members of the Interurban. But a purely cynical reading of the text may prevent us from observing some of the texture of the experience of intellectually oriented medicine refining and recreating itself in the Flexner era. Clinicians faced some critical issues because of the tension between bedside and bench. Academic clinicians faced the question of how to support themselves on a full-time academic basis—and whether to do so. The clinic here took on a new economic, as well as a new social and intellectual meaning.[25] Clinicians also faced pressing questions raised by the Flexnerian program for the reform of medical education. A generation of nascent medical scientists were arriving in the medical schools and house-staff training programs of the elite institutions, a generation soon to be sent off to war, a generation which would be the first to learn all of its science at home. The Interurban educators' charge, as they saw it, was to inculcate the pure culture of an indigenous scientific medicine and to keep its focus in the clinic.

How far, then, to accede to the exigencies of the laboratory? This issue, as well as the other associated issues just enumerated, boiled up in the fourteenth meeting of the Interurban Clinical Club, held in New York in December of 1911. Lewellys F. Barker, Rufus Cole, William S. Thayer, and Theodore C. Janeway mulled over the implications of determining the locus of science in medicine from the economic, intellectual, and social point of view. Their lack of consensus was perhaps the most modern feature of their discourse.[26]

Of the participants in the 1911 debate, Cole, in particular, was a telling figure, one who recognized the need to reduce the strains in the perceived meaning of "medical science." As director of the Johns Hopkins Hospital from 1910 and the Hospital of the Rockefeller Institute when it opened in 1914, Cole was a passionate advocate of the ideal of clinical investigation. His notion was to create a hybrid, crossing the English model of hospital-based research with the German laboratory model, providing ancillary laboratory space in the hospital for clinicians who would carry ongoing responsibilities for patient care. Cole hoped to take the concept of clinical investigation at least one full step beyond Osler's rather rigidly distanced stance: he would attempt to ease the laboratory back toward the bedside. The extent of his success was mirrored first at the Rockefeller Institute.[27]

SAMUEL MELTZER, SPECIALISM, AND THE SCIENTIFIC IDEAL

The figure who most clearly internalized and hence best typified the tensions I have described was not a member of the Interurban Clinical Club at all. Samuel J. Meltzer was a Lithuanian Jew who had studied in Berlin and Königsberg before immigrating to New York. He had come closest to finding a mentor in the person of a clinical scientist, the German medical educator and prototypic gastroenterologist, Hugo von Kronecker.

The year 1904 was as much as a critical point in Meltzer's career as it was in American scientific medicine. In addition to the appearance of Rosenbach's diatribe against the laboratory, 1904 saw the recently reorganized American Medical Association summoning its energies to form an influential new Committee on Medical Education. In Germany, Paul Ehrlich was beginning the line of research which would lead to his therapeutic "magic bullet." And in New York City, Samuel Meltzer, fresh from his role in the founding of the Society for Experimental Biology and Medicine (soon dubbed the "Meltzer Verein"), heeded Simon Flexner's entreaties to join the staff of the Rockefeller Institute. In the same year he assumed the presidency of the fledgling (and still rather sickly) American Gastroenterologic Association, founded in 1897, and proceeded to use it as a platform from which to extol the virtues of specialist medical science. Those virtues rested, he felt, on a balance between bench and bedside—with the fulcrum nearest the latter.

Never reluctant, when it was a matter of joining (and leading) organizations, Meltzer went on successfully to promote, at the 1907 Atlantic City meeting of the AMA, his idea of an American Society of Clinical Investigation. The society which Meltzer thus proposed was convened for the first time in 1908. Less than a year later, he ascended to yet another presidency, that of the newly formed Association for the Advancement of Clinical Research.[28]

Meltzer's addresses to his several overlapping constitutencies—scientists, specialists, and clinical academicians—survived to become exceptionally useful historical tools. They serve collectively as a practically transparent window on the aspirations and self-perceptions of a generation of physicians who were in the process of inventing a new social form: something identifiable as clinical science, something which might

distance them from both the general practitioner and the laboratory researcher. The thread running throughout Meltzer's programmatic statements was the strain between the two potential spheres of the scientific
physician's work. This tension had both creative and destructive possibilities. It cut across every issue relating to the social and economic
organization of medical work. In 1904, speaking to the gastroenterolo-
gists, for example, Meltzer noted that "there can be some discussion as
to the division of labor in the practice of medicine, but there can be
no doubt as to the desirability of the division of labor in the . . . *science* of medicine."[29] Perhaps his most impassioned plea, however,
came in a remarkable address presented in Washington on 10 May,
1909:

> With the development of scientific methods . . . heavy branches grew out of the
> stem of medicine, broke off and obtained an independent existence. . . . Bacteri-
> ology tore off the branches of etiology and established itself as an independent
> growth. . . . What is left of the old stem is clinical medicine. What is the
> character of this residuum . . . who should be the man to carry on the research
> in this field, what should be their qualifications? In the first place, they must have
> a training fitting them to carry out investigations in conformity with the require-
> ments in all pure sciences. . . . However, after all these preparations they must
> select clinical research as the main field of their scientific activity. Clinical
> science will not thrive through chance investigations by friendly neighbors from
> the adjoining practical and scientific domains. . . . for such a purpose we need
> the service of a standing army of regulars.[30]

THE POSTWAR GENERATION: CLINICAL INVESTIGATION

World War I was, in many ways, a turning point, as Americans veered away
from the German experience and sought to fashion an indigenous medical
research establishment. After 1918, the American Society for Clinical
Investigation gathered strength in slow, sure steps. By 1924, its leaders were
ready to publish an official journal. In the first issue of the *Journal of
Clinical Investigation*, its editor, Alfred E. Cohn, was again at pains to
distance himself from the bacteriology laboratory:

> On account perhaps of the social importance of epidemic diseases, bacteriologists
> apart from physicians have, it is true, busied themselves with the communicable
> affections. But the diseases due to microbic agents have after all a curious external
> relation not common to other disease groups; their prevention, their manage-
> ment as hygiene prevents and manages them, requires no necessary contact with

infected individuals. Management so far as cure is concerned naturally involves an equipment different from that of the bacteriologist. . . . [M]edicine is indebted for [its] advance to bacteriologists. . . . [But such a] dependence on the outside world for the solution of its problems is in part a reproach to medicine. [Needed, then, to fill the breach, is a cadre of physicians] properly trained and supplied with adequate equipment. . . . This, then, is the task which academic medicine in the United States, now become self-conscious, has set itself; it is the task of Clinical Investigation.[31]

Cohn, based at the hospital of the Rockefeller Institute, had a keen sense of disciplinary boundary conditions and "near neighbor" relations. He both wrote and spoke often from his stance of an accomplished ideologue of clinical science. Matching phrases with the best of a generation of postwar apologists for applied science, Cohn time and again showed himself keenly aware of the strains and demands placed on the careers and institutions of those whom he called simply "the new men." In a particularly prescient 1929 address to the New York chapter of the medical honorary society, Alpha Omega Alpha, he looked back over the years since the heyday of Abraham Flexner and Samuel J. Meltzer.

There were many who unfortunately believed that what was chiefly wanted was to discard whatever was old; there were others who thought that it was necessary only, alongside the old, to introduce representatives of the new; they believed that what was required was to import, into the clinic, where the occasion offered, a friendly scientist. . . . [T]here were, furthermore, those who believed that what was wanted was to add to the old going concern co-ordinate enterprises that were new, as for instance, departments of research medicine. It is scarcely remarkable that there were finally those who believed that all change was undesirable.[32]

Cohn went on to liken clinical medical science to physics, and the medical "art" to engineering. Entitling his lecture "The Hierarchy of Medicine," he examined realistically the social and economic roots of the financial hierarchy and the intellectual conflicts still current in academic medicine. Clearly, he found the clinical investigator embattled on two sides: on the one hand by the bench scientist, and on the other by the "grand old men." Later, in the 1940s, he looked back on his thoughts of 1929 and mused that "many a grand old man of medicine felt put upon. He resisted dislocation. And so there *was* strife. Being a man of peace I wrote 'The Hierarchy of Medicine.' I should now call that address . . . 'Careers in Medicine.' "[33]

In 1919, Knud Faber, a Dane, whose interests lay in the clinical manifestations of bacterial exotoxins, had written a short history of clinical investigation.[34] Such an effort may be viewed as the type of crucial legitimating device which is frequently found between the first and second generations of a growing discipline. Faber, concerned with the neglected scientific contributions of a pantheon of nineteenth- and twentieth-century internists, entitled his book *Nosography*. It was a telling touch. The classification and description of disease, the old natural-historical mode, was, in fact, rather irrelevant by now to much of the substance of the book. But it was a device to which clinicians, uniquely, still clung.

The very title of what remains a unique history of clinical science was designed, then, to distance clinical science from the laboratory, as was Faber's emphasis on men like Frerichs, Traube, and Rosenbach. And when, in 1923, an American translation was published, a new English introduction was provided by the director of the Hospital of the Rockefeller Institute, Rufus Cole.

CONCLUSION

I have sketched a sequence of positions assumed by medical leaders in Germany and the United States on the question of how science and medicine should interact in an era of new institutional forms. The paradoxical relationship between bedside and bench did not, however, reflect an irreparable split between the two. The fissures and fault lines separating them did not, and indeed could not, deepen into chasms. Laboratory and clinic were interdependent from the outset, and, in research-oriented institutions, evolved toward ever more symbiotic relationships. But they could never feel the same instrumentally, in terms of the physician's daily work. Nor could they ever generate analogous types of financial patronage, because of the clinician's readier access to clinical sources of support. University-based physicians were thus confronted, after World War I, with the prospect of perceiving their economic and social center of gravity in basic science, clinical, or "research medicine" departments.

The tensions which I have discussed were superimposed upon, and indeed fed, the symbiosis between the two contexts. A few individuals, in America and abroad, were able fruitfully to investigate problems growing up at the interstices of clinic and laboratory by moving back and forth from one to the other. Examples abound. In the United States, for example, Simon Flexner was able to carry out his polio work at the Rockefeller Institute only by applying his expertise in both clinic and laboratory.[35] In continental Europe, Clemens von Pirquet's investigations of serum sickness were clearly dependent on the intellectual, instrumental, and institutional symbiosis of the two loci.[36]

This essay is thus every bit as much about physicians' self-perceptions as it is about the outcome of their career choices in 1885, or indeed in 1915. That is just the point, for such is the stuff of which scientific ideologies are made: programmatic statements about how the actor sees him- or herself fitting into larger social forms.

But if the ideology of scientific medicine reflected physicians' notions about the texture of their experience, then some current interpretations of the role of "scientism" in late nineteenth- and early twentieth-century medicine are somewhat simplistic and reductionist.[37] The contention that "science," as a monolithic value system, was grafted onto medicine by physicians wishing to shore up their own claims to legitimacy, or to dominate the medical marketplace, requires a great deal more careful scrutiny.

"Science," in medicine, came to mean different things to different people. Clinicians mistrusted it or tried to tame it; some, indeed, may have ultimately followed its lead to higher status. That there was an ideology of scientific medicine operating in the medical community is revealed by the existence of strains and fissures within the sensibilities which defined that ideology. At the same time, this more complex view impels us to set aside the revisionist notion of science as simply the great legitimator, the engine of domination and "medicalization." The superimposing of science onto medicine added not brute force, but new complexities, new strains, and new possibilities. That configuration persists in the third century of American medicine.[38]

NOTES

I thank Dr. Bonnie Blustein and Profs. Alvan Feinstein, David Hollinger, and Charles Rosenberg for their critical readings and suggestions regarding drafts of this chapter.

1. The disciplinary boundaries of these intellectual spheres of activity were probably clearer in Germany than in the United States, where even pathology was only fully professionalized and institutionalized in the early years of the twentieth century. On this process, and on the emergence of bacteriology in America from its parent discipline of pathology, see R. Maulitz, "[The Education of the American Physician in] Pathology," in Ronald Numbers, ed., *The Education of American Physicians* (Los Angeles: University of California Press, 1979). With respect to neighboring disciplines in medical and physiological chemistry, Robert E. Kohler is preparing an institutional and social history of biochemistry that promises to be comprehensive in its comparative view of national contexts.

2. One suspects that such changes obtained elsewhere in Europe as well; I have

confined the compass of the study on which this paper draws, however, to the German-American axis.

3. On this period see Owsei Temkin, "The Era of Paul Ehrlich," *Bulletin of the New York Academy of Medicine* 30 (1954): 261–68; on the texture of bacteriology in one major U.S. city see Jonathan Liebenau, "Bacteriology in Philadelphia," (unpublished manuscript, University of Pennsylvania, fall 1977). An excellent overview of the American experience in this period is Barbara Rosenkrantz, "Cart before Horse: Theory, Practice, and Professional Image in American Public Health, 1870–1920," *Journal of the History of Medicine* 29 (1974): 55–73.

4. By *modern* I refer simply to that which is recognizable in terms of the canons of twentieth-century medical care and medical research.

5. A similar point can be made regarding the socioeconomic location of a parallel development, that of specialization; there is, as yet, no adequate historical typology of specialism, though two standard sources remain serviceable and suggestive: George Rosen, *Specialization: with Special Reference to Ophthalmology* (1944; reprint ed., N.Y.: Arno Press, 1972), and Rosemary Stevens, *American Medicine and the Public Interest* (New Haven: Yale University Press, 1971).

6. Few historical treatments deal with the central role of technique in the laboratory as a critical determinant of the formation of medical disciplines; but see Liebenau, "Bacteriology," n. 3, and Lewis Rubin, "Leo Loeb's Role in the Development of Tissue Culture," *Clio Medica* 12 (1977): 33–56.

7. On the importance of the routine, the texture of the individual's quotidian work experience, see Fernand Braudel, *Afterthoughts on Material Civilization and Capitalism* (Baltimore: Johns Hopkins University Press, 1977).

8. Charles E. Rosenberg, "Martin Arrowsmith: the Scientist as Hero," *American Quarterly* 15 (1963): 447–58; reprinted in his *No Other Gods* (Baltimore: Johns Hopkins University Press, 1976).

9. See Thomas Gariepy, "The Acceptance of Antiseptic Surgery in the United States," (M.A. thesis, Notre Dame University, 1976), and J. Liebenau, "Antisepsis in the United States," paper presented to the American Association for the History of Medicine, Kansas City, Mo., May 1978. A useful starting place is Gert H. Brieger, "American Surgery and the Germ Theory of Disease," *Bulletin of the History of Medicine* 40 (1966): 135–45.

10. Edward H. Clarke, "Practical medicine," in E.H. Clarke *et al. A Century of American Medicine* (1876; reprint ed., Brinklow, Md.: Old Hickory Bookshop, 1962), pp. 3–72.

11. There were, no doubt, exceptions to this generalization, one of which may have been cellular pathology: see n. 14 below.

12. On the German background and the American connection, a useful recent article is that of Saul Benison, "The Development of Clinical Research at the Rockefeller Before 1939," in *Trends in Biomedical Research, 1901–1976, Proceedings of the 2nd Annual Rockefeller Archives Center Conference* (10 December 1976), pp. 35–45; see esp. p. 36.

13. The best general source on the history of this aspect of internal medicine remains Knud Faber, *Nosography in Modern Internal Medicine* (New York: Hoeber, 1923); see also Temkin, "Era of Paul Ehrlich," n. 3, and Bernhard Naunyn, *Erinnerungen, Gedanken und Meinungen* (Munich: Bergmann, 1925).

14. Russell C. Maulitz, "Rudolf Virchow, Julius Cohnheim, and the Program of Pathology," *Bulletin of the History of Medicine* 52 (1978): 162–82.

15. See Faber, *Nosography*, n. 13, and a brief but useful work, Kenneth Keele, *The Evolution of Clinical Methods in Medicine* (London: Pitman, 1963).

16. The others were Francis Delafield, William Draper, Robert Edes, George Peabody, James Tyson, and William Pepper.

17. My discussion of the AAP owes much to Daniel Todes, "Scientific Medicine in the Minority: the Birth of the Association of American Physicians," unpublished manuscript, University of Pennsylvania, 1975.

18. Todes, ibid., points out that six of the seven founders were elite both socially and intellectually (judging membership in the intellectual elite on the basis of graduation from elite medical schools: Columbia, 3; Harvard, 1; McGill, 1; Pennsylvania, 2).

19. See Lewis Rubin, "The Dreaded Scourge of Childhood: the Impact of New York City's Antidiphtheria Campaign upon American Medicine," paper read before American Association for the History of Medicine, Kansas City, Mo., May 1978. See also Rosenkrantz, "Cart before Horse," n. 3.

20. Only Faber (n. 13), in the secondary literature, deals to any extent with Rosenbach; the importance of this neglected and rather contradictory life has been made clearer to me in several conversations with Gert H. Brieger and George Rosen. Thomas Bonner, whose book on German-American medical relations remains, in many ways, the standard source, mentions Rosenbach only in passing: *American Doctors and German Universities* (Lincoln, Neb.: University of Nebraska Press, 1963), p. 35.

21. Ottomar Rosenbach, *Physician versus Bacteriologist* (N.Y.: Funk and Wagnalls, 1904), pp. vii–ix, 208–9.

22. Ibid., p. xiv.

23. See, for example, J.J. Lawrence, M.D. [Review of] Rosenbach, in *Medical Brief* 32 (1904): 713–14.

24. David Riesman, ed., *History of the Interurban Clinical Club, 1905–37* (Phila.: Winston, n.d.). This *History* reprints, with few emendations, an earlier (1927) history of the club, along with the organization's exceedingly useful minutes and a group of individual members' biographical sketches. The four cities were Baltimore, Philadelphia, New York, and Boston.

25. The controversy over "full-time" academic employment of clinicians remains a pivotal topic awaiting its historian.

26. By now I trust that the reader will have discerned my contention that it is this very ambiguity, the "spread" of options between the career of physician, or bacteriologist, or in some other laboratory role that characterizes the peculiar modernity of the scenario depicted here. After this paper was prepared, Prof. David Hollinger kindly directed me to an analogous treatment of the ideology of science in engineering by Edwin Layton, "American Ideologies of Science and Engineering," *Technology and Culture* 17 (1976): 688–701.

27. Cole was not alone in assuming this posture. See the other papers, especially those by A. McG. Harvey and Pauline Mazumdar, in *Trends in Biomedical Research, 1901–1976* (n. 12).

28. Meltzer published extensively on the specificity of bacterial infections in the clinical context. Often his argument rested on a demonstration of the complexity of the host-parasite relationship, one which he felt bacteriology tended to oversimplify: see "Some of the Physiological Methods and Means Employed by the Animal Organism in Its Continual Struggle against Bacteria from Maintenance of Life and Health," *Transactions of the American Congress of Physicians & Surgeons* 5 (1900): 12–25. The argument from complexity could indeed lead him into an outright indictment of physicochemical reductionism, tarring the biochemists with the same brush: see, e.g., *Science*, N.S. 19 (1904): 18–27. Prior to his move to the Rockefeller in 1904, Meltzer had for years pursued the private practice of medicine in New York. While in practice he had gained access to William H. Welch's laboratory at Bellevue Hospital, thus increasing his familiarity with both bedside and bench.

29. S.J. Meltzer, "Our Aims," Presidential Address, American Gastro-Enterological Association, Atlantic City, 6 June 1904, *Medical News* (1 October 1904), pp. 1–7.

30. S. J. Meltzer, "The Science of Clinical Medicine: What it Ought to Be and the Men to Uphold It," in J. M. Cattell, ed., *Medical Research and Education* (N.Y.: Science Press, 1913), vol. 2, *Science and Education,* pp. 428–39.

31. Alfred E. Cohn, "Purposes in Medical Research: an Introduction to the Journal of Clinical Investigation," *Journal of Clinical Investigation* 1 (1924): 1–11; repr. in Alfred E. Cohn, *Medicine, Science and Art* (Chicago: University of Chicago Press, 1931), pp. 120–37.

32. Cohn, "The Hierarchy of Medicine," repr. in Cohn, *Medicine,* n. 31, pp. 170–212; p. 191.

33. Alfred E. Cohn, *No Retreat from Reason* (New York: Harcourt, Brace and Co., 1948), p. x.

34. Faber, *Nosography,* n. 13.

35. Saul Benison, "Poliomyelitis and the Rockefeller Institute: Social Effects and Institutional Response," *Journal of the History of Medicine* 29 (1974): 74–92.

36. Erna Lesky, "Viennese Serological Research c. 1900," *Bulletin of the New York Academy of Medicine* 49 (1973): 100–11.

37. See, for example, H.S. Berliner, "A Larger Perspective on the Flexner Report," *International Journal of Health Services* 5 (1975): 573–92.

38. This is not to say that science did not, in some ways, genuinely lend "legitimacy" to medicine in this period. The most lucid demonstration of the persistence of the phenomena I have described is provided in Alvan Feinstein, *Clinical Judgement* (Baltimore: Williams and Wilkins, 1967), passim.

Note added in proof: Since I submitted the final text of this article, two pertinent additional works by an "insider," A. McG. Harvey (n. 27) have come to my attention: "Samuel J. Meltzer: Pioneer Catalyst in the Evolution of Clinical Science in America," Perspectives in Biology and Medicine *21 (1978): 431–40; and* The Interuban Clinical Club *(1905–1976) (N.p.: Interuban Clinical Club, 1978), which extends the Riesman volume (n. 24).*

5 DOCTORS, BIRTH CONTROL, AND SOCIAL VALUES: 1830–1970

JAMES REED

The history of medical attitudes toward birth control in the United States provides a stark example of the extent to which social values sometimes shape medical practice regardless of the knowledge and technology available to the profession. From the 1830s, when the practice of family limitation first became a subject of broad public debate, until the marketing of the birth control pill in the early 1960s, the majority of doctors viewed the desire for fewer children as a problem rather than as an opportunity to provide a medical service. They associated birth control with threats to the social order that they served and to their profession.[1]

Beginning in the late eighteenth century, generation after generation of Americans had progressively fewer children despite the wails of social leaders that they were shirking their patriotic duty, committing "race suicide," sinning against nature.[2] Before the 1960s, "the population problem" in the United States was a dearth of people of the "right kind."[3] Doctors, like other social arbiters, persistently complained of the low birth rate among the middle classes, a result, they claimed, of the selfish hedonism of the socially ambitious. While the "best" people too often avoided parenthood, the poor and foreign born seemed to multiply with abandon, raising the spectre of a tragic decline in the quality of the population. By the early 1930s, Americans were reproducing at a rate that would have resulted in a stationary or declining population, if it had continued. The end of population growth seemed to be at hand, and with it the prospect of economic stagnation and national decline. Americans regained the will to multiply with wartime prosperity, but in 1960, as in 1830, the healthy woman was defined as a willing mother who wanted to do her part to bolster the sagging population growth rate. The unwilling mother was sick or confused, and her reluctance to procreate a sad commentary on social conditions.

Despite the dominant pronatalist values of American culture, large numbers of married Americans learned to control their fertility. Their restrictive behavior reflected decisions made within the family, for private reasons, in the absence of broadly recognized social justification or public sanction for family limitation. The great majority of would-be contraceptors succeeded or failed without the aid of a doctor. Businessmen who promoted powders and appliances for "feminine hygiene," marginal physicians, and quacks filled the void left by the indifference of medical leaders to the widespread, if semi-licit, demand for contraceptive advice. Birth control became associated with the patent medicine business and irregular practice, and with the threat which they posed to the economic and social status of the ethical physician. The reluctance of physicians to provide contraceptive services was not, however, a result of the association of birth control with quackery. Rather, medical leaders left birth control to the second-rate and the disreputable because of their commitment to the maintenance of social order as they understood it. The association of birth control with quackery was a result, rather than a cause, of the physicians' reluctance to provide services.[4]

If nineteenth-century medical men had wanted to provide reliable contraceptive means to the public, the requisite technology and knowledge of the process of conception were available. Historians have sometimes asserted that there were no "scientific" birth control methods available in the nineteenth century, but by 1865 rubber condoms, vaginal diaphragms, spermicidal douches, and the "infertile period" had all been described in popular medical manuals that were sold to the public.[5] Although Margaret Sanger led a successful campaign to popularize the spring-loaded diaphragm in the 1920s, there were no fundamental advances in contraceptive technology from the middle of the nineteenth century until the marketing of the birth control pill in 1960.[6] Sanger's crusade for birth control was necessary because the great majority of physicians did not perceive contraception as an important problem. Their attitudes had little to do with the birth control means available. Birth control methods were damned as unreliable and unsafe because of their association with apparent threats to stable family life—specifically, the growing hedonism of a consumer society, the dissatisfaction of middle class women with the social roles assigned to them, and the decline in birth rates among the "fit."

While attitudes toward sex, women, and the family were the most important determinants of medical opinion on contraception, doctors shared these attitudes with the great majority of respectable people. Since the integrity of any profession depends on public support, doctors could not have taken radical public positions on any sexual question without endangering their status. Before the rise of modern medicine, the physician's central role was to comfort and to reassure by interpreting the natural order, by explaining the sources of disease in the individual's failure to observe the laws of nature and of society.[7] Since his professional position depended on this essentially priestly function, he could hardly question the prevailing standards of sexual morality. Duty dictated, in fact, that he provide disease sanctions for them.[8]

The development of a somatic pathology, anesthesia, antisepsis, and bacteriology during the nineteenth century improved the physician's ability to prevent and to cure disease, but these gains did not lessen his profession's dependence on community support. If the new doctor was to be a scientist, then huge sums of money would have to be raised to subsidize medical education, and the new university-affiliated medical schools would need access to public hospitals and to the patients who provided subjects for both student and researcher. The newly rich found medical education and research especially attractive because these endeavors seemed to be unquestionable public benefits, philanthropies that minimized the risk of criticism for misusing the power represented by money. The continuing flow of philanthropic dollars into the new medical establishment depended, however, on a reputation for social service rather than criticism, especially not criticism of "civilized morality." It was appropriate that "the" man in gynecology at Johns Hopkins, during its era as the symbol of scientific medicine, was Howard Kelley, a Christian gentleman, well known for his piety and prudery, who had no interest in contraception or any kind of sex research.[9]

The demands of Margaret Sanger and other sexual reformers that physicians learn contraceptive technique and engage in contraceptive research were anathema to most physicians on two counts. First, they offended the sensibilities of medical men as social arbiters who wholeheartedly shared their society's values and who were reticent about birth control, not because of moral cowardice, as Sanger claimed, but because they, along with other respectable people, thought that women needed to have more children. Second, sexual reform threatened physicians as professionals who were dependent on the public's good will for the legislation and institutional support required if standards of education and practice were to be raised.

The career of James Marion Sims, the founder of American gynecology, illustrates the close relationship between the social attitudes of medical leaders and the services that they offered. Sims gained international fame in the 1850s by developing an operation for repair of tears in the bladder (vesicovaginal fistula), a common childbirth injury that had formerly doomed thousands of women to live out their lives continuously soaked with urine. He devoted a large part of his practice, however, to the treatment of sterility, and most of his classic *Clinical Notes on Uterine Surgery* (1866) was devoted to the dozens of elaborate, ingenious, and sometimes painful methods that he developed to help women conceive. He shared the prevailing sexual ideology which viewed all healthy women as willing mothers, and he ignored contraceptive technique. In an age when hysterectomy was a high-risk procedure, even the great surgeons like Sims relied heavily on pessaries in the treatment of uterine prolapse, and Sims described dozens of pessaries for various purposes, including a spring-loaded rubber ring that resembled in all but contraceptive intent the vaginal diaphragms used in twentieth-century birth control clinics. The popular medical journalist Edward Bliss Foote provided his lay readers with a description of a contraceptive "womb veil" (essentially a diaphragm) in *Medical Common Sense* (1864), but Sims, like most specialists in women's diseases, devoted himself solely to helping women become mothers, leaving contraception to the second-rate or the quack. As an expert in the fitting of pessaries, Sims was, if anything, more capable of designing and fitting a contraceptive diaphragm than physicians of the 1920s, when this device began to be widely used by American women. He chose not to, largely, it appears, because he did not feel that his society needed efficient contraception.[10]

After the passage of the Comstock Act (1873), it was illegal to give contraceptive advice, and the subject was omitted from post-1873 editions of many books in which it had originally been given space. Some physicians were prosecuted under the Comstock Act, but the suppression of birth control information was but a small part of a great crusade to make American cities safe for middle class families through the suppression of commercial vice.[11] Some medical leaders were in sympathy with the purity crusaders. Others clashed with them, suffered humiliating defeats, and learned that it was the duty of their profession to defend the highest moral standards of the community. In 1874, Sims, president of the American Medical Association (AMA), recommended a national system of regulation for prostitution as a means of controlling venereal disease, but the effort to mobilize the medical profession for regulation was defeated by purity lobbyists who argued that the only acceptable venereal disease prophylaxis was a moral one, a single high standard for all, male and female. By 1894 the president of the New York Academy of Medicine endorsed efforts to collect physicians' signatures on a petition stating that chastity was in accord with the laws of health. The "new abolitionists" had taught doctors that sexual matters were to be treated with great seriousness.[12]

It is difficult, however, to estimate just how large an impact Comstockery had on medical behavior. Physicians seem to have been much more concerned over the apparently rising tide of marital unhappiness that they witnessed and by the low birth rate among their paying customers than with either the safety or legality of birth control.[13] In 1898, the Physicians Club of Chicago sponsored a symposium on "sexual hygiene" in order to provide a forum for a frank exchange of information that would help local doctors to become better marriage counselors. One of the participants explained, "Outside the medical profession it is taken for granted that the doctor knows all about these things [sex]. But within our ranks we are aware that this is not true. The text-books omit this department." The public increasingly turned to physicians instead of to the clergy for sex advice, but some doctors were willing to admit, at least among themselves, that they had insufficient knowledge of the subject. An edited transcript of the symposium was published as a "for doctors only" handbook, entitled *Sexual Hygiene*, in an effort to meet the need for information.[14]

The editors of *Sexual Hygiene* believed that husbands bore a major share of the blame for the marital unhappiness that seemed to be reaching epidemic proportions. Too many of them were ignorant of, or ignored, the sexual needs of their wives. Husbands had to be taught that "the god-given relation is two-sided, and that without harmony and mutual enjoyment it becomes a mere masturbation to the body and mind of the one who alone is gratified." Perhaps better marital sex would lower the divorce rate and keep both husbands and wives at home, where they belonged.[15]

One chapter of *Sexual Hygiene* was devoted to contraception. Contributors ignored the illegality of contraceptive advice and accepted birth control as a necessary means, in some cases, of reconciling the economic and personal interests of husbands and wives. They knew of numerous methods, but birth control information had to be given with discretion. There were situations in which it should be kept from patients. "We all know perfectly

the difference between the dragged-out woman on the verge of consumption . . . and the society belle who mistakenly thinks she does not want
babies when every fiber of her being is crying out for this means of bringing
her back to healthy thought."[16]

This ambiguous attitude toward birth control was most strikingly revealed in a long discussion of contraceptive methods. The strong-willed
might try "limiting intercourse to the period from the sixteenth day after
menstruation to the twenty-fifth." Men could practice withdrawal or use
condoms. The condom was very effective, "if the best are used, but we all
know that rubber is a non-conductor of electricity, and this is a factor that
I think should not be lost sight of. They are not the easiest thing in the
world to put on either."[17]

While a highly effective and safe contraceptive was mocked because it
interfered with male pleasure, female methods received indiscriminate
endorsement. "The little sponge in a silk net with string attached is a
familiar sight in drug stores. If this is moistened with some acid or anticep-
tic solution before use and rightly placed it is very safe and harmless." In
addition to the sponge, would-be female contraceptors might choose either
douching, or "a vaginal suppository of cocoa butter and ten per cent of
boric and tannic acids," or "the womb veil with eighty grams of quinine
mutate to an ounce of petrolatum." All seemed to work well enough. The
chief complaint against intrauterine stem pessaries was that "there are
many women who cannot place them." A final bit of advice was offered
for the woman who wanted to avoid having children without good reason.
"Get a divorce and vacate the position for some other woman, who is able
and willing to fulfill all a wife's duties as well as to enjoy her privileges."[18]

Although these physicians knew of many female methods, they expressed
no concern with making distinctions between them or for the problems
that women might have in using them. Systematic clinical evaluation of
birth control would not begin until the 1920s, when minor improvements
in the "womb veil" or vaginal diaphragm would provide the most effective
female method available until the marketing of the anovulant pill in 1960.
Serious study of birth control methods might have begun in the late
nineteenth century, since, as the discussion of birth control methods in
Sexual Hygiene makes clear, both the necessary technology and knowledge
of sexual anatomy were available, but doctors did not make any major
efforts to improve contraceptive means. Since the family might be weakened if sex was too easily separated from procreation, doctors believed that
they had a social obligation to carefully manage the dissemination of birth
control. Indeed, in the case of the "society belle" or other healthy woman
who did not want children, their duty was to force "her back to healthy

thought." In this context doctors were not greatly concerned over the failure rates of birth control regimens.[19]

The major impetus for change in the status of contraception came during the first half of the twentieth century from lay women rather than from within the medical profession, but they were aided by some allies among medical men, most notably Robert Latou Dickinson.[20] Organized medicine could never accept demands from lay women, especially not from Margaret Sanger, a sexual reformer and biting critic of the profession. Dickinson played the role of mediator through whom organized medicine finally made its peace with the birth control movement. His personal lobbying led to a 1937 AMA resolution recognizing that informing patients about contraceptive methods was an important medical subject that should be taught in medical schools.

While Dickinson enjoyed considerable success in the role of medical educator, his own efforts to organize contraceptive research failed. Ironically, he was forced to depend on data from clinical investigations organized and directed by Margaret Sanger in his campaign to change medical opinion on birth control. His unsuccessful efforts during the 1920s to organize contraceptive research revealed the deep antagonism among his colleagues toward sexual reform and the barriers that even a distinguished gynecologist faced in attempting to study contraception.

Dickinson's social background and personal contacts were important sources of strength in his campaign to win medical support for birth control. His parents were prominent members of Brooklyn's social elite during the Gilded Age. He attended private schools in Europe, finished high school at Brooklyn Polytechnic, and began medical study at Long Island College Hospital in 1879, at the age of nineteen. He became the protégé of Alexander Skene, the modern discoverer of the paraurethral ducts in women ("Skene's glands"). Dickinson's artistic ability led to a job as illustrator for Skene's textbook, *Treatise on Diseases of Women* (1888), which dominated the American textbook market in gynecology for a decade.

Educated at a proprietary medical school in a pre-Flexner-Report system, Dickinson plunged into the business of ordinary practice upon graduation from Long Island College Hospital, in 1881, and found time to write only through driving self-discipline. He gradually won recognition as one of the country's leading specialists in the diseases of women and published prodigiously on questions of concern to the working practitioner of the art of medicine. He shed light on topics ranging from surgical technique to how to keep office records, but made no important contributions to the new science of obstetrics championed by J. Whitridge Williams of Johns Hopkins.[21]

Dickinson's lasting contributions to his specialty were made not as a surgeon or clinician, however, but as a sex researcher and reformer. Early in his career he became concerned over the contrast between his culture's genteel code of sexual morality and the behavior that he daily encountered as a doctor. In one of his early case histories, he wrote, "Pregnant, have not asked particulars. I would never have believed it of this girl. My mother often praised her. . . ." He noticed frequent enlargements of the labia minora among his patients and traced these deviations from normal sexual anatomy to masturbation, a practice that he found to be present among women of all classes and ages and not necessarily associated with any kind of antisocial behavior. Experience taught that there were probably as many induced abortions as live births in Brooklyn and that sexual incompatibility destroyed many marriages even when it did not lead to divorce. Dickinson responded to this sexual nightmare as a Christian gentlemen with an empirical bent, by gathering information, consulting colleagues, and cautiously reporting his opinions through the proper channels. The correctness of his social and professional attitudes helped him to obtain a tolerant reception for his unorthodox work. His sex research always kept the goal of happy marriage in view. If sexual adjustment could be improved, then the family might be strengthened.[22]

Before he retired from active practice Dickinson published relatively little on sex, but the records he made of female sex anatomy in its diverse normal and pathological forms were unique in their quantity and accuracy. He recorded his observations in minute detail and then carefully compared and classified the specimens. Eventually providing a series stretching over forty years of practice, these records were a medical natural history and the essential source on which he later drew in founding American medical sex research.

Dickinson boasted that he always kept the perspective of the family physician, and his 1920 address as president of the American Gynecological Society (AGS) provides a sharp contrast with the scathing presidential rebuke delivered to the society by J. Whitridge Williams in 1914.[23] During the first decades of the century specialists in what Dickinson liked to call "uterology" (obstetrics and gynecology) were much concerned over the future of their group. The obstetrician had to compete with midwives and general practitioners, while general surgeons were performing the operations pioneered by gynecologists. Williams argued that the future of the speciality lay in basic research, in developing knowledge upon which a specialist's therapeutics could securely rest. Williams's attack on the generally "casuistical" and "sometimes puerile" publications of AGS members was self-conscious propaganda for the Johns Hopkins ideal and might be read as an attack on the tradition of education and practice that Dickinson exemplified. Dickinson lacked training in basic research but admitted no need to apologize for a career of healing and sexual counseling. He had devoted his life to "the study of womankind," and, like all great naturalists, he knew what could be discovered by the naked eye about his subject. In his 1920 presidential address, Dickinson argued that the future of the speciality depended on informed sexual counseling, and on modernizing the physician's traditional priestly role. He already had data in his own records to answer the rhetorical questions that he posed. What about the "distasteful" but burning issue of contraception? "What, indeed, is normal sex life?" He made a new career for himself. Retiring from active practice in 1920, Dickinson lived his own recommendation that "uterologists" take an "interest in sociological problems" falling within their domain and give serious attention to the social pathology caused by the conflict between the ideal and the real in the sexual realm.[24]

In 1916, Dickinson had urged a group of Chicago physicians to begin a clinical investigation of the safety and effectiveness of birth control methods. "We as a profession should take hold of this matter and not let it go to the radicals, and not let it receive harm by being pushed in any undignified or improper manner." When Margaret Sanger asked for his endorsement, he politely refused, but he believed that contraception was essential if normal marital relations were to be improved, so birth control was first on his agenda of topics that needed him. Having secured a grant from one of Sanger's disaffected supporters, in 1923 he began a search for institutional sponsorship for contraceptive research. The New York Obstetrical Society turned him down, but he was able to recruit some distinguished colleagues to serve on a Committee on Maternal Health, with temporary headquarters in Dickinson's apartment.[25]

Dickinson hoped that his Committee on Maternal Health would conduct authoritative investigations that would command the respect of the medical and philanthropic establishments and provide guidelines for ordered change. In January of 1923, Sanger opened the first physician-staffed birth control clinic in the United States, next door to the offices of the American Birth Control League, but the medical community was militantly opposed to the delivery of health care in "special" or extramural clinics, and Dickinson believed that the most efficient source for clinical data would be hospital outpatient departments. He hoped that the Committee on Maternal Health could provide contraceptive supplies and honorariums to hospital clinic directors and then simply collect the records that would surely exceed those of Sanger's clinic in both quality and quantity.[26]

The first hitch in Dickinson's plan came when the diaphragms which he had ordered from Germany were confiscated by United States Customs despite a "gentlemen's agreement" that they would be allowed to pass. Sanger smuggled hers in. Since the committee forswore illegal activity, it could not provide clients with the most promising female contraceptive device. Finally, Sanger agreed to sell the committee diaphragms at cost from her own meagre supply.[27]

The second problem that stymied Dickinson's research was a lack of patients. His committee made up a rigid set of procedures that met all of the requirements of the New York law, which, thanks to a 1919 court decision engineered by Sanger, permitted contraceptive advice by a physician, but only "to cure or prevent disease." Thus, the committee required that all patients treated under its auspices have a written description from a gynecologist of the medical indications justifying contraceptive advice. This requirement caused hospital physicians who were being paid by the committee to refer patients to them to send their patients to the Sanger clinic. One doctor explained, "However positive he might be that a certain patient would be in very grave danger if she conceived, yet he doubted whether he would be willing to put his name to a recommendation for contraceptive advice to be handed the patient, for fear of the use that might be put to such a paper." The committee even decided not to give slips of printed instructions to patients because they "might be copied or lost or other-wise convey information where it should not be available."[28]

Even with these stringent safeguards, hospital doctors refused to cooperate, despite generous monthly honorariums. One doctor received $125 and handed in six cases. In all, $1500 brought only twenty-three patient records. Fitting diaphragms was just difficult enough to require special training and a willingness to devote time to work from which no professional prestige would result. With no glamor and some risk attached to this work, it was much easier to refuse advice or to send patients to the Sanger clinic, where female general practitioners were developing considerable skill in contraceptive technique.[29]

Dickinson finally gave up the effort to collect his own records and began a campaign to get Sanger to give control of her clinic to the committee. Sanger had never been able to obtain a dispensary license for the Birth Control Clinical Research Bureau, and she agreed to allow Dickinson to take over the bureau if he could obtain a license. The Rockefeller-funded Bureau of Social Hygiene provided a $10,000 grant for the first year of this arrangement. Dickinson recruited a staff of eminent medical men to serve as directors of the proposed Maternity Research Council, and only a dispensary license from the State Board of Charities was lacking to put the

plan into effect. The Board of Charities admitted that all standard requirements had been met for a license but demanded a waiver from representatives of the Jewish, Protestant, and Roman Catholic faiths. Dickinson
obtained waivers from Jewish and Protestant leaders but could get no
response from the Catholic hierarchy of New York.[30]

Dickinson tried to get the Committee on Maternal Health to go ahead
with the plan without a license, but the whole purpose of taking over the
Sanger clinic had been to conduct a completely legal and ethical investigation, and the committee voted not to pursue further the plan to cooperate
with Sanger. Sanger, however, had only agreed to cooperate on the condition that Dickinson provide what she could not—a license.

Although the clinic, staffed as it was by female general practitioners, had
no specialists in gynecology, it did provide good records for analysis. By
1927, Dr. Hannah Stone, the clinic's medical director, had data to prove
that the vaginal diaphragm was a safe and effective contraceptive. Dickinson was instrumental in getting these records published in 1928, although,
characteristically, he promised more than he could deliver when he guaran-
teed Sanger that, if she would delay private publication, he would get
Stone's article on "Therapeutic Contraception" into either the *Journal of
the American Medical Association* or the *American Journal of Obstetrics
and Gynecology.* Both journals refused the article because the research was
sponsored by Sanger. Stone's article finally appeared in the *Medical Journal
and Record,* with a preface by Dickinson.[31]

Under Dickinson's direction it is doubtful that the Sanger clinic would
have been able to find many women in the certified mortal danger required
to meet the letter of the New York law. It was fortunate in this respect that
Dickinson failed in his effort to capitalize on Sanger's good will with the
fertile women of New York by taking control of her clinic. His frustrated
adventure in clinical research under the auspices of the Committee on
Maternal Health demonstrated, however, that it was impossible to conduct
a clinical investigation of contraception that met all of the requirements
of the law and of medical ethics.[32]

The rejection of Dr. Stone's pioneering analysis of the Birth Control
Clinical Research Bureau's records by the AMA's *Journal* and by the
leading journal in gynecology is not surprising, in view of the social values
of their editors, Morris Fishbein and George Kosmak. Fishbein had included an intemperate attack on birth control advocates in his *Medical
Follies* (1925). In the shrill tone characteristic of his treatment of all
heresy, from faith healing to the Sheppard Towner Act (1923), a law which
provided modest federal subsidies for state programs to improve infant and
maternal health, Fishbein unequivocally asserted that "no method of birth

control is physiologically, psychologically and biologically sound in both principle and practice." One historian has explained Fishbein's diatribe against the "ardent economists, biologists, sociologists and philosophers who favor birth control" as part of his larger concern with the defense of a profession just coming into its own after years of struggle with quackery and with public indifference to the needs of the ethical practitioner. Yet Fishbein's categorical rejection of contraception was logically, if not emotionally, inconsistent with the brand of medicine which he claimed to be defending in *Medical Follies*.[33]

One of the most objectionable traits of quack systems of medicine, in Fishbein's view, was the oversimplification of complex issues, the a priori rejection of empirical treatment, and the exaggeration of the effectiveness of simplistic therapeutics. Fishbein stood for a sane positivism based on both science and common sense. Contraception certainly represented an area of social and medical practice which needed the empirical, common sense treatment provided by Hannah Stone, and in which Fishbein claimed to believe. Fishbein, however, justified his rejection of birth control on the grounds that the effectiveness of the known methods ranged from 10 to 90 percent. "Moreover some of them may have produced irritation of the tissues and grave consequences, including cancer. Little need be said of their psychological effects." Having raised the spectre of cancer and refused to distinguish between methods, or to recognize that medicine might have a responsibility to improve what was available, Fishbein saw sterilization by X ray or the development of a spermatoxin as possible future sources of relief, but concluded that the only safe birth control method was continence.[34]

The inconsistency in his attitude was pointed out by James F. Cooper, the medical director of the American Birth Control League, in *Technique of Contraception* (1928). Cooper noted that there was a "great deal of thoughtless talk about 'no one hundred per cent method.' "

> It is fair then to ask, have we any one hundred per cent methods in medicine, or surgery, or serum, or vaccine therapy? . . . . The only ethical attitude a physician can take is to guarantee nothing. He can only promise to do his best.
>
> This being true, how clearly absurd it is to single out one department of medical practice, namely contraception, for criticism on the ground that it is not one hundred per cent perfect and for that reason to regard it with indifference! If all physicians had adopted the same general attitude toward every other brand of medicine and surgery, their profession long since would discontinued its activities.
>
> As a matter of fact, there are very few fields indeed in the practice of medicine

where such uniformly good results can be obtained as in contraception. It is a fact that the method recommended . . . in this book [vaginal diaphragm with spermicidal jelly] is safe, simple, and when properly followed, almost uniformly reliable.[35]

Fishbein's treatment of birth control had less to do with "professionalism" than with his attitudes toward women. He was reacting not as a scientist or physician but as a conservative who despised feminists almost as much as medical socialism.[36]

George Kosmak, editor of the *American Journal of Obstetrics and Gynecology,* also rejected Stone's "Therapeutic Contraception." Dickinson recruited his old friend Kosmak for the Committee on Maternal Health because he wanted it to be representative of medical opinion, but Kosmak was a practicing Catholic and proved a difficult ally. In 1936, he candidly admitted, "whenever a young wife fails in her contraceptive practice one thanks God that she did."[37] An inveterate foe of socialized medicine, whether in the form of national health insurance or birth control clinics, Kosmak fretted constantly over the low birth rate among the middle classes, believed that most women who could legally qualify for contraception were in such bad health that they should not have sex anyway, and, in 1939, told the delegates to the AMA convention that birth control propaganda was responsible "for the lack of sexual restraint which has become so evident."[38]

Kosmak agreed to join Dickinson's committee, in 1923, because it provided an opportunity to investigate and to condemn Sanger's activities. He wanted medical control of the dissemination of birth control information because that, he felt, was infinitely better than its free availability in any form. Proponents of birth control aroused public sympathy through tales of gravely ill women who could not obtain contraceptive advice, and Kosmak wanted contraception taught in medical schools, so that no woman with serious medical reasons for avoiding pregnancy would be unable to obtain advice from a private practitioner. In this way, charges of negligence could be disproved and the justification for clinics sponsored by lay groups undermined. But most important, medical students would learn "proper" attitudes toward contraception, along with techniques.[39]

If the antagonism toward birth control of two key leaders such as Kosmak and Fishbein was at all representative of their constituency, how did an affirmative resolution on birth control finally get through an AMA convention in 1937? It was not easy, but Dickinson managed, through persistent lobbying in a changing social context. Lay birth control advocates, with the cooperation of a few medical allies, had established a nationwide chain of several hundred birth control clinics, by the middle of the 1930s. The data from these clinics, reported in many authoritative publications, including Dickinson's *Control of Conception* (1931), demonstrated that safe and effective contraceptive practice was possible. Vague references to contraceptive-induced cancer and to psychological trauma had gradually lost their credibility.[40]

Social conservatives found contraception less offensive as supporters of birth control began to exploit the issue of skyrocketing welfare costs during the Depression; the reformers now talked less of women controlling their bodies and more of the need to "democratize" contraceptive practice. Since the middle classes were clearly not going to stop practicing contraception, many of those who were concerned over differential fertility between classes believed that their best hope for altering dysgenic population trends lay in birth control for the poor.[41]

By the early thirties the "feminine hygiene" racket, supported by unscrupulous advertising, and flourishing in the absence of any medically recognized standards for discriminating among methods and products, began to arouse public attention, including that of doctors. Birth control was a $250 million-a-year business, "slightly bigger than the barbershop business and very slightly smaller than the jewelry business," but a business without any rational public regulation. In 1937, Americans spent an estimated $200 million for douche powders and other "feminine hygiene" products, $38 million on condoms, and less than $1 million on diaphragms. Concern over this situation led to the creation of an AMA Committee on Contraception in 1935.[42]

Dickinson's initial optimism turned to chagrin when this committee, which included George Kosmak, issued its first report in 1936. The report denied that any safe or effective birth control methods existed; found no evidence that the federal or state Comstock laws had "interfered with any medical advice which a physician has felt called upon to furnish his patients"; and criticized the lay birth control leagues and "the support of such agencies by members of the medical profession." The AMA House of Delegates instructed the committee to continue its investigation.[43]

At this point, federal appeals court judge Augustus Hand and Robert Dickinson, acting independently, took decisive actions that led to a 1937 AMA report on contraception which seems hardly compatible with the 1936 document. Judge Hand confronted the task of making sense of the Comstock Act's prohibition of contraceptives in the changed social environment of the 1930s. A shipment of experimental diaphragms intended for Dr. Hannah Stone had been seized by United States Customs. Stone sued. Hand ruled that while the language of the Comstock Act was uncompromising with regard to contraceptive devices and information, if Congress had had available in 1873 the clinical data on the dangers of pregnancy and the safety of contraceptive practice that were available in 1936, birth control would not have been classified as obscenity. As Morris Ernst, Stone's lawyer, observed, "the law process is a simple one, it is a matter of educating judges to the mores of the day." Judge Hand's decision opened the mails to contraceptive materials intended for physicians and definitely established their right to give information, at least as far as federal law was concerned.[44]

Dickinson seized the opportunity provided by the Hand decision. Several key members of the AMA Committee on Contraception attended the American Gynecological Society meeting at Atlantic City in May 1936, where Dickinson spent three days with committee chairman Carl Davis, member E. D. Plass, and Kosmak, refuting the committee's report point by point. The committee requested that he provide it with a detailed brief. Before the next meeting of the Committee on Contraception in February 1937, Dickinson's Committee on Maternal Health supplied "a voluminous amount of data . . . bearing on clinical prescription and success of contraception in this country."[45]

The committee on Maternal Health also received a request for information on the "safe period" from another member of the AMA committee, John Rock, a Harvard gynecologist. Rock was a devout Catholic, and his views on contraception were far from those he later expressed in *The Time Has Come* (1963), where he argued that the pill was the "natural" contraceptive that Catholics had been waiting for, and that the population explosion provided another compelling reason for a liberalization of Catholic doctrine on birth control. Dickinson invited Rock to a dinner sponsored by the Committee on Maternal Health and a round table discussion on the topic "Should the Newly Married Practice Contraception?" in December 1936.[46]

Rock happily accepted the invitation because he "objected to the emphasis on *contra-*ception" and wanted "a more positive approach to fertility." There was, Rock stated at the meeting, only one valid reason for birth control: definite medical contraindications to pregnancy. But such situations should not arise, for "those with medical contraindications should not get married." The purpose of sex was procreation. Marriage existed to provide support for woman so that she could fulfill her nature. "Nature intended motherhood to be woman's career, and her proper career, she should start right away. . . . Anything which diverts her from her prime purpose is socially wrong." Economic arguments about the burden of children were "9/10s subterfuge and distortion of value. . . . Cases come to mind of wives supporting husbands' scholastic activities; far better to let the man take off [leave school] so that she can have her baby, and then go back to his educational work." Finally, sex could not "be made an end in itself without dire consequences," yet that was the result of most decisions to postpone pregnancy in early marriage.[47]

Some sarcasm had crept into earlier discussions by the Committee on Maternal Health of Catholic doctrine on birth control. When told of support for the rhythm method at the 1934 AMA convention, Dickinson wanted to know, "Did they give out jelly with the calendars?"[48] But when Dr. Rock came to call, all was sweetness and light. His views were politely received and criticism was gentle. The eugenicist Frederick Osborn pointed out that birth control was "an accomplished fact which will not disappear, but which will spread." Regina Stix, of the Milbank Memorial Fund, argued that her studies with Raymond Pearl showed that contraception had "very little to do with the . . . advice of physicians," and that medical influence in this area waited on a better-informed profession. Another participant in the meeting observed that Rock's "view was, of course, not a biological but a philosophical one." Rock, he said, "failed to mention that his view makes of the physician a deus ex machina controlling the masses through enforced ignorance. Decisions should not be based upon ignorance, but upon knowledge." Dr. Sophia Kleegman made it clear that there was "no evidence that the early use of contraception leads to a diminution in desire for children," or the functional inability to have them when medically supervised. Finally,

> Dr. Dickinson pointed out that the National Committee on Maternal Health thirteen years ago stressed the positive side of birth control. When the first child comes too soon, the second may come never. Early marriage and shorter period of engagement are necessary; yet they are impractical unless contraception may be employed. Anyone who thinks young people do not want children is wrong.[49]

The Committee on Contraception's second report of February 1937 is all the more remarkable in that Rock and Kosmak remained on the committee. An AMA-sponsored study of techniques and standards was recommended, along with the promotion of instruction in medical schools. Significantly, criticism of lay-backed organizations in the field, and of their medical allies, was omitted. Finally, the committee declared that contraceptive advice should be given by the physician "largely on the judgment and wishes of individual patients."[50]

Although proponents of birth control were able to organize some major experiments in the mass delivery of contraceptives between 1937 and 1960, the prospect of spreading contraceptive practice beyond the middle class seemed to be profoundly limited by a lack of technology for birth control methods that required less motivation from the user than the diaphragm or condom. Clarence James Gamble, a Harvard M.D. (1920) and researcher in experimental pharmacology at the University of Pennsylvania from 1923 to 1937, devoted a large part of his considerable ingenuity and wealth (from the soap fortune) to a search for a better contraceptive. Under the auspices of the Committee on Maternal Health, Gamble conducted a number of pioneer experiments in the mass delivery of simple contraceptives such as lactic-acid jelly, but few medical men shared his interest in improving birth control techniques and technology.[51] Most first-class investigators, such as Earl Engle and Howard Taylor, Jr., both members of the Committee on Maternal Health, and colleagues on the Columbia medical school faculty, believed that real progress would have to wait for fundamental advances in knowledge of human sexual physiology. They opposed further experimentation with simple methods by the committee. As Engle bluntly explained in 1946, "We don't give a damn about contraception. We want a study of basic factors in human reproduction."[52] Basic researches were being conducted which would eventually make technological innovation possible, but it is significant that when Dr. George Corner of the University of Rochester, who in 1930 had been, along with his colleague Willard Allen, the first to demonstrate the specific effects of progesterone, reviewed the prospects for clinical use of the hormone in 1947, he did not mention suppression of ovulation as one of its potential uses.[53]

In the middle 1950s, the average physician had little more interest in contraception than in the 1930s. Only one doctor in five, among a sample interviewed by Columbia's Bureau of Applied Social Research in 1957, thought that most married couples got contraceptive advice from medical sources. A majority of Americans still learned about birth control from their relatives or friends.[54] The major movers in the campaign to spread contraceptive practice and to improve contraceptive technology during the 1950s were lay birth control advocates and social scientists.[55] Physicians reported that more married women complained of infertility than asked for contraceptive advice, and until the public demanded better contraceptive services, doctors were unlikely to take much more interest in providing them. A medical editor spoke for a good part of the general public as well as his profession when he declared, "Caustic self-analysis leads to only one honest conclusion: candid physicians are ashamed of these messy makeshifts . . . there is a sense of relative inadequacy . . . nourished by the contemplation of these disreputable paraphernalia." "The messy little gadgets, the pastes, and creams and jellies" were simply "an embarrassment to the scientific mind."[56]

The renewed "sex appeal" of condoms, diaphragms, jellies, and foams during the 1970s illustrated the point that social values played a significant part in the "embarrassment of the scientific mind" in the jelly/diaphragm/condom days of contraception. Christopher Tietze and Sarah Lewit, long-time research associates of the Population Council, recall that it was impossible to continue a large-scale study of the relative effectiveness of barrier methods of contraception once the public learned that an oral contraceptive was available. Hundreds of patients suddenly developed "the hurting diaphragm syndrome" and could only be restored to health with a pill.[57] The eagerness with which physicians embraced this new wonder of modern science reflected their common assumption with the lay public that many of life's most personal problems could be solved with a technological fix. Their patients could now have "spontaneous sex," and doctors had a birth control method which lent the prestige of science to them and did not require them or their patients to touch genitalia, or to fumble with "messy little gadgets."

John Rock played an important role in the pill's development. The biologist Gregory Pincus chose Rock to test on women the synthetic hormone regimen that Pincus believed would work because of the animal studies conducted by his staff at the Worcester Foundation for Experimental Biology. Rock's odyssey, as he developed from a critic of birth control in the 1930s to an outspoken champion of population control in the 1960s, illustrates some of the forces that were reshaping medical attitudes toward contraception.[58]

Margaret Sanger originally opposed bringing Rock into the pill project, arguing that "he would not dare advance the cause of contraceptive research and remain a Catholic." Pincus insisted that Rock was the right man. He explained his view of Rock to his financial angel Katharine McCormick, and McCormick reported to Sanger that Rock was a "reformed Catholic whose position is that religion has nothing to do with medicine or the practice of it and that if the Church does not interfere with him he will not interfere with it—whatever that may mean!" Sanger eventually changed her mind about Rock and marveled at his ability to win support for her cause. "Being a good R.C. and as handsome as a god, he can just get away with anything."[59]

Some Catholic officials were outraged by Rock's habit of proclaiming his faith while he was violating Catholic dogma in his medical practice. In telling the world that the Pope would surely accept a "natural" contraceptive of synthetic hormones as soon as he was able to review the facts, Rock provided a rationale for Catholic contraceptors. By the time Catholic authorities decided that the pill was no more natural than other contraceptives, many Catholic laymen had found the pill acceptable to them, regardless of the hierarchy's attitude. Rock sincerely believed himself a good Catholic, however, and his changing attitudes toward contraception were those of a conservative seeking to preserve stable family life.[60]

He first spoke out on the issue of contraception in a 1931 article criticizing the poor obstetrical training of Massachusetts physicians. The Harvard associate professor of obstetrics cited laws prohibiting contraceptive advice as a minor factor in the state's high maternal mortality rate, but he was quick to distinguish "medical contraception," prescribed only when a woman's life would be endangered by pregnancy, from "birth control." Indeed, all efforts to separate sex from procreation were fraught with social risk, he thought, since only child-rearing provided the discipline and purpose essential to happy marriage.[61] As late as 1943, in an article advocating repeal of Massachusetts laws that restricted "medical birth control advice," Rock noted:

> I hold no brief for those young or even older husbands and wives who for no good reason refuse to bear as many children as they can properly rear and as society can properly engross. Ignorant of the fact that sustained happiness comes only from dutiful sacrifice, such deluded mates are perhaps doing society a backhanded favor. Whatever genetic trait may contribute to the intellectual deficiency which permits them selfishly to seek more immediate comfort, is at least kept from the inheritable common pool, and in time their kind is thus bred out.[62]

Thirty years later Rock told a reporter, "I think it's shocking to see the big family glorified."[63] Despite the apparent contradiction in his views at different periods, Rock's attitudes toward the family and its place in society were consistent. He considered himself a humanist, in contrast to the contemplative "egoist" who saw man as part of a transcendental unit, or the hedonist-naturalist who believed that life had no spiritual purpose. In Rock's view, life's meaning derived from social interaction, and especially from service to others. Man was an animal, evolved from lower forms of life. Cultural values, derived from centuries of trial and error, made man human.

Sexuality was an immutable part of man's biological heritage. "Unprejudiced observation of so-called civilized man discloses that his fundamental coital pattern . . . is that of other primates, however his coital behavior may appear to be modified by social and spiritual factors." The family provided an essential social focus for sexual expression. For centuries society had needed all the young that women could bear. Thus, the immutable coital urge, when expressed in marriage, had been compatible with, if not essential to, social well-being.[64]

Rock, the father of five, shared the pronatalist values that were one of the givens of American culture during the first half of the twentieth century. By 1943, his experience as a gynecologist made it clear, however, that human fertility would have to be curbed in some situations if the family was to remain a strong institution in an industrial society. Rock did not believe that sexual repression was an acceptable solution for the great majority of Americans. Like the physicians who participated in the Physicians Club of Chicago symposium on "sexual hygiene" in 1898, he had learned that social order depended on satisfying sexual expression within marriage, but good sex without contraception would lead to more children than most American breadwinners could support. Gradually, Rock was coming to the view that physicians should provide the contraceptive advice necessary to protect the family from the economic burden of too many children.[65]

Rock associated his respect for the family with a Catholic heritage, but his views were widely shared by Protestants and Jews. Having gradually accepted contraception as an aid to marital sexual adjustment, while disapproving of those who were able to raise large families but refused to do so, Rock was ready to alter his position when his perception of social needs changed. As demographers like Princeton's Frank Notestein began after World War II to publicize their conviction that rapid population growth was a threat to social order in the Third World and ultimately in the West, social and professional leaders began to advocate population control and to treat the small family with more sympathy. Changes in Rock's views mirrored the redefinition of "the population problem" that was taking place among social scientists and the educated public. Rock was an invaluable ally for family planners because his background and competence gave him an aura of objectivity that they lacked. But his presence in their ranks in the 1960s was symbolic of a broad change in social attitudes, the decline of pronatalism as a more critical attitude toward population growth developed. Rock was no less a humanist in 1973 than he had been in 1931. His view of what mankind needed had simply changed.[66]

Medical attitudes toward contraception, in 1830 or in 1970, were primarily conditioned by the social values which physicians shared with other citizens, rather than by the state of contraceptive technology or by internal scientific standards for judging the usefulness of therapeutic procedures. One could hardly have expected the physicians to behave differently. They were chosen by a process that reflected ability to internalize the values of a professional culture which depended on public confidence and support. Their function was to comfort and to explain, and sometimes to cure—not to question the basic structure or justice of the social system. Contraceptives were not therapeutic means in a narrow sense, since they were usually sought by healthy women for social, as opposed to medical, reasons. From the era of James Marion Sims to the era of John Rock, physicians were increasingly confident, with good reason, of their ability to manage difficult pregnancies and to repair birth injuries. Healthy babies delivered of willing mothers represented a congenial challenge to their improving art. In contrast, birth control was, as Howard Taylor, Jr., complained more than once, a banal topic for the first-class clinician.[67] The medical profession would only take an interest in contraceptive practice when the fertility of healthy women began to seem a clear and present danger to the moral and economic order that it served.

NOTES

Most of the research upon which this paper is based was conducted in the Countway Library of Medicine, Boston, Mass. I am indebted to Richard Wolfe, the rare books librarian at Countway, for bringing a number of collections to my attention and for numerous professional favors that made working in the Countway a pleasure as well as a privilege.

1. There were some important changes in medical attitudes toward birth control between 1830 and 1960. One milestone was a 1937 AMA resolution which recognized contraception as a legitimate service to be provided to patients on request. This victory for birth control was the direct result of an intense lobbying effort by Dr. Robert L. Dickinson and a few allies. Their efforts are described in this paper. The 1937 resolution did not mark the end of medical reluctance to provide contraceptive services, however. Rather, it reversed a ludicrous 1936 report by the AMA Committee on Contraception which denied that safe and effective contraceptive means existed, and which denounced lay birth control supporters and their medical allies, who had been lobbying for recognition of contraception as a routine part of practice. For the 1937 resolution and the 1936 report, see *Journal of the American Medical Association* 106 (1936): 1910–11 and 108 (1937): 2217–18. For a fuller discussion of American attitudes toward birth control, see James Reed, *From Private Vice to Public Virtue: The Birth Control Movement and American Society since 1830* (New York: Basic Books, 1978).

2. Early nineteenth-century birth rates must be constructed from inadequate sources, but the best projections available indicate that native-born white women averaged 7.04 children in 1800; 5.21 in 1860; 3.56 in 1900; 2.10 in 1936. The low fertility of the 1930s should not be viewed primarily as a result of the Great Depression, since fertility had been declining for 150 years. The rate of this long-term trend varied with geographical location and social class. The native-born white women of New England, for example, had ceased to reproduce themselves by the late nineteenth century. By the middle 1930s, however, the fertility of the whole population hovered around a level barely adequate to maintain the existing popula-

tion, despite the dramatic declines in mortality during the preceding forty years. See Ansley Coale and Melvin Zelnik, *New Estimates of Fertility and Population in the United States* (Princeton: Princeton University Press, 1963), pp. 33–37; Alan Sweezy, "The Economic Explaination of Fertility Changes in the United States," *Population Studies* 25 (July 1971): 255–67; Maris Vinovskis, "Demographic Changes in America from the Revolution to the Civil War: An Analysis of the Socio-Economic Determinants of Fertility Differentials and Trends in Massachusetts" (Ph.D. diss., Harvard, 1975).

3. Reed, "Birth Control in American Social Science, 1870–1940," chap. 14 in *Birth Control Movement*, pp. 197–210.

4. For a contrasting interpretation, see David M. Kennedy, *Birth Control in America: The Career of Margaret Sanger* (New Haven: Yale University Press, 1971), pp. 176–79.

5. Reed, *Birth Control Movement*, pp. 3–18. I concluded that these contraceptive practices worked for highly motivated users. The problem in assessing their impact on fertility is to determine their "psychological availability."

6. The substitution of latex, for rubber, in condoms during the 1930s was a significant advance in contraceptive technology, but, like the improvement of the spring-loaded diaphragm in the 1920s, the latex condom was simply a refinement of a contraceptive that had been available for some time. The development of plastic intrauterine devices followed the marketing of the birth control bill.

7. See "The Search for Professional Order in 19th Century American Medicine," a working paper made available to me by Barbara Rosenkrantz of Harvard University; Charles E. Rosenberg, "The Practice of Medicine in New York a Century Ago," *Bulletin of the History of Medicine* 41 (1967): 223–53.

8. The use of disease sanctions to reinforce female sex roles is discussed by Carroll Smith-Rosenberg and Charles Rosenberg in "The Female Animal: Medical and Biological Views of Woman and Her Role in Nineteenth-Century America," *Journal of American History* 60 (September 1973): 332–56. For a discussion of the attitudes of French doctors toward contraception which emphasizes the prescriptive nature of medical advice, see Angus McLaren, "Doctor in the House: Medicine and Private Morality in France, 1800–1850," *Feminist Studies* 2 (1975): 39–54, and "Some Secular Attitudes toward Sexual Behavior in France, 1760–1860," *French Historical Studies* 8 (Fall 1974): 604–25.

9. The standard biography is Audrey Davis, *Dr. Kelly of Hopkins: Surgeon, Scientist, Christian* (Baltimore: Johns Hopkins University Press, 1959). Donald Fleming provides a vivid portrait of Kelly in *William H. Welch and the Rise of Modern Medicine* (Boston: Little, Brown, 1954), pp. 90–91. For an interesting exchange of views between Kelly and Robert Dickinson on the problem of genital changes related to masturbation, see Reed, *Birth Control Movement*, p. 160.

10. Seale Harris describes the development of the operation in *Woman's Surgeon: The Life of J. Marion Sims* (New York: Macmillan, 1950), chaps. 10–11. For the spring-loaded pessary, see James Marion Sims, *Clinical Notes* (New York: W. Wood and Co., 1871), p. 269, and fig. 11. On Foote, see Vincent J. Cirillo, "Edward Foote's *Medical Common Sense:* An Early American Comment on Birth Control," *Journal of the History of Medicine* 25 (July 1970): 341–45, and Cirillo, "Edward Bliss Foote: American Advocate of Birth Control," *Bulletin of the History of Medicine* 47 (September–October 1973): 471–79.

11. On Comstock's arrest of physicians, see Heywood Broun and Margaret Leech, *Anthony Comstock: Roundsman of the Lord* (New York: A and C. Boni, 1927), pp. 160, 167, and Comstock's reply to criticism of his activity in *Frauds Exposed* (New York: J.H. Brown, 1880), p. 542. Broad interpretations of the war on commercial vice are provided by David Pivar, *Purity Crusade: Sexual Morality*

and Social Control, 1868–1900 (Westport, Conn.: Greenwood, 1973), and R. Christian Johnson, "Anthony Comstock: Reform, Vice, and the American Way" (Ph.D. diss., University of Wisconsin, 1973).

12. Pivar, *Purity Crusade,* pp. 88–99. See also the dissertation version of Pivar's work, "The New Abolitionists: The Quest for Social Purity, 1876–1900" (University of Pennsylvania, 1965), pp. 108, 267, 264, where the following source is quoted: Charles H. Kitchell, *The Social Evil* (New York: privately printed, 1886).

13. The 1937 resolution on birth control did follow the "One Package" federal court decision of 1936 which exempted physicians from the Comstock Act's ban on contraceptive information. In the 1950s, state and local Comstock laws were still having an effect on the prescription of diaphragms by physicians. On the decision, see C. Thomas Dienes, *Law, Politics, and Birth Control* (Urbana: University of Illinois Press, 1972), pp. 112–13. Medical prescription of contraceptives in the 1950s is analyzed in Mary Jean Cornish *et al., Doctors and Family Planning* (New York: National Committee on Maternal Health, 1963); see especially pp. 56–58.

14. The Editorial Staff of the Alkalodia Clinic, eds., *Sexual Hygiene* (Chicago: privately printed, 1902), "Preface," and pp. 10–15. There are two copies of *Sexual Hygiene* in the Countway Library of Medicine.

15. Ibid., p. 95.

16. Ibid., p. 184.

17. Ibid., pp. 188, 190.

18. Ibid., pp. 186–87, 189–90.

19. The attitudes of many influential physicians toward higher education for women closely paralled their stance on birth control. See, for example, Alexander J. C. Skene, *Education and Culture as Related to the Health and Diseases of Women* (Detroit: G.S. Davis, 1889), in which Skene denounces both higher education and attempts to avoid pregnancy as violations of the natural order. See my analysis of literature of this genre in "The Suppression of Contraceptive Information," chap. 3, *Birth Control Movement.*

20. I provide a biography of Dickinson in *Birth Control Movement,* pt. 3. The Dickinson Papers (hereafter cited as RLD-CL), are in the Countway Library of Medicine, Boston, Mass.

21. J. Whitridge Williams, "Has the American Gynecological Society Done Its Part in the Advancement of Obstetrical Knowledge?" *Transactions of the American Gynecological Society* 39 (1914): 3–20.

22. Robert L. Dickinson and Lura Beam, *The Single Woman: A Study in Sex Education* (New York: Williams and Wilkins, 1934), p. 4; Dickinson, "Hypertrophies of the Labia Minora and Their Significance," *American Gynecology* 1 (1902): 225–54; "'Urethral Labia' or 'Urethral Hymen': Pathological Structures Due to Repeated Traction," *American Medicine* 7 (1904): 347–49; "Marital Maladjustment: The Business of Preventive Gynecology," *Long Island Medical Journal* 2 (1908): 1–5; interview with Dorothy Dickinson Barbour, Cincinnati, Ohio, 2 June 1971.

23. See n. 21 above.

24. Robert L. Dickinson, "Suggestions for a Program for American Gynecology," *Transactions of the American Gynecological Society* 45 (1920): 1–13.

25. *Surgery, Gynecology, and Obstetrics* 23 (1916): 185–90; Dickinson to Sanger, 7 November 1945, Margaret Sanger Papers, Sophia Smith Collection Smith College, Northampton, Mass., (hereafter cited as MS-SS); Sanger to Dickinson, 9 November 1945, RLD-CL. These letters were exchanged when Dickinson was preparing an article on the early history of the birth control movement and wanted to check some of his dates with Sanger. For Dickinson's unsuccessful attempt to gain backing from the New York Obstetrical Society, and the early

activities of the Committee on Maternal Health, see Reed, *Birth Control Movment*, chap. 21, "Clinical Studies."

26. "Origins of National Committee on Maternal Health," undated, unsigned memo, RLD-CL.

27. Minutes of the Committee on Maternal Health, 28 November 1925; 28 May, 1924; 13 June 1924; 1 February 1928; 12 March 1926, in RLD-CL (hereafter cited as CMH).

28. 9 March 1923; 10 May 1923; 10 January 1924, CMH.

29. 7 December 1923; 11 December 1924; 10 December 1925, CMH. On the history and influence of Sanger's Birth Control Clinical Research Bureau, see Reed *Birth Control Movement*, chap. 9, "Providing Clinics."

30. 21 January and 10 December 1928, CMH; "Report of the Conference of the Maternal Health Committee and the Clinic Committee of the American Birth Control League, November 29, 1925"; "Minutes of the Public Hearing: January 15, 1926," Margaret Sanger Papers, Library of Congress (hereafter cited as MS-LC); Dickinson, "England and Birth Control," RLD-CL.

31. Sanger to Edward M. East, 28 May 1925, MS-LC; 17 January 1927 CMH; Clarence Little to Dickinson, 26 October 1925, MS-LC; Committee on Maternal Health, *Biennial Report: 1928*, pp. 5–6, RLD-CL; Hannah Stone, "Therapeutic Contraception," *Medical Journal and Record* 127 (1928): 9–17.

32. In 1956 the Clinical Research Bureau was still operating without a license, on advice of the Planned Parenthood Federation of America's counsel, Morris Ernst, in candid recognition of the fact that a dispensary license was unattainable. See Mary Calderone to Ethel Wortis, 25 October 1956, Mary Calderone Papers, The Schlesinger Library, Radcliffe College, Cambridge, Mass., and the transcript of my interview with Dr. Calderone, Schlesinger-Rockefeller Oral History Project, Schlesinger Library, pp. 9–10.

33. Morris Fishbein, *Medical Follies* (New York: Boni and Liveright, 1925), p. 125; Kennedy, *Birth Control in America*, pp. 176–79; Reed, *Birth Control Movement*, pp. 144–46.

34. Fishbein, *Medical Follies*, pp. 56–58, 218–20, 142–49.

35. (New York: Day-Nichols, 1928), pp. 23–24.

36. For discussion of a revealing attempt by Fishbein to impose his views on woman's proper social role on a woman author, see my interview with Emily H. Mudd, Ph.D., Schlesinger-Rockefeller Oral History Project, pp. 124–27.

37. "Notes on the Round Table Meeting of December 4, 1936," RLD-CL.

38. George Kosmak, "The Broader Aspects of the Birth Control Propaganda," (discussion of paper) *American Journal of Obstetrics and Gynecology* 6 (1923): 351–53; George Kosmak, compiler, "Newspaper Clippings on Birth Control, Child Birth Deaths, etc.: 1917–1941" (hereafter cited as Kosmak Clippings), vol. 2, New York Academy of Medicine; Kosmak, "What Shall Be the Attitude Toward the Percent Propaganda," *Medical Record* 91 (1917): 268–273; Kosmak Clippings, 18 May 1939; Reed, *Birth Control Movement*, pp. 168–71.

39. Kosmak, "The Broader Aspects."

40. Reed, *Birth Control Movement*, pp. 181–90.

41. Ibid., chaps. 15–17, pp. 211–38.

42. "The Accident of Birth," *Fortune* (17 February 1938): 83–86, 108–14; "The Lay Press Looks at Birth Control," *Journal of Contraception* 3 (March 1938): pp. 60–61; Reed, *Birth Control Movement*, chap. 18, "Policing the Market Place," pp. 239–46.

43. Reed, *Birth Control Movement*, pp. 186–87; *Journal of the American Medical Association* 106 (1936): 1910–11.

44. Dienes, *Law, Politics, and Birth Control*, pp. 112–113.

45. "Notes on Informal Meeting at Atlantic City . . .," CMH; 24 February 1937, CMH.

46. 24 February 1937, CMH; "Notes on the Round Table Meeting of December 4, 1936," RLD-CL.

47. "Notes on the Round Table Meeting of December 4, 1936," RLD-CL.

48. "Report of the Round Table Meeting, October 5, 1934," ibid.

49. "Notes on the Round Table Meeting of December 4, 1936," ibid.

50. *Journal of the American Medical Association* 108 (1937): 2217–18.

51. Reed, *Birth Control Movement,* part 5, "Birth Control Entrepreneur: The Philanthropic Pathfinding of Clarence J. Gamble."

52. 14 June 1946, CMH; Reed, *Birth Control Movement,* p. 243.

53. George Corner, *The Hormones in Human Reproduction* (Princeton: Princeton University Press, 1947; [first edition, 1942]), p. 87; Reed, *Birth Control Movement,* pp. 313–16.

54. Cornish *et al., Doctors and Family Planning,* passim.

55. Reed, *Birth Control Movement,* chaps. 21, 23, "The Population Explosion" and "The Failure of Simple Methods: The IUD Justified."

56. Editorial, *Western Journal of Surgery, Obstetrics, and Gynecology* 51 (September 1943): 381–83.

57. Interview with Sarah Lewitt Tietze and Christopher Tietze, Schlesinger-Rockefeller Oral History Project, p. 10.

58. Reed, *Birth Control Movement* pp. 351–54.

59. Sanger to Marion Ingersoll, 18 February 1954; McCormick to Sanger, 19 July 1954; Sanger to Mrs. John D. Rockefeller, Jr., 19 February 1960, MS-SS.

60. Rock stated his views on oral contraception in *The Time Has Come: A Catholic Doctor's Proposals to End The Battle Over Birth Control* (New York: 1963). For criticism of Rock by a Catholic spokesman, see remarks by Msgr. George Kelly, *New York Times,* 6 May 1963, p. 20. For criticism by a more liberal Catholic, see J. S. Duhamel's review of *The Time Has Come* in *America* 108 (27 April 1963): 608. For criticism of Rock's rationalization of "the pill" by a fellow physician and birth control advocate, see Robert Hall's review in the *New York Times Review of Books* (12 May 1963), p. 30.

61. John Rock, "Maternal Mortality: What Must Be Done About It," *New England Journal of Medicine* 205 (1931): 902.

62. "Medical and Biological Aspects of Contraception," *Clinics* 1 (April 1943): 1601–2.

63. "Dr. John Rock at 83: An Interview," *Boston Globe Sunday Magazine* (19 July 1973), pp. 6–8.

64. "Medical and Biological Aspects," 1608–9.

65. Ibid., 1599–1601.

66. Ibid.

67. Interview with Howard Taylor, Jr., New York City, 27 April 1971; 24 September 1936; 2 April 1937; 27 April 1937; 6 October 1938, CMH.

6 REDISCOVERING ASYLUMS: *The Unhistorical History of the Mental Hospital*

GERALD N. GROB

During the last two decades there has been unending controversy in the United States over how to deal with the mentally ill. There are those who argue that confinement in hospitals is the worst possible policy; others urge greater public expenditures to upgrade institutional care and treatment; still others deny that there is any such thing as mental disease; and finally, there are those who insist that only a totally new approach involving the entire community can resolve painful dilemmas. Most individuals attempt to "prove" the validity of their own position by drawing on the experiences of the past.

As a historian I am pleased that those involved in policy decisions do turn to the past. What troubles me, however, is the quality of the historical data used in legitimating or opposing particular policies. Let me be more specific. Anyone concerned with the development of mental hospitals (or, for that matter, of schools, prisons, almshouses, houses of refuge, to cite only a few examples) immediately confronts a scholarly controversy. On one side stand those who celebrate these institutions as evidence of human progress, humanitarianism, and liberal sentiment. Although these scholars concede that there are serious flaws and imperfections in these institutions, they operate on the assumption that with additional effort and funding, most societal defects could have been eliminated. On the other, there are those scholars who denigrate these same institutions, viewing them as the agencies by which dominant elites restrained deviant groups, or largely lower class elements, thereby ensuring their own hegemony. Although I have deliberately set forth these two general approaches in dichotomous terms, I do not believe such a conceptualization about the ways in which scholars have dealt with the problem is far from the truth, even though many individual studies do not fit within such a framework.[1]

Interestingly enough, both interpretations reflect in large part the professional orientation of their formulators. The first (or traditional) position represents a fusion of the beliefs of two groups: institutional psychiatrists and liberal historians, who tend to take an optimistic view, and interpret American history in terms of continuous progress toward a more ideal social order. Ira Van Giesen, the influential first director of New York State's pioneering Pathological Institute, for example, once divided the history of psychiatry into four distinct periods. The first was dominated by a spirit of revenge; any transgression by insane persons was met with immediate retaliation. The second stage was marked by indifference; insane persons were sequestered by themselves in institutions. The third period, on the other hand, marked a fundamental reversal of attitudes and perceptions; it was characterized by altruisitc intervention by society "in behalf of the welfare of the insane through legislation and the founding of hospitals for beneficent care and medical treatment." During this era medical treatment tended to be empirical, in that it emphasized the material welfare and comfort of the mentally ill. In Van Giesen's view, the establishment of mental hospitals reflected an important turning point, for they institutionalized these new attitudes and practices. Indeed, he optimistically predicted, in 1897, that the history of psychiatry and of the insane was entering its fourth, and presumably final phase. In this last stage, modern scientific inquiry would finally reveal the etiology and distinctive pathology of mental disease and thus make possible its eventual eradication and prevention.[2]

Van Giesen's optimistic views (which were quite typical) were reflected in subsequent studies by liberal historians. Albert Deutsch, in his classic and still valuable work, accepted at face value the optimistic claims of psychiatrists and their definitions of mental diseases. Conceding that institutional care of the mentally ill was far from successful and left much to be desired, he placed responsibility for past failures squarely upon American society, which had not provided sufficient material resources.[3] Even in his devastating exposé of public mental hospitals published shortly after the close of the Second World War, Deutsch did not despair, or conclude that institutional care and treatment was predestined to fail. On the contrary, he upheld the *theory* of institutional practice and urged his fellow citizens to band together "to participate in the common drive toward improved mental hygiene facilities" and to insist that government at all levels provide appropriate funding.[4]

The second (or revisionist) interpretation emerged in its most mature form in the 1960s. One of the major sources of revisionism was a view that had its intellectual origins in the social and behavioral sciences. In those disciplines a number of scholars explicitly rejected as unproven the allegation that mental diseases were comparable to diseases like pneumonia or smallpox. They developed instead a "societal reaction model" of mental illness that shifted the focus from the individual to the social group. The concept of mental illness, they insisted, was a creation of social groups applying their own standards to judge what was normal and abnormal behavior. Hence mental illness, instead of resulting from physiological processes or learned pathological behavior, was, in fact, largely defined by applying certain specific behavioral norms. Behavior which violated the norms was defined as "mental illness." Within this framework, mental diseases lost their presumably objective character and became simply labels given to certain forms of behavior by dominant, elite social groups. Similarly, the mental hospital was the characteristic institution in which society placed individuals whose peculiar behavior threatened public order and stability.[5]

Despite differences between disciplines, it did not take long before certain historians—especially those interested in the application of new methodologies and the use of conceptual models developed in the social and behavioral sciences—incorporated revisionist concepts into their analyses of American history. These "new" social historians were concerned with illuminating the experiences of the mass of inarticulate and lower class groups as well as those institutions that touched their lives. Critical of the traditional preoccupation of earlier historians with social and political elites, they insisted that an analysis of crime, dependency, illness, and the response to these problems would reveal the prevailing values of American culture and illuminate internal social relationships. Consequently, they undertook detailed investigations of the experiences of a variety of groups, including—but not limited to—ethnic and racial minorities.[6]

Part of the scholarship of what is now designated as the "new social history" was also influenced by the disillusionment which followed the social and political activism of the 1960s. Indeed, a number of younger scholars implicitly justified their work by arguing that the study of history could not be separated from politics and ideology. Critical of American society, they interpreted the proliferation of many institutions as further evidence of fundamental flaws within the social order which could be eradicated only through either a process of deinstitutionalization or radical economic change. Whether they dealt with schools, prisons, or mental hospitals, the message was the same; such institutions served mainly to perpetuate the hegemony of dominant social elites, rather than the interests of their clientele.[7]

Curiously enough, there were some striking similarities between the traditional and the revisionist approaches. Both began at precisely the same starting point, namely, the assertion that many institutions failed to achieve their purposes. However, whereas the former saw this failure as only transitory, the latter saw it as an inevitable consequence of institutional solutions. Influenced by the critics of orthodox psychiatry, and the sociological concept of the total institution,[8] the revisionists came up with quite a different interpretation. Mental illness, some of them argued, was not an appropriate category; it was a concept designed to penalize disruptive and aberrant behavior rather than to describe physiological malfunctions. Similarly, mental hospitals grew out of the fear of social disorder; consequently, they eventually served custodial and penal functions, rather than therapeutic roles. Although there are significant differences in the outlooks and historical methods of such commentators as Michel Foucault, Thomas S. Szasz, and David J. Rothman, it is a point of view which they have in common—a critical stance toward psychiatry and mental institutions—which largely accounts for their popularity and widespread influence.[9]

Although historians may fight among themselves over opposing interpretations, why should other scholars be concerned with the recreation of a perhaps irrelevant past? Was not Voltaire right when he remarked that history was simply a trick that the living played on the dead? Whether we like it or not, however, such historical debates do influence the present, as well as the future. Innumerable public debates and decisions rest upon a particular reading of the past. In his study of American foreign policy after 1945, for example, Ernest R. May convincingly demonstrated how decision-makers employed their understanding, or misunderstanding, of earlier events both to formulate and to justify postwar diplomatic policies.[10] Our interpretation of the past, therefore, may very well influence our understanding of the present (just as the present can influence our view of the past.

The literature dealing with mental illness and institutions illustrates in a graphic manner the intimate relationship between historical interpretations, on the one hand, and contemporary policy positions, on the other hand. Deutsch's demand for increased funding for mental health was dependent upon his belief that Americans had never given a sufficiently high priority to this problem. Rothman's provocative analysis of the origins of the asylum was linked with his conviction that contemporary solutions had to take a very different direction. "The [Jacksonian] reformers' original doctrines," Rothman observed in the conclusion of his influential book,

> were especially liable to abuse, their emphasis on authority, obedience, and regularity turning all too predictably into a mechanical application of discipline. And by incarcerating the deviant and the dependent, and defending the step with hyperbolic rhetoric, they discouraged—really eliminated—the search for other solutions that might have been less susceptible to abuse. . . .
>
> Still, there are alternative perspectives that can dispel some of this gloom. The history of the discovery of the asylum is not without a relevance that may be more liberating than stifling for us. We still live with many of these institutions, accepting their presence as inevitable. Despite a personal revulsion, we think of them as always having been with us, and therefore as always to be with us. We tend to forget that they were the invention of one generation to serve very special needs. . . . In this sense the story of the origins of the asylum is liberating. We need not remain trapped in inherited answers.

Even Thomas S. Szasz, perhaps the most articulate and influential critic of orthodox psychiatry and mental hospitals, usually employed historical data to strengthen his argument. In *The Manufacture of Madness*, he attempted to demonstrate, through an examination of the past, that the "ethical convictions and social arrangements" based upon the concept of mental illness constituted "an immoral ideology of intolerance."[11]

Insofar as historical scholarship is concerned, of course, the issue is not whether we should move toward or away from institutional solutions. Policy issues are too complex for any single discipline to attempt to provide definitive answers, no matter how competent and informed its practitioners may be. Moreover, democratic theory militates against the transfer of authority to alleged experts; few issues can or should be isolated from the political arena. What the historian can offer, however, is an informed analysis of the past, based upon wide research in the primary sources, avoiding polemical tone and inaccuracies. Historians, after all, are especially well equipped to bring to the forefront some of the basic facts all too often disregarded in the heat of battle.

To understand the history and evolution of institutional care and treatment of the mentally ill in America is by no means an easy task. Mental hospitals were complex, rather than simple institutions; they served a variety of purposes, some of which were inadvertently thrust upon them by a society seeking solutions to novel problems which grew, in part, out of rapid social and economic change. Indeed, to ask whether mental hospitals were designed to treat or to incarcerate patients is to force a polarization that denies many realities.

All too often historians and other scholars have remained within the confines of the treatment/incarceration paradigm, and have taken sides. The outcome was predicatable. Those who accepted the definition of insanity as illness saw hospitals in therapeutic terms. The fact that such institutions were unable to provide therapy, they insisted, was due to a shortage of competent staff, inadequate facilities, and a lack of material resources. Conversely, the critics who denied the existence of mental disease maintained that hospitals were repressive institutions which violated basic civil liberties and destroyed individual dignity.

Much of the contemporary debate, however, rest upon an ahistorical analysis of medicine and disease. Consider, for example, the controversy over the definition of "mental disease." Critics of psychiatry often point to an inability to identify physiological processes as causes of mental illness, as proof that persons designated as insane are in fact being punished for their violation of conventional social norms. It then follows that mental hospitals perform a penal function in isolating deviants from the rest of society. Neither the premise nor the conclusion, however, is necessarily valid. The fact of the matter is that the way in which psychiatry historically defined mental illness was (and is) not fundamentally different from the way in which medicine historically defined disease. Viewed in this light, there may be fewer differences between the definitions of somatic and mental diseases than is commonly assumed.[12]

A brief discussion of the history of medical thought may help to clarify the problem. By the late eighteenth century, medicine was influenced by the prevailing receptivity toward taxonomy, which, in turn, reflected the Baconian conviction that general laws could be derived from the collection and analysis of particular facts. The underlying assumption of taxonomical science was that genera and species had a natural and independent existence, apart from the subjective perceptions of the human observer. Just as plants and minerals could be classified, so, too, could diseases. The goal of nosological medicine, therefore, was twofold: first, to give clear and precise definitions of diseases; and secondly, to exhibit the relationships and inner nature of disease states by grouping together states with similar characteristics. Once this process was accomplished, it might then become possible to identify the conditions which determined health and disease, and then to alter them. Unable to establish the etiology of diseases, physicians developed a nosology based on external symptoms, in the belief that they would be able to infer causation, usually by employing a statistical nosology.[13]

Thus, prior to the specific germ theory of disease, all physicians—psychiatrists and generalists—defined pathological states by describing them in terms of external and visible symptoms. This process was inevitable, if only because neither the prevailing technology nor theory could establish a relationship between biological mechanisms and external symptoms. To be sure, a classification system based on external symptoms created serious intellectual and scientific problems. Was fever, for example, one disease state or many? While often disagreeing on specifics, few physicians questioned the practice of defining disease by observing symptoms; no other alternative was available. Nor was there any tendency to argue that individuals with a high fever were social deviants because their immediate condition (mental as well as physical) differed significantly from that of the population at large. Indeed, there are numerous contemporary examples in medicine where physicians define pathological states even when patients appear to feel in perfect health. The classic illustration, of course, is hypertension; an individual with high blood pressure may be designated as being sick even in the absence of any conscious symptoms.

The similarity between medical and psychiatric definitions of disease was well illustrated by the career of Philippe Pinel, who is generally regarded as one of the founding fathers of modern psychiatry. Although best remembered for his classic treatise on insanity, he was also the author of the equally important *Nosographie philosophique ou méthode de l'analyse apliquée à la médicine.* In this treatise he sought to redefine medical theory by applying to it an analytically empirical method. Pinel emphasized that medicine should employ the same methods "commonly used in all other branches of natural history." Psychological concepts could be broken down into original sensations; clinical data could be studied in a similar manner; and changes in human organs could be further investigated in order to analyze the entire pathological picture.[14] Thus Pinel rejected theorizing about the ultimate nature of disease; he confined himself to the accumulation and analysis of data. He did so in the hope that medicine would be able "to assume its proper dignity, to establish its theories on facts alone, to generalize these facts, and to maintain its level with other departments of natural history."[15]

To maintain that psychiatric and medical definitions of disease are not fundamentally dissimilar is not in any way to reject the view that the concept of disease is dependent partly on a series of nonscientific or external variables. Obesity, for example, has been defined in other cultures as a symbol of beauty and health, whereas our society views it as evidence of disease. The same is true of drug addiction and alcoholism.[16] With the possible exception of a number of infectious diseases, most pathological states are still described in terms of symptoms, rather than etiology.[17] Admittedly, there is a difference between defining disease in terms of behavioral symptoms on the one hand and physiological symptoms on the other, but the difference may not be of fundamental significance (particularly if little or no distinction is made between behavior and physiological processes). In fact, we know relatively little about what is designated as mental illness, making it difficult to prove or to disprove its existence. Moreover, in many cases it is not feasible at the present time to establish the validity of psychiatric disease categories. Schizophrenia, to cite one example, may be, in fact, what "fever" was before 1870—a general inclusive category describing a multiplicity of diseases. Assertions about the existence or nonexistence of mental illness represent, largely, acts of faith which reflect commitments to particular courses of action. Historians who begin with an acceptance of either proposition are developing interpretations which are, at best, forms of social criticism.

To concede that psychiatric thought and practice are shaped by external and nonmedical factors is only to repeat a truism which can, with justification, be applied to all other branches of medicine, as well as of science. There are relatively few areas of medicine which remain unaffected by external variables. Even where science and technology have provided clinical medicine with some understanding of pathological mechanisms and defined effective therapies, clinicians have been unable to discount social, economic, and psychological variables in etiology, diagnosis, and treatment.

Psychiatry admittedly faces perhaps more difficult and complex problems than most medical specialities. Although there are large areas of agreement in general medicine on certain basic diagnostic categories—virtually no one, for example, would deny the reality of diabetes, or smallpox, or pneumonia—such agreement on basic disease categories is generally lacking in psychiatry. If physiological processes are responsible for psychiatric diseases we cannot identify them. Nor is it possible at present to identify the role played by either genetic or environmental factors in producing what is designated as mental disease.[18] Although these problems exist, in some degree, in all branches of medicine, past and present, they are particularly acute in psychiatry. There is even precedent for applying the medical model to certain diseases which have traditionally fallen within the jurisdiction of psychiatry. By the nineteenth century, the care of persons afflicted with general paresis—the tertiary stage of syphilis—had been assigned to institutional psychiatry, even though the specific etiology of the disease had not been conclusively demonstrated. This came about because of the inability of persons with the characteristic symptoms of paresis to care for themselves, and the fact that their aberrant behavior created grave problems for their families. In time, clinical and experimental medicine demonstrated the existence of a clear relationship between an invading organism, damage to the central nervous system, and a certain constellation of behavioral characteristics. Whether or not general paresis (or comparable somatic diseases with accompanying behavioral symptoms, including pellagra or cretinism) is or should be a model for psychiatry, of course, remains an unresolved problem.

If the contemporary debate over the legitimacy and function of academic psychiatry has had limited consequences, the same cannot be said about the related controversy concerning the role of mental hospitals. Here the revisionist point of view, both in its historical and contemporary formulations, has had a major influence on public policy. Mental hospitals, once viewed as the fruits of humanitarian reform, and evidence of the progress of mankind, are now widely perceived as political instruments designed to suppress deviancy and to promote a general conformity. Thomas S. Szasz put the issue very simply. "To maintain that a social institution suffers from certain 'abuses,' " he wrote, "is to imply that it has certain other desirable or good uses. This, in my opinion, has been the fatal weakness of the countless exposés—old and recent, literary and professional—of private and public mental hospitals. My thesis is quite different: Simply put, it is that there are, and can be, no abuses *of* Institutional Psychiatry, because Institutional Psychiatry *is*, itself, an abuse."[19]

Influenced by the opponents of institutionalization, a number of state legislatures, during the 1960s and 1970s, passed laws the goal of which, at least in theory, was to discharge as many involuntarily committed patients as possible from mental hospitals and thereby to restore to them their rightful liberties. An unstated objective of some advocates of this legislation, perhaps, was the eventual abolition of all public mental hospitals. Contributing to the attack on institutional care was the growing activism of both the federal and state judiciary. In *Rouse v. Cameron* (1966) David L. Bazelon, chief judge of the United States Court of Appeals for the

District of Columbia, insisted that if the purpose of involuntary hospitalization was treatment (as distinguished from preventing some real danger to self or others), then the absence of treatment called into doubt the constitutionality of confinement. In an equally famous decision Federal District Judge Frank M. Johnson, in Alabama, established minimum constitutional standards for adequate treatment of the mentally ill. With the support of various groups and organizations, the amount of such litigation has increased dramatically during the 1970s. These judicial decisions involved such issues as the right to least restrictive treatment, compensation for labor within hospitals, freedom from cruel and unusual punishment, and due process.[20]

Underlying these attacks on the legitimacy of mental hospitals have been several parallel interpretations of the past. To individuals like Szasz, the mental hospital, from its very inception, was an example of institutional failure. If hospitals did not provide the therapeutic care for which they were intended, their raison d'etre no longer existed.

To clarify this issue, let us begin with the allegation that mental hospitals were designed, consciously or not, to control individuals (generally from a lower class background), whose behavior threatened the stability of society or indirectly endangered the dominance of particular social elites. If this statement is valid, it ought to be possible to demonstrate that most individuals who were involuntarily committed to mental hospitals were perceived as threats to the community, which then responded by using judicial procedures leading to incarceration. Unfortunately, there is relatively little historical data to support such an interpretation, even though some individuals were institutionalized because their behavior seemed to pose a threat to others.

A cursory analysis of those individuals institutionalized in the nineteenth and twentieth centuries provides little evidence to support the claims of the critics of mental hospitals. Who, for example, commenced the commitment process? If fear of social disorder was the paramount motive in judicial proceedings, we might expect to find public authorities or social elites taking the lead in such a process. This, however, was hardly the case. The majority of commitment proceedings, as a matter of fact, originated within the family. In a recent analysis of commitment proceedings in San Francisco during the first three decades of the twentieth century, Richard W. Fox found that 57 per cent of commitment proceedings were begun by relatives, 21 per cent by physicians, and only 8 per cent by the police.[21] That public institutions also received a clientele from lower class or lower-middle-class backgrounds is not at all surprising; such families lacked the necessary funds to pay for private home or institutional care.

Although historical studies about the internal conditions which led families to send members to mental hospitals are still lacking, we do know something of the characteristics of institutional populations during the last century or so. These characteristics do not sustain the view that hospitals were intended as instruments of control (or, for that matter, as therapeutic institutions). Nearly 18 per cent of all "first admissions" to New York State mental hospitals in 1920, for example, were diagnosed as psychotic, either because of senility or cerebral arteriosclerosis. By 1940, this group accounted for nearly 31 per cent of all first admissions. Similarly, in the mid-1930s, aged persons constituted between 18 per cent and 21 per cent of the total admissions at the Dayton State Hospital in Ohio. The practice of using mental hospitals as a home for older persons suffering from some sort of physical and mental impairment was widespread. In 1900, to offer another illustration, the 880 patients over sixty-five years of age constituted nearly 13 per cent of the total population of public institutions in Massachusetts. Of this number, 127 (14.4 per cent) were confined to bed; 211 (24 per cent) were unable to maintain minimal personal hygiene; 215 (24.4 per cent) were helpless and had to be cared for like young children; and 272 (27.5 per cent) had no friends.[22]

Although the number of aged persons in state mental hospitals varied by period and geographical locale, there is no doubt that this group always constituted a substantial proportion of the total institutionalized population. Indeed, by the late nineteenth century, age-specific admission rates of older persons began to rise markedly, as compared with admission rates for younger persons. In their classic study of rates of institutionalization, covering more than a century, Herbert Goldhamer and Andrew W. Marshall found that the greatest increase occurred in the age group of those sixty years old or older. In 1885, age-specific first admission rates in Massachusetts for males sixty and over was 70.4, and for females 65.5 (per 100,000); by the beginning of the Second World War, the corresponding figures were 279.5 and 223.0.[23] (see table 1)

Why were aged persons committed to mental hospitals? There is little evidence that the community perceived them as threats to their security. Nor can it be said that the function of institutionalization was to alter the behavior of such persons or to provide restorative therapy. "The question of the care of the aged is one that will confront us always," noted one superintendent who conceded that no proper treatment was available.[24] In point of fact, mental hospitals assumed the responsibility for caring for older people partly because of the absence of alternatives. In addition, decline in mortality rates among younger groups also led to a relative and absolute increase in the size of older groups, thereby exacerbating the social

Table 1

Male and Female Age-Specific First-Admission Rates,
Massachusetts, 1885 and 1939–41

Age	1885		1939–41	
	Male	Female	Male	Female
10–19	22.0	15.0	57.2	42.8
20–29	96.4	75.0	124.2	91.1
30–39	111.0	107.9	159.9	108.2
40–49	110.0	108.1	164.0	106.0
50–59	102.9	78.8	174.5	117.3
60–	70.4	65.5	279.5	223.0

Source: Herbert Goldhamer and Andrew C. Marshall, *Psychosis and Civilization: Two Studies in the Frequency of Mental Disease* (Glencoe, Ill.: The Free Press, 1953), p. 54.

problems arising from an aged population. Between 1900 and 1940, the number of persons age sixty-five and over increased from 3,080,498 to 9,019,314 (as compared with a population rise from 75,994,575 to only 131,669,275).[25] Older persons ended up in mental hospitals for a variety of reasons. Some had no family to provide basic care. Others were institutionalized because of the inability or unwillingness of relatives to assume responsibility. Still other senile individuals obviously exhibited the kind of behavior which was difficult for a family to cope with. Finally, the increasing frequency of commitment of aged persons to mental hospitals may have in part reflected a shift of population from almshouses and other welfare institutions, which were declining in number.

Psychiatrists and public officials were well aware of the practice of committing older persons to mental hospitals. Unhappy with this situation, but not lacking in compassion, they went along with the idea of confining such persons, because there seemed to be no other alternative. Dr. Charles C. Wagner, superintendent of the Binghampton State Hospital in New York, defined the issue in simple, yet moving terms. "We are receiving every year a large number of old people, some of them very old, who are simply suffering from the mental decay incident to extreme old age," he wrote in 1900. "A little mental confusion, forgetfulness and garrulity are sometimes the only symptoms exhibited, but the patient is duly certified to us as insane and has no one at home capable or possessed of means to care for him. We are unable to refuse these patients without creating ill-feeling in the community where they reside, nor are we able to assert that they are not insane within the meaning of the statute, for many of them, judged by the ordinary standards of sanity, cannot be regarded as entirely sane."[26]

The secretary of the Pennsylvania Board of Public Charities expressed a similar sentiment a few years later. "In ordinary parlance," he noted,

> this [senile dementia] is known as the childishness of old age, a condition so frequently attendant upon those who have exceeded the "three score and ten" limit. After a life of activity and probably of usefulness, after having nurtured and cared for their offspring, and often at the sacrifice of their own comfort fitted them for future success and prosperity; when the tired and worn brain loses its power and the "grasshopper becomes a burden" these children unwilling to inconvenience themselves will shirk a duty by placing the wearied parent in a hospital to tarry with the insane until the golden chord shall be broken. Harmless are these old people, prone to wander, living perhaps in the past and vainly seeking the friends of other days; continuity of thought broken, sometimes incoherent in speech and occasionally causing by their own actions mortification, they are not insane although, of course, not normal. Selfishly neglected by those who owe to them every thing they are thrust into seclusion in order that they may not be burdens, and too frequently forgotten and neglected by those through whose veins flows the same blood, they must helplessly and hopelessly wait, receiving kindness and care from those who are neither kith nor kin, until the coming of the Great Messenger shall mercifully relieve and release them. A crime has been committed and yet a legalized crime and this will be repeated again and again until medical examiners shall more wisely discriminate in their certification of insanity.

The secretary's observations were exaggerated, no doubt, but the intent of his message was unmistakable. Nor were such sentiments confined to the early part of the century. In 1938, another superintendent repeated much the same words. "There is no excuse whatsoever for their commitment," he wrote, "and it can be explained only on the basis of a loosening of natural family ties and a desire to be relieved of dutiful responsibility."[27]

Senility was by no means the only source of admissions of persons whose behavioral peculiarities were related to underlying physiological processes. Before the widespread use of penicillin and other antibiotics limited the course of venereal disease, insanity resulting from syphilis accounted also for substantial numbers of admissions to mental hospitals. Between 1911 and 1920, about 20 percent of all male first admissions to mental hospitals in New York State were cases of general paresis (the comparable rate for women during this same period was about one-third that of men). New York State, once again, was not unique in this respect. The superintendents of the Western State Hospital in Washington and the Dayton State Hospital in Ohio estimated that syphilis accounted for between 16 per cent and 20 per cent of all new admissions during the 1930s.[28] These statistics were by no means unrepresentative for the rest of the country. It must also be remembered that after 1906, the Wassermann test (which was routinely administered in virtually all mental hospitals) provided a fairly reliable (although not infallible) serological technique for determining whether the *treponema pallidum* (the organism responsible for causing syphilis) was present in the blood, thus adding an element of reliability to twentieth-century institutional statistics.

Admittedly, to most Americans in the prepenicillin era, syphilis was more than a physical disease; it symbolized, in part, the penalty for moral corruption. By the early twentieth century, syphilis and prostitution were often regarded as merely different sides of the same coin. In his famous study of European prostitution, Abraham Flexner (who helped to transform the shape of medical education in the United States) denied that the European effort to regulate prostitution was an appropriate example for Americans. Prostitution, he insisted, grew out of a corrupt and decadent culture; Americans could only be contaminated if they attempted to regulate, rather than suppress, the evil practice.[29] Nevertheless, we should not conclude that syphilitic patients committed to mental hospitals were being punished for their transgressions. In the tertiary stage of this disease, massive damage to the central nervous system resulted not only in bizarre behavior but in dramatic neurological symptoms, paralysis, and eventually death. For such cases, institutional care was almost a sina qua non; few households were prepared to cope with such problems. Since general hospitals did not have separate facilities to care for patients in the tertiary stage (who could live from one to five years), responsibility devolved upon the mental hospital.

Overall, at least one-third (and probably more) of all first admissions to state mental hospitals represented cases where behavioral symptoms were probably of somatic origin. In 1922, for example, 52,472 persons were admitted for the first time into state mental hospitals. Of this number, 15,916 were sent there either because of senility, cerebral arteriosclerosis, general paresis, cerebral syphilis, Huntington's chorea, pellagra, brain tumor or other brain disease, and other somatic illnesses. The statistics a decade later showed much the same pattern.[30] There were, of course, some significant regional differences. Pellagra (a disease caused by a dietary deficiency, often accompanied by behavioral symptoms), for example, was generally confined to the South. Between 1930 and 1932, the State Hospital at Goldsboro, North Carolina, (which was limited to black individuals only), reported that no less than 19 per cent of its admissions were due to pellagra. In northern hospitals, the disease was virtually unknown.[31]

Mental hospitals, in other words, cared for a variety of patients. Some individuals were institutionalized because of physical disability. In other cases, hospitals served as asylums for persons, who, for one reason or another, seemed to require a structured environment. Noting that it was often alleged that public mental hospitals cared for persons who could just as easily have been sent home, the Pennsylvania Commission on Lunacy warned of the dangers of generalizing on such issues. The Commission concluded that no doubt many could be sent home, "provided that the home existed, or that conditions at home were suitable for the patient's return"; unfortunately, these necessities did not always exist. Frederick H. Wines, one of the most influential figures in late nineteenth-century public welfare, observed that many mental hospitals were imposed upon in "that patients are sent to them who should not be so sent, because their friends wish to avoid the responsibility of keeping and caring for them at home."[32]

Aside from the problems presented by contradictory data, the thesis that mental hospitals were instruments of social control presents logical and semantic difficulties. Institutions and organizations (by definition) to some extent perform functions of social control. But is control a primary element, or is it a necessary by-product or concommitant? A school clearly controls the behavior of the student, in that it mandates the exclusion of certain activities (e.g., sleeping, mowing grass, fighting) and emphasizes others (reading, writing, etc.). That the establishment of schools—or mental hospitals—came about because of a desire to institute controls does not logically follow. What those with an affinity for the "social control" mode of explanation have done is to confuse at times the by-product with the primary intention. In addition, these scholars also fail to recognize that it is not social control in general that they are rejecting, but specific forms of control with which they disagree. From a purely logical point of view, the very definition of society presupposes the existence of controls. Indeed, only an absolute anarchist rejects the very idea of any social controls.

Viewed in the light of the past, and of logical analysis, therefore, a good part of the debate dealing with mental illness becomes irrelevant. Mental hospitals were not intended to function only as therapeutic institutions, nor were they established primarily because of fear that abnormal behavior threatened public safety or the social order. And to discuss the issue of involuntary commitment solely in terms of abstract individual rights is to avoid the far more difficult task of evaluating theory in the light of concrete situations which rarely offered clearcut moral choices. In many instances the application of a single general principle often has the inadvertent consequence of invalidating another general principle which may be equally compelling. An absolutist definition of freedom, for example, may very well negate other humanitarian or ethical principles and rights. It is entirely possible to honor the absolute right of persons in an advanced state of senility to liberty by not hospitalizing them, while denying their right to care from society by not hospitalizing them, and allowing them to die from exposure, starvation, and neglect.

Nor have the revisionists been alone in misinterpreting the functions of mental hospitals. Twentieth-century orthodox psychiatrists, by way of contrast, generally applied a therapeutic standard in evaluating institutional care. Reflecting their own image of themselves as physicians, such psychiatrists rejected the legitimacy of custodial care in hospitals (which their nineteenth-century predecessors had accepted). To do otherwise would have been to modify the traditional psychiatric goals of prevention and therapy, and to place themselves in the role of mere caretakers. Ironically, much of the criticism of mental hospitals came from the ranks of institutional psychiatrists, who repeatedly condemned the practice of committing aged and physically infirm persons to their care. Even more significant, claims about the importance of therapy resulted in a gross distortion of the functions which many institutions were, in fact, performing. Also, in seeking greater public financial support, psychiatrists posited a direct relationship between resources and cures which could not be realized, even under the best of circumstances.

There is considerable evidence, then, to indicate that the familiar therapy/incarceration theme is misleading as a framework for understanding the development of mental hospitals. Even a superficial analysis of the composition of patient populations renders this dichotomy untenable. A substantial proportion of patients were hospitalized neither for therapeutic reasons nor because of any alleged dangers to the community. We need to know much more about the characteristics of these patients, the reasons for institutionalization, and the ways in which such patients influenced the character of hospitals.[33] In addition, we must also be aware that statistics dealing with hospital populations can easily be misinterpreted. Many prominent native-born Americans in the late nineteenth and early twentieth century continuously pointed to the overrepresentation of the foreign-born in hospitals, as compared with their proportions in the general population. Such data were then used to justify racial interpretations of culture, or the passage of legislation designed to curtail unrestricted immigration to the United States of certain undesirable groups. Yet when the data dealing with institutionalized foreign-born patients are corrected by taking into account the dissimilar age distributions of native and immigrant, the differential between them narrows sharply. Moreover, the introduction of other variables, such as sex, income, and urban or rural residence, alters the results still further and discredits the allegation that immigrants and their children, for genetic reasons, were liable to become mentally ill at a rate significantly higher than native-born persons.[34]

Nor can we easily disregard the broader social context within which psychiatrists and mental hospitals functioned. To maintain that aged and senile groups, as well as persons suffering from physical impairments with accompanying behavioral symptoms, did not belong in mental hospitals, or to insist that individual rights were ignored, is in part to misunderstand the nature of social change in the nineteenth and twentieth centuries. In point of fact, high rates of geographical mobility, a rapid increase in the size of urban areas, and the inability of traditional means of alleviating distress and dependency by reliance on familial and community traditions and practices, led Americans increasingly to turn to quasi-public or public institutions to act in surrogate capacities. Although advocates may debate the wisdom or desirability of the shift in social policy toward institutional solutions, historians would be better advised to illuminate the sources of change, policy formulation and administration, and the dynamics of institutional growth and elaboration.

Mental hospitals never were the monolithic institutions portrayed by critics. During the nineteenth century, for example, there was considerable experimentation with various institutional forms—including the establishment of decentralized hospitals which attempted to move patients from a structured setting to an environment approximating the community from which they came. Nor was traditional psychiatry monolithic in its attitudes; dissent and conflict existed alongside consensus.[35]

Some of the more traditional approaches to the history of psychiatry and mental hospitals suffer from many of the same defects as do the works of revisionists.[36] There has been a disconcerting tendency to see the past in terms of progress. Thus the replacement of the category of dementia praecox by schizophrenia becomes a sign of advance; the dominance of Freudian and neo-Freudian patterns of thought is applauded; and the emphasis on mental hygiene is viewed as a symbol of maturity. Such interpretations tell us far more about the hopes and aspirations of those individuals and groups connected with the mental health professions than they do about historical realities. We need to know much more about both the internal and external factors which governed the evolution of psychiatry and mental hospitals. The development of nosological systems was both a medical and a social phenomenon; to emphasize one and neglect the other leads to a skewed and inaccurate view. Moreover, there is considerable evidence demonstrating the irrelevance of diagnostic categories to institutional practice. In my own research on the history of mental hospitals from the late nineteenth century to the Second World War, for example, I have found little or no evidence that Freudian concepts affected psychiatric practice in public mental hospitals in the least. To assume that Freud influenced the treatment of the majority of institutionalized patients is to misread the past.

In future historical research dealing with mental hospitals and psychiatry, it will be essential to separate intentions from subsequent developments; the two often had little to do with each other. It is, after all, extraordinarily difficult to infer motives from outcome without adopting a viewpoint which makes events the result of strictly rational, logical, and conscious behavior. Nor can we assume, with any degree of confidence, that undesirable consequences resulted simply from callous behavior or malevolent intentions, even though such elements were by no means absent. Knowledge about individual behavior, social behavior, and institutions remains limited, despite claims to the contrary. Few human beings, no matter how well informed, can predict with any degree of reliability the actual results of their actions. And to argue that there "had to be a better way of doing things" is only to repeat a truism and a cliché.[37]

That historical knowledge conditions attitudes and behavior in the present to some degree is obvious. The issue, therefore, is not whether historical knowledge will be employed to influence decision-making and public policies, but what kind of history will be used. Recently Ernest R. May observed that most policy-makers and policy advocates employ history badly, rather than well. "When resorting to an analogy," he noted, "they tend to seize upon the first that comes to mind. They do not search more widely. Nor do they pause to analyze the case, test its fitness, or even ask in what ways it might be misleading. Seeing a trend running toward the present, they tend to assume that it will continue into the future, not stopping to consider what produced it or why a linear projection might prove to be mistaken."[38] May's observations are equally applicable to the history of institutional care and treatment of the mentally ill.

It would be a tragedy if a misunderstanding of the past guided our responses to the problems presented by mental illness in the present and future. The history of psychiatry and mental hospitals has for too long been determined, at least in part, by contemporary concerns and by personal commitments to specific policies. The result has been a history which is often poor, not because of its didactic qualities, but because the data employed has either been incomplete or biased in a particular direction, while other data was simply ignored because it failed to fit a particular conceptual framework.[39] It is easy, of course, to attribute the fact that the overwhelming majority of mental hospitals fell far short of their stated objectives to evil and shortsighted human beings, or to a society lacking in sympathy or compassion. Yet a careful analysis does not substantiate such interpretations. Indeed, the most impressive fact is the relative absence of malevolence, or for that matter, consistency of behavior. What may very well emerge from a careful and scholarly study is more akin to a tragedy in which most participants, to a greater or lesser degree, were well intentioned, but whose efforts gave rise to a series of unintended results, because of unforeseen circumstances. For the history of the care and treatment of the mentally ill in America is surely fraught with all of the elements of tragedy. Within such a perspective, any definitive judgment must contain some room for a measure of understanding and even compassion for all concerned—patients, psychiatrists, and the larger society. Perhaps the accomplishments of mental hospitals fell far short of expectations, but surely they achieved certain goals not necessarily undesirable or inherently evil. In this respect mental hospitals were not fundamentally dissimilar to most human institutions, the achievements of which usually fall far short of the hopes and aspirations of the individuals who founded and led them.[40]

NOTES

The author wishes to acknowledge that the research for this paper was supported by a grant from the Public Health Service (HEW), National Library of Medicine, No. 2306. A slightly different version was published in the Hastings Center Report 7 *(August 1977): 33–41.*

1. For examples of work which do *not* fit a dichotomous conceptual framework see Norman Dain, *Concepts of Insanity in the United States, 1789–1865* (New Brunswick: Rutgers University Press, 1964); Charles E. Rosenberg, *The Trial of the Assassin Guiteau: Psychiatry and Law in the Gilded Age* (Chicago: University of Chicago Press, 1968); Nathan G. Hale, *Freud and the Americans: The Beginnings of Psychoanalysis in the United States, 1876–1917* (New York: Oxford University Press, 1971); and John C. Burnham, *Psychoanalysis and American Medicine: 1894–1918; Medicine, Science, and Culture* (New York: International Universities Press, 1967).

2. Van Giesen's discussion of the history of psychiatry appeared in his second annual report as Director of the Pathological Institute, which was published in the New York State Commission in Lunacy, *Annual Report* 9 (1897): 92ff.

3. Albert Deutsch, *The Mentally Ill in America: A History of Their Care and Treatment from Colonial Times,* 2d ed. (New York: Columbia University Press, 1949); first edition, 1937.

4. Albert Deutsch, *The Shame of the States* (New York: Harcourt, Brace and Co., 1948), p. 187 et passim.

5. For a brief summary of this approach see Robert Perrucci, *Circle of Madness: On Being Insane and Institutionalized in America* (Englewood Cliffs, N.J.: Prentice-Hall, Inc., 1974), chap. 1.

6. For a discussion of the "new social history," see Samuel P. Hays, "A

Systematic Social History," in *American History: Retrospect and Prospect,* ed. George A. Billias and Gerald N. Grob (New York: The Free Press, 1971), pp. 315–66.

7. The historiography of education is particularly revealing of this trend. See, for example, the following: Michael B. Katz, *The Irony of Early School Reform: Educational Innovation in Mid-Nineteenth Century Massachusetts* (Cambridge: Harvard University Press, 1968), and *Class, Bureaucracy, and Schools: The Illusion of Educational Change in America* (New York: Praeger Publishers, 1971); Carl F. Kaestle, *The Evolution of an Urban School System: New York City, 1750–1850* (Cambridge: Harvard University Press, 1973); Colin Greer, *The Great School Legend: A Revisionist Interpretation of American Public Education* (New York: Viking Press, 1973); Joel Spring, *Education and the Rise of the Corporate State* (Boston: Beacon Press, 1972); and Raymond E. Callahan, *Education and the Cult of Efficiency: A Study of the Social Forces That Have Shaped the Administration of the Public Schools* (Chicago: University of Chicago Press, 1962).

8. The concept of the "total institution" was implicit in Bruno Bettelheim's famous study of behavior in Nazi concentration camps, "Individual and Mass Behavior in Extreme Situations," *Journal of Abnormal and Social Psychology* 38 (October 1943): 417–52. The most mature development of this theme was Erving Goffman's *Asylums: Essays on the Social Situation of Mental Patients and Other Inmates* (Garden City: Doubleday and Co., 1961). Goffman defined a total institution "as a place of residence and work where a large number of like-situated individuals, cut off from the wider society for an appreciable period of time, together lead an enclosed, formally administered round of life" (p. xiii).

9. Michel Foucault, *Madness and Civilization: A History of Insanity in the Age of Reason* (New York: Pantheon Books, 1965); Thomas S. Szasz, *The Myth of Mental Illness: Foundations of a Theory of Personal Conduct* (New York: Hoeber-Harper, 1961), *Law, Liberty, and Psychiatry: An Inquiry into the Social Uses of Mental Health Practices* (New York: The Macmillan Co., 1963), *The Manufacture of Madness: A Comparative Study of the Inquisition and the Mental Health Movement* (New York: Harper and Row, 1970), and *The Age of Madness: The History of Involuntary Mental Hospitalization, Presented in Selected Texts* (Garden City: Anchor Books, 1973); David J. Rothman, *The Discovery of the Asylum: Social Order and Disorder in the New Republic* (Boston: Little, Brown and Co., 1971). For a penetrating discussion of the differences between critics of psychiatry and of mental hospitals, see Peter Sedgwick, "Illness—Mental and Otherwise," *Hastings Center Studies* vol. 1, no. 3 (1973): 19–40.

10. Ernest R. May, *"Lessons" of the Past: The Use and Misuse of History in American Foreign Policy* (New York: Oxford University Press, 1973).

11. Deutsch, *Shame of the States,* passim; Rothman, *Discovery of the Asylum,* pp. 294–95; Szasz, *Manufacture of Madness,* p. xv.

12. Unfortunately, the history of the concept of disease has yet to be written. But even a cursory analysis shows that psychiatrists were not engaging in a unique practice when they in effect identified symptoms as pathology. For some interesting (but fragmentary) general discussion, see the collection of papers "Concepts of Health and Disease," ed. F.C. Redlich, in the *Journal of Medicine and Philosophy* 1 (September 1976).

13. Lester F. King, *The Medical World of the Eighteenth Century* (Chicago: University of Chicago Press, 1958), chap. 7. For the affinity between statistics and medicine in the nineteenth century, see Gerald N. Grob, *Edward Jarvis and the Medical World of Nineteenth-Century America* (Knoxville: University of Tennessee Press, 1978), passim.

14. George Rosen, "The Philosophy of Ideology and the Emergence of Modern Medicine in France," *Bulletin of the History of Medicine* 20 (July 1946):

332–33; Richard H. Shryock, *The Development of Modern Medicine: An Interpretation of the Social and Scientific Factors Involved* (rev. ed.; New York: Alfred A. Knopf, 1947): 151–53.

15. Philippe Pinel, *A Treatise on Insanity*, trans. D.D. Davis (Sheffield, England: W. Todd, 1806), pp. 2, 45.

16. For a fascinating contemporary discussion of the concept of disease, see Rene Dubos, *Mirage of Health: Utopias, Progress, and Biological Change* (New York: Harper, 1959), and *Man Adapting* (New Haven: Yale University Press, 1965).

17. It should be remembered that even in the case of infectious diseases where the most significant therapeutic advances have occurred, it cannot be argued that the presence of a particular organism "explains" or "causes" the disease. It is by no means uncommon, for example, for an individual carrying the tubercule bacillin to develop the characteristic symptoms of tuberculosis, while another individual carrying the very same organism remains free from disease, or the symptoms of disease.

18. For a perceptive analysis of psychiatry, see Charles E. Rosenberg, "The Crisis in Psychiatric Legitimacy: Reflections on Psychiatry, Medicine, and Public Policy," in *American Psychiatry: Past, Present, and Future*, ed. George Kriegman, Robert D. Gardner, and D. Wilfred Abse (Charlottesville: University Press of Virginia, 1975), pp. 135–48.

19. Szasz, *The Manufacture of Madness*, pp. xxix–xxv.

20. *Rouse v. Cameron*, 373 F. 2d 451 (1966); *Wyatt v. Stickney*, 344 F. Supp. 373 (1972). For a general discussion of psychiatry and policy see Ralph Slovenko, *Psychiatry and Law* (Boston: Little, Brown and Co., 1973).

21. For a broad statistical analysis of commitment proceedings and of the social background of persons designated as mentally ill in San Francisco during the early twentieth century, by a scholar who accepts the social control thesis, but in a modified form, see Richard W. Fox, *So Far Disordered in Mind: Insanity in California, 1870–1930* (Berkeley: University of California Press, 1978), p. 84 et passim.

22. New York State Department of Mental Hygiene, *Annual Report* 52 (1939–40): 174–75; Ohio Department of Public Welfare, *Annual Report* 15 (1936): 303–4; Massachusetts State Board of Insanity, *Annual Report* 2 (1900): 32. For additional data on the confinement of aged people in mental hospitals, see the following: Michigan State Board of Corrections and Charities, *Biennial Report* 15 (1898–1900): 210; New York State Commission in Lunacy, *Annual Report* 12 (1900): 23–36, 19 (1907): 161–68; Oklahoma Commissioner of Charities and Corrections, *Biennial Report* 6 (1917–18): 41; Colorado State Board of Charities and Corrections, *Biennial Report* 11 (1911–12): 29–30; Maryland Board of Welfare, *Annual Report* 4 (1926): 62–63; Kentucky Department of Public Welfare, *Biennial Report* 1931–33; 36, 70. For a study of institutionalized patients in New York State since the mid-nineteenth century, see M. Harvey Brenner, *Mental Illness and the Economy* (Cambridge, Harvard University Press, 1973).

23. Herbert Goldhamer and Andrew W. Marshall, *Psychosis and Civilization: Two Studies in the Frequency of Mental Disease* (Glencoe, Ill.: The Free Press, 1953), pp. 54, 91. For another discussion of the relationship between mental disease and age, see Benjamin Malzberg, *Social and Biological Aspects of Mental Disease* (Utica: State Hospitals Press, 1940), chap. 2.

24. Ohio Department of Public Welfare, *Annual Report*, 15 (1936), 303–4.

25. United States Bureau of the Census, *Historical Statistics of the United States: Colonial Times to 1970*, 2 vols. (Washington, D.C.: Government Printing Office, 1975), part 1, p. 15.

26. New York State Commission in Lunacy, *Annual Report* 12 (1900): 29–30.

27. Pennsylvania Committee on Lunacy, *Annual Report* 22 (1904): 8–9, in Pennsylvania Board of Commissioners of Public Charities, *Annual Report* 35 (1904); Topeka State Hospital, *Biennial Report* 31 (1936–38): 9, in Kansas Board of Administration, *Biennial Report* 11 (1936–38).

28. New York State Department of Mental Hygiene, *Annual Report* 52 (1939–40): 176; Washington (State) Department of Business Control, *Biennial Report* 7 (1933–34): 27; Ohio Department of Public Welfare, *Annual Report* 15 (1936): 304. For other examples, see Ohio Board of Administration, *Annual Report* 1 (1912): 43–44, 3 (1914): 183; Ohio Department of Public Welfare, *Annual Report* 11–12 (1932–33): 349, 358–60; Oregon State Board of Control, *Biennial Report* 4 (1919–20): 47; Illinois Department of Public Welfare, *Annual Report* 12 (1928–29): 310; North Carolina Charitable, Penal, and Correctional Institutions, *Biennial Report* 1930–32: 48.

29. Abraham Flexner, *Prostitution in Europe* (New York: The Century Co., 1914).

30. United States Bureau of the Census, *Mental Patients in State Hospitals: 1926 and 1927* (Washington, D.C.: Government Printing Office, 1930), p. 9, and *Mental Patients in State Hospitals: 1931 and 1932* (Washington, D.C.: Government Printing Office, 1934), p. 6.

31. North Carolina Charitable, Penal, and·Correctional Institutions, *Biennial Report* (1930–32): 48.

32. Pennsylvania Committee on Lunacy, *Annual Report* 16 (1898): 44–45, in Pennsylvania Board of Commissioners of Public Charities, *Annual Report* 29 (1898); *Proceedings of the National Conference of Charities and Correction* 17 (1890): 431.

33. For an interesting study of the ways in which prison inmates influence their institutional environment, see Gresham M. Sykes, *The Society of Captives: A Study of a Maximum Security Prison* (Princeton: Princeton University Press, 1958). There is no retrospective study of the ways in which patients influenced the development of mental hospitals.

34. Malzberg, *Social and Biological Aspects*, pp. 143–76; Malzberg, "Are Immigrants Psychologically Disturbed?" in *Changing Perspectives in Mental Illness*, ed. Stanley C. Plog and Robert B. Edgerton (New York: Holt, Rinehart and Winston, 1969), pp. 395–421; Neil A. Dayton, *New Facts on Mental Disorders: Study of 89,190 Cases* (Springfield: Charles C. Thomas, 1940), chap. 8; United States Bureau of the Census, *Insane and Feeble-Minded in Institutions: 1910* (Washington, D.C.: Government Printing Office, 1914), pp. 25ff. Richard W. Fox (in *So Far Disordered in Mind*, pp. 107–8) appropriately points out the fallacies in some of the data relating to immigrants in my *Mental Institutions in America: Social Policy to 1875* (New York: The Free Press, 1973), and Rothman's *Discovery of the Asylum*. It must be kept in mind, however, that many individuals believed that there was a clear relationship between certain immigrant groups and the incidence of mental disease, and acted accordingly; data to the contrary were simply ignored.

35. For a summary and analysis of the debates over appropriate institutional forms among psychiatrists see Grob, *Mental Institutions in America*, chap. 8.

36. Cf. Gregory Zilboorg, *A History of Medical Psychology* (New York: W.W. Norton and Co., 1941), and Franz G. Alexander and Sheldon T. Selesnick, *The History of Psychiatry: An Evaluation of Psychiatric Thought and Practice from Prehistoric Times to the Present* (New York: Harper and Row, 1966).

37. Put in simple terms, I am not fully persuaded that the modern confidence in the ability of human beings to control their environment is completely warranted. It is important to recognize that there may be no solutions which are themselves

not the source of further problems. The history of disease is a case in point. Public policy and attitudes in America seem to be based in large measure upon the belief that it is possible to conquer disease; the result has been a phenomenal increase in the resources allocated to treatment and research. The actual record, on the other hand, hardly warrants such optimism. When infectious diseases (which killed large numbers of infants and children) declined in importance (partly as a result of public health innovations and changes in the standard of living in the late nineteenth and early twentieth centuries), more people survived to adulthood. Consequently, there was an increase in degenerative disease (e.g., cardiovascular disease and cancer), the incidence of which is proportionately higher in nations with aged populations. The decline in one set of illnesses, therefore, was in part the occasion for a corresponding increase in a different group.

The introduction of the widespread use of antibiotics during the 1940s provides another illustration of this theme. Before penicillin, the infections that played a major role in morbidity were caused by pneumococci, streptococci, tubercle bacilli, and staphylococci. By about 1958, with the exception of staphylococci, these bacteria were rarely a factor in fatal disease; they had been replaced by fungi and gram-negative rods. Moreover, certain species, hitherto relatively harmless, now assumed an infectious nature, since other microorganisms which had competed with them had been suppressed by the introduction of antibiotic drugs. Finally, resistance to antibiotic drugs can be transferred under specific kinds of conditions. For a discussion of these points, see Harry F. Dowling, *Fighting Infection: Conquests of the Twentieth Century* (Cambridge: Harvard University Press, 1977), pp. 191–92.

38. May, *"Lessons" of the Past,* p. xi.

39. Rothman's influential book, *The Discovery of the Asylum,* is a case in point; his use of sources raises some serious methodological questions. By consistently italicizing certain words in quotations from his sources, he altered their meaning. He italicized phrases like "order," "obedience," and "regularity" (presumably because they proved that hospitals were repressive institutions), while ignoring words like "kind," "humane," and "considerate" (perhaps because they ran counter to his thesis). A number of his quotations were selectively edited; a reading of the entire source reveals that the evidence in question confirms an opposite hypothesis. Contrary evidence was often omitted. In attempting to refute the high curability rates claimed by mid-nineteenth-century psychiatrists, for example, Rothman cited Pliny Earle, but ignored other sources which seemed to validate at least some of the curability statistics. His research was deficient. In his bibliography he conceded that he had not, for the most part, examined a large mass of rich manuscript material; he defended his procedure by insisting that there were few differences between the private and public statements of psychiatrists. Such a statement, however, is justified only if both classes of material have been examined; it is not possible to offer a judgment about an unexamined class of sources. Finally, Rothman's assertions about the uniqueness of American psychiatric thought cannot be supported, at least in the manner in which he presents the subject. For a lengthy analysis of the ways in which Rothman uses historical evidence, see the review article by Jacques M. Quen, in the *Journal of Psychiatry and Law* 2 (spring 1974): 105–22. In offering these criticisms of Rothman's book, I want to make it clear that I am not expressing a judgment about his conceptual framework. I am criticizing his use of sources, which involves more than questions of judgment or disagreements over interpretations.

40. This paragraph is based on the conclusion of my book, *Mental Institutions in America: Social Policy to 1875,* pp. 341–42.

7 MACHINE POLITICS AND MEDICAL CARE: The City Hospital at the Turn of the Century

MORRIS J. VOGEL

Resident physicians and lay officials shared the responsibility for admitting patients to Philadelphia's Blockley Hospital in the late nineteenth century. Residents rotated the chore of representing the medical staff in screening applicants at the institution's downtown office; the lay officials were political appointees, members of the machine-dominated local government that controlled the city hospital. Participants in the admissions process often brought differing values to their tasks and applied different standards in judging the suitability of patients. The admissions process therefore sometimes highlighted conflicting definitions of the hospital.

Arthur Ames Bliss participated in the admissions process during his tenure as a resident physician in 1883–84. In an introspective memoir, Bliss appreciated his role as advocate for the hospital's medical interests. Medical admissions officers, he noted tongue-in-cheek, "were ever mindful that our colleagues do not excuse any errors that the man on duty may make in admitting unimportant and uninteresting cases." Bliss confessed that while on admissions duty, "the young medical man was too often disposed to be sarcastic, cynical, suspicious, and anxious to drive away every applicant who did not bear in his or her body the symptoms of being an interesting medical or surgical case." While the physician applied the test of medical significance to each applicant and found many wanting, the politician was more sympathetic. Facing "wretched, broken men and women," whom Bliss might have dismissed as "not sick enough," the politician not infrequently "would find some excuse for admitting the subject to the Outwards—the Almshouse Department,—or would mildly set aside my verdict and make out a pass for the hospital." The politician considered the prospective patient within his social context, as an applicant for care and shelter; the primary concern of the physician was with the medical facts of the case.[1]

Conflicting views of the hospital—as a site for social care, on the one hand, and a setting for medical treatment, on the other—were not peculiar to the city institution. This dichotomous definition, expressed differently, had characterized the voluntary hospital, the dominant form of the institution in the United States, throughout its history. The physicians and lay boards of trustees associated with these facilities were generally members of the same social elites, and thus had more in common with each other than did Bliss and his political antagonists. Yet the physicians and trustees of voluntary hospitals did not agree entirely on institutional policy. This tension stemmed from the nature of the nineteenth-century hospital.

The first American hospitals established the basic pattern. The Pennsylvania Hospital and the New York Hospital, which date from the second half of the eighteenth century, and the Massachusetts General Hospital, founded at the beginning of the nineteenth century, were private institutions. Each represented a joint effort on the part of medical men and dominant lay figures, often substantial merchants. From the outset, each had both social and medical goals. But the nature of the patient class, the orientation of lay donors and their domination of governing boards, and the intellectual content of medical practice, taken together, emphasized social purposes.

Patients were not a cross section of the sick and injured in the community at large, but were drawn disproportionately from the unfortunate classes. Medical care within the context of home and family remained the norm for most Americans. The very act of seeking hospitalization—going among strangers for care when ill—was often an act of desperation; the applicant for admission to one of the hundred or so general hospitals in this country in 1870 in effect acknowledged that his social situation was deficient. Through the mid-nineteenth century, general hospital care meant food and shelter for the needy and incidentally ill.[2]

The stewardship of the well-to-do supported most general hospitals. The motivations of the hospital's lay supporters were mixed; generally present to some degree was a pietistic desire to do good and a concern for social order. This latter motivation was intertwined with the expectation that the hospital could act as an agency of individual betterment and social control. Donors hoped that patients would be impressed by the good efforts of their betters. Easing the burden of illness for the poor could serve as an antidote against embitterment, a prophylaxis for social discontent. The lay trustees who represented the donor class felt themselves responsible for the personal character of their patients.

While sometimes submerged before the last quarter of the nineteenth century, the medical purpose of the hospital was always significant. Laymen financed the institution, partly in order to advance the work of medical men with whom they shared ties of class and social outlook. And though the doctrine of stewardship was invoked to explain the unremunerated treatment physicians rendered in their part-time service to the institutionalized poor, hospital practice had an entirely medical rationale. The small minority of physicians associated with hospitals formed a self-conscious group, aware that their interests, training and aspirations set them apart from the profession at large.[3] This group shared most dramatically in the nineteenth-century revolution in medical knowledge. Hospitals furnished these practitioners the opportunities to enhance their skills by observing and treating large numbers of cases in clinical settings. While hospital physicians continued to acknowledge home treatment—where the patient would be diagnosed and managed holistically, within the context of family—as the best medical care, these same practitioners eagerly devoted some of their time to the hospitalized poor. Within the institution, they could perceive their charges as abstractions, closely follow their symptoms, correlate symptoms with lesions, and compare the course of disease in one patient with other cases close by.[4] This seeming contradiction explains why conflicts between hospital trustees and physicians were muted. For much of the nineteenth century, the growth of science had more impact on medical perception than on therapeutics. Hospital practitioners might wish that their institutions devoted more beds to the more interesting acutely ill, and so excluded the chronically ill and debilitated, but their treatment did not challenge the dominant conception of good medicine. Even among the most scientifically attuned practitioners, medical treatment remained broadly defined; environmental manipulation—advice about career and family choices, and personal habits—was as much the province of the physician as any narrow, physiologically-oriented therapeutics. Hospital doctors and donors shared a view of their patients as moral and social beings. Further, the condition of the patient class seemed to cry out for social therapeutics.

Given its moral, social, and medical purposes, the hospital was a mixed blessing for its patients. For the poor and immigrants who supplied the bulk of the patients, the hospital's creature comforts were probably no worse— and presumably better—than what was available in their homes. But as was the case with other late nineteenth-century charities, the attitudes of those who controlled the institution toward their charges was not completely benign. The humane feelings of the social elite which supported and managed the hospital, and the medical elite which served it were lessened by the cultural and social distance that divided patient from patron and practitioner. It was within this context that the order and control necessary for the functioning of the hospital were instituted.

Herbert Gutman, in an essay on "Work, Culture, and Society in Industrializing America, 1815–1919," has shown how successive waves of immigrants had to be disciplined into the habits and virtues necessary for their industrial roles.[5] The same argument is made elsewhere for rural migrants and urban roles. The late nineteenth-century hospital provides an exaggerated example of this "disciplining" process. In Boston's hospitals, at least, the great majority of patients in the 1870s was of rural origin, largely foreign born, though also including Americans.[6] His often foreign origin tainted the hospital patient; so too did his reliance on charity. The continuing stream of literature about "medical abuse" addressed the fear that institutions were making free medical care so readily available that much of it was going to the "undeserving." No matter how much this literature might attempt to distinguish the worthy from the unworthy patient, the presumption remained that any hospital patient not paying his own way (that is, the great majority) was suspect.[7] Hospital rules reflected this interpretation of the patient. Rules instructed the patient to behave himself. Rude language was forbidden, as was card playing. When physicians made ward visits, patients were to sit up silently in bed. Severely restricted visiting hours limited the patient's contact with friends and family, potential sources of moral corruption. The high masonry walls surrounding hospital yards did the same. Necessary to enforce appropriate behavior within the institution, rules, practices, and even institutional design could result in petty tyrannies and oppressive discipline. While the sources for documenting patient response to the moralistic and authoritarian hospital regimen are limited, there can be little doubt that the interaction of lower class patients with upper class perceptions and proscriptions added to the discomfort of a hospital stay. Confronted by an environment he perceived as hostile, the hospital patient underwent an experience similar to that of the peasant in an industrializing society and the foreigner in a new country. But the hospital patient of the 1870s was often peasant and immigrant as well as patient. And in his status as patient he was injured or weakened, less able to protect himself than those in parallel roles who had their full strength. It is no wonder that contemporaries realized that hospital admission evoked a "dread" among the poor that the same kind of medical treatment outside the institution did not.[8] The hospital signalled that it was providing its patients with "favors to which they had not a shadow of a claim."[9]

The dependency role fostered by the hospital patient experience today is also degrading.[10] But it is not produced by the same institutional perception of the patient that prevailed in the mid-nineteenth century. The complementary medical and moral definitions of the patient became unsynchronized in the last decades of the nineteenth century. As medical science expanded the range of effective, narrowly medical therapies, broader, socially-oriented treatment modalities lost their professional legitimacy. A series of conflicts distrubed the voluntary hospital as physicians sought to recast the institution to fit their professional agenda. In the process of replacing the lay trustees as the dominant force in the management of the hospital, physicians lifted the burden of moralistic judgment from the patient class and replaced it with the weight of scientific absolutism.[11]

It is at this point that the independent history of the municipal hospital largely begins. At voluntary institutions, the conflict accompanying the shift in institutional rationale peaked in the last decades of the nineteenth century.[12] Medical domination—or at least lay acquiesence in medically established priorities—ensued. Contributing to this phenomenom was the broadening of the hospital's patient constituency to include the middle classes, for whom moral therapeutics were not as appropriate as medical and surgical intervention. Up to the late nineteenth century, the handful of city hospitals financed by public taxation had resembled their private counterparts more than they differed from them. Though the patients of public hospitals came from lower down on the socioeconomic scale than the patients of voluntary hospitals, the boards of institutions like Blockley, Bellevue, and Boston City Hospital had generally sought to have treatment at their institutions adhere to the same perception of the patient as a social being that obtained at voluntary hospitals. But in the closing decades of the century, municipal hospital trustees were caught between physicians and representatives of the patient class. Both groups questioned the almshouse tradition out of which the municipal hospital had grown. Physicians wanted to follow the lead of their colleagues at voluntary hospitals and establish a medical version of the earlier authoritarianism. Representatives of the patient class wished to continue the broad, socially-oriented definition of good medicine—but they advocated an end to the view of patients as morally suspect. At the same time that hospital physicians became increasingly aggressive in asserting their claims on the institution, political change raised a challenge to their authority at city hospitals.

In the closing decades of the nineteenth century, the hegemony of traditional American urban elites was challenged by new forces associated with the rising political power of ethnic groups. The political machines that resulted, while generally charged as corrupt, effectively championed the interests of the immigrant groups out of which they developed. The machines provided not simply jobs, but a cultural defense of the way of life and self-image of these urban peoples. Where once social and economic inferiors had either passively accepted or tolerated the discipline of their betters, the class- and ethnically-based political machine enabled them to resist and reshape the public city to their own needs. This new ethnic politics affected city hospitals no less than other urban institutions. It took issue with the political and medical upper class coalition that had held effective control over the municipal hospital. Both politics and professionalism had been extensions of the elite social order in the mid-nineteenth century, and hospital practitioners and political patricians of similar social origins had shared the same perceptions of the hospital patient class, and thus shared many of the same expectations of the institution's role. The first president of the Boston City Hospital was succinct in explaining how he thought that the hospital should relate to its patients: "Its decrees may often involve considerations not to be explained or communicated, and should be final without question or appeal."[13] The ethnic ward bosses, as political representatives of the hospital's patients, challenged the municipal hospital's identity as an instrument for grudging and inexpensive relief to the sick poor, an agency of social control, and an arena for the professional aspirations of elite physicians.

Ethnic politics forced a redefinition of the general hospitals most stigmatized by their association with the poorest patients. Since the growing responsiveness of municipal institutions to their patients coincided with the medical revolution and the legitimation of the hospital, ethnic politics was especially significant in recasting the institutional attitude of the hospital toward its traditional patient population. It is clear, in retrospect, that the lower classes did not share fully in the benefits of the redefined hospital; that, in other words, the hospital did not become a classless institution. It is also clear that some ethnic groups—those closest to the new politics— shared more fully than others. In the long run, the political challenge to medical domination failed. The hospital today is characterized by medical absolutism, but the demands of patients expressed through the political machines were not without impact. Partial successes gaining humane treatment for the poorest patients helped create the expectations against which many hospital patients today measure their treatment.

Hospital practitioners resisted attempts to shift authority over the municipal hospital away from the traditonal elite in the late nineteenth century. In Boston, city hospital physicians responded to the increased political assertiveness of representatives of the patient class by seeking state legislation to insulate the institution from the local political process. They were dissatisfied with the nine-member hospital governing board because it was drawn directly from the city council and hence contained some ward leaders. Fearful that new additions made to the board in 1879—an Irish Catholic and a Jew—boded ill for the future composition of the governing body, hospital practitioners sought to reform the board. They advocated a board appointed by the mayor, a figure responsible to a city-wide constituency and thus more respectable than the local bosses. The hope was that such a board would not be drawn from among the city's politicians, but would be composed of "gentlemen who have time . . . to devote to such an institution." The new board was to be smaller; its members were to serve staggered five-year terms rather than the one-year terms of the old board. Staggered terms precluded sudden change in board personnel or policy, minimizing the disruption that might be wrought by the political process. Longer terms of service would allow outsiders greater opportunity to identify with the institution and understand its needs—particularly the needs of its medical practitioners. The Massachusetts legislature, dominated by rural and small town Protestants, was sympathetic to Boston's traditional Protestant elite and incorporated Boston City Hospital in 1880.

The desire for incorporation manifested a siege mentality, an attempt to prevent newly potent political forces from defining the hospital in terms of its patients rather than in terms of the medical and social elite. It duplicated the process which in 1878 had removed the Boston Public Library from the control of the city council and put it under a blue ribbon mayoral board. An Irish witness testifying against change in the status of the hospital complained that the newly incorporated library board was serving as a model for the hospital reformers. He noted that the new library board had made proposals "the like of which have never been presented before. In the last annual report of the trustees they say there should be two libraries in two places, one where the literary men could frequent it, and one in another place—to use the words of the trustees—where the masses could go." According to the ethnic ward bosses, it was essential to the masses that the city hospital "be kept under the immediate control of the people." These democratic forces suffered a temporary setback in 1880. This was, however, less crippling a blow to the popular redefinition of the hospital than parallel changes in Boston's police department were to local control of that agency. In 1878, the legislature had removed the police from city council authority, and vested control in a mayoral board; in 1885, a state authority removed control of the police from Boston altogether.[14]

Because the hospital budget remained subject to city council appropriations, the influence of democratic politics on the management of the institution could not be wholly avoided.[15] Formal city council resolutions replaced the informal influence of overlapping council and governing board membership, making more visible (to the historian, at least) the intermediation of politicians representing their constituents before the hospital authorities. Fearing rejection when applying for admission, for example, potential patients carried letters from ward leaders or other persons they considered powerful or well connected. In some cases, elected officials personally contacted trustees—a difficult task, according to Alderman Martin Lomasney, both because Boston's upper classes had deserted other sections of the city for the Back Bay, and because they deserted the city entirely for summer vacations. In the face of mounting demands that patients pay something for their care, politicians broadened their patronage with requests to excuse individual patients from whatever charges the hospital might assess.[16] In securing admission or the remission of fees, ward leaders, in effect, duplicated the function of wealthy donors to voluntary hospitals. At the same time, politicians were more accessible and perceived as more benign than elite subscribers to hospital free-bed funds.

Those dissatisfied with the medical standards for hospital admissions also sought to use the political process and the weight of public opinion to change those policies. Opposition to the hospital's restrictive admissions policy sometimes crystallized around the difficulty encountered in gaining hospital admission for the inebriated or apparently drunk. The police, who often found themselves responsible for such cases, either could not secure their admission to the city hospital, or else did not attempt to do so. The police judged admission improbable on the basis of prior experience with medical admissions officers. Hospital practitioners objected that the admission of drunkards would clutter their wards and exclude medically significant cases. It was not uncommon for poor drunkards, picked up by the police, to die unattended in station house lockups. Such incidents might be followed by public investigations or inquests finding that obvious drunkenness had masked pneumonia or serious injury. Inebriates died in police custody when medical care might have saved their lives.[17] The poor were also suspicious of the use of the diagnosis of alcoholism as an excuse for withholding medical services, a suspicion reinforced by the way that legitimate medical complaints in an "unappealing" person might be mistaken for alcoholic stupor and denied hospital admission. As the incorporated governing board adopted increasingly restrictive admissions policies for Boston City Hospital in the 1880s, the city council sponsored investigations of individual cases and asked the trustees to consider changing their procedures to effect a more generous policy toward intoxicated persons who were injured or sick.[18]

The admissions policy was part of the larger issue of accessibility. By the 1890s, politicians had forced the hospital to consider whether the needs of medical practitioners or the demands of the public should determine the location of services and the hours of their availability. This had not heretofore been a seriously debated question. Hospital outpatient facilities, for example, were designed primarily to offer experience to young physicians and to serve as clinics for medical schools. Traditionally, hospitals had not taken into account the convenience of patients in setting the hours for outpatient care. In 1890, Boston City Hospital provided outpatient care between 9 and 11 A.M. on weekdays, for surgical cases, and between 9 and 11 A.M. on Tuesday, Thursday, and Saturday for medical cases, with specialty clinics on various weekday mornings. For those most likely to resort to outpatient care, attendance at a free clinic involved the loss of work and pay, and jeopardized job security. Confronted by demands for evening clinic hours, the trustees responded favorably, but sought the advice of the hospital staff before announcing their answer. The institution's senior physicians and surgeons urged a negative decision. The medical men noted that the real purpose of a clinic was instruction. An evening clinic, coming after the fatigue of a long day, would be useless for teaching and learning. In the end, the issue was compromised. Morning medical clinics were expanded from three to six days each week, and a new outpatient building, opened in 1897, housed interns available for emergencies on a twenty-four-hour basis.[19]

The 1890s witnessed a parallel discussion about the physical growth of the hospital. There was a consensus that the institution would respond directly to Boston's growth by growing along with the city, but this agreement did not extend to the site for hospital expansion. The city council, responding to local demands for small neighborhood facilities, asked the hospital trustees to develop a comprehensive plan for the institution's continued growth. The council favored a series of branches, or "cottage" hospitals in various areas of the city. The trustees turned the issue over to the medical staff for comment. Hospital practitioners advised that providing Boston's neighborhoods with basic, general practice services—medically uninteresting in themselves—would dissipate the scientific energies of the institution. Modern medicine and the specialization it implied required large centralized institutions. The hospital submitted to the city government a long-range plan that argued for the continued consolidation of hospital services at a single site.[20] Ultimately, the political system compromised this conflict as well. The hospital built and staffed two emergency relief stations: one, located in the central business district, at least promised the excitement of medically significant trauma; the other, in remote East Boston, was a medical Siberia through which junior physicians rotated, looking after runny noses and bandaging skinned knees.[21]

Clashes over admissions and accessibility highlighted differing perceptions of the hospital's role. Physicians might think one type of service appropriate to the institution, patients might prefer another. "Good medicine" as doctors understood it was sometimes not the supportive and personal care that the public seemed to want. When councilman William Whitmore had opposed incorporation in 1880, he had acknowledged these contradictory—and equally valid—conceptions of the hospital: the practitioners wanted "to make it a great institution, . . . to create a great scientific school and do other things in their own way"; Whitmore's constituents wanted "a simple charity [for] the poor needing it."[22]

There were other debates over how the hospital should serve its patients. In accident cases, for example, was the hospital to facilitate the victim's right to sue for damages, or was it to side with employers and property owners? The first inclination of the trustees was to benefit employers, or those who might be held responsible for accidents, by limiting the in-hospital activities of patients. When it was learned that lawyers and law students were "visiting patients with the purpose of instigating suits," the trustees ordered the superintendent to "take particular care to prevent others than friends visiting patients on visiting days."[23] These attorneys may have appeared unscrupulous in soliciting cases, but their ambulance-chasing activities could also promote settlements for injured patients who might otherwise not have pursued their claims with the same vigor.

While patients were constrained, those who might be called upon to defend their suits were not. Physicians, retained by insurance companies and employers to provide expert testimony, were free to consult the hospital's medical records to prepare cases. Though the surgical staff asked the trustees to restrict access to medical records to hospital staff members only, the action was undertaken not to secure the privacy of patients, but to further the monopoly of Boston City Hospital staff members on lucrative insurance company positions. The trustees complied.[24] When Dr. Edwin

Wells Dwight asked permission to consult the files to obtain information on behalf of the Employers Liability Insurance Company, he was refused; within a year he was appointed to the hospital staff, giving him and the company he represented unlimited access to all of the hospital's records.[25] Finally, popular pressure mounted by politicians representing immigrant wards caused a change in policy. The trustees informed the staff that "recent criticisms have been made relative to the alleged use of the Medical Records of the Hospital, by some members of the Medical and Surgical Staff, in matters of settlement and in suits in Court, and it has been said that this use has been more especially made against the interests of patients whose records are given." Patient records were ordered to be held confidential and released only by authority of the patient concerned, the trustees, or a subpoena. Doctors serving corporations in obtaining such information were told that such action was "inconsistent" with their holding hospital positions.[26]

Popular dissatisfaction did not end there. In 1909, Alderman James Michael Curley complained of the abuse that resulted from the employment of hospital doctors by insurance companies and corporations in the defense of accident claims. The problem did not lie with medical men making records available, but rather with the kind of entries which they made in those records. As Curley explained,

> Quite often, where a man, either in the employ of some public service corporation or while at work on a building, meets with an accident and is rendered unconscious it is customary to give him a little drink of brandy, and if it happens that the physician who attends him when he arrives at the hospital is in close touch with the corporations in whose employ the man has met with the accident it is customary to give him a little brandy in order to bring him around to consciousness and then to mark his card at the hospital "Alcoholism."

Physicians and surgeons did well under the system, receiving, Curley charged, large retainers and witness fees of fifty dollars a case from corporations (railroads and street railways, in particular). Patients suffered, however, as their cases were prejudiced by a medical record that indicated that they had been injured while intoxicated.[27] The trustees responded by changing the hospital rules to require that notation be made in the medical record if alcohol were administered to an accident case.[28]

In the case of patient records, regulations were tightened at the behest of patient spokesmen. In other areas, the same forces succeeded in loosening rules to benefit patients. This was most evident in the policy of visiting hours. During the debate over incorporation in 1880, advocates of a hospital responsive to the popular will contrasted the ease of access to patients at the city hospital with the situation at the Massachusetts General Hospital. Councilman P. F. McGaragle noted his constituents' feelings that "the latter was so private that one might as well attempt to get into the vaults of the savings banks as into it, even to see a friend." Before incorporation, the hospital trustees had already refused Sunday visiting, necessary if workingmen were to visit family and friends. But there was fear that an incorporated hospital board, like the incorporated library board which refused to open the public library on Sunday, would be even more adamant in refusing to accede to the request for Sunday visiting.[29]

Original policy allowed one visitor per patient every day, with visits to occur during one afternoon hour on each of four weekdays. Intensive city council pressures, in the 1880s and 1890s, led to a more generous policy. Two visitors were allowed each day, instead of one; the number of days with visiting hours was expanded from four to six; and city councilmen won the right to issue passes to admit visitors outside of regular hours. In 1902, the hospital instituted Sunday visiting and also added an early evening visiting period on weekdays.[30]

The hospital was further humanized by its increasing responsiveness to the wishes its users expressed through the political system. The trustees went along with a common council request that they no longer charge messenger fees for notifying relatives of the death of a patient. The trustees heeded the wishes of the board of aldermen in making it easier for relatives to collect corpses by reducing the waiting period after death and lengthening the hours during which bodies could be removed from the hospital. The rule against card playing was dropped, making it easier for patients to pass time in the hospital. When a Father Mahoney complained of some unspecified behavior of a hospital physician toward a patient, the trustees, increasingly sensitive to the Catholic community, ordered the physician discharged immediately. And when the Boston Central Labor Union complained that one of its members had received inadequate care at the outpatient department, the trustees arranged a meeting between representatives of the union and the staff. Though the trustees decided that most of the charges aired at the meeting were unsubstantiated, they did agree that the original complaint had merit and took steps to more closely monitor the work of the outpatient department and cut down the time that patients had to wait for medical attention.[31] To further safeguard the interests of the working classes, the Central Labor Union asked the mayor, in 1903, to appoint one of the city hospital trustees from the ranks of labor, for "inasmuch as working men are the chief patrons of the institution, they should have a voice in its managment." In practice, the board consisted of one physician, one lawyer, and three businessmen. Protecting the already tenuous position of the elite in the direction of the hospital, organized medicine opposed the labor union request: "The fallacy and possible danger of such a principle of representation is apparent."[32]

By the turn of the century, the very composition of the hospital elite, the professional staff, was no longer beyond the influence of the political system. In the same way that ward heelers had brought many of the hospital's workers under the patronage system (turning election day, St. Patrick's Day, and the Jewish high holidays into paid days off, in the process), city politicians championed the claims of certain kinds of practitioners for medical-staff appointments. As at most other hospitals in Boston, medical and surgical positions at the city hospital were dominated by Brahmin physicians in the nineteenth century. The use of Boston City Hospital for teaching purposes by the city's elite medical school at Harvard University emphasized the social composition of the institution's medical staff.

According to city hospital rules, new staff members were nominated by the senior staff and then appointed by the trustees. Trustees and politicians responsive to groups not usually represented in hospital staffs used their positions to encourage the nomination of physicians from these outside groups. By the 1890s, Jewish politicians were urging the claims of their medical coreligionists. The process had begun earlier with Irish politicians and Irish-Catholic medical men. Among the Irish there even appeared physician-politicos who used their personal involvement in city politics to advocate hospital appointments for themselves.[33] The advocacy of non-elite physicians by politicians helped to create among their own people a sense that the hospital was not an alien institution. The presence of Irish-Catholic and Jewish doctors made the hospital less threatening to others of those groups and reinforced their feeling that Boston City was the people's hospital.

The democratic process worked for medical schools no less than for individual practitioners. Because its medical staff was drawn from the city's elite practitioners in the nineteenth century, the city hospital staff contained a significant proportion of the Harvard Medical School clinical faculty. Harvard thus monopolized teaching opportunities at the hospital. By the mid-1880s women medical students, a homeopathic school, and other regular but less favored medical schools were petitioning that the hospital's wards be opened for clinical instruction on an equal basis. Over strenuous protests from the staff, these requests seem to have been granted, at least formally, on a limited basis. Instruction, however, remained under the control of the Harvard-dominated staff. Meager though this victory was, it contrasted starkly with the situation at the Massachusetts General Hospital. In an unsuccessful plea for a limited teaching affiliation with that institution, the Tufts Medical School felt compelled to volunteer the promise that none of its female or black students would enter the hospital.[34]

The changing needs of medical education in the twentieth century forced a more definite solution to the problem of medical school affiliation with the city hospital. As schools sought hospital services to which they could control appointments, the presence of Harvard men on the city hospital staff led naturally to arrangements for Harvard medical, surgical, and specialty teaching services in the hospital. Such special treatment for one school could not be defended. In the pursuit of additional staff appointments and its own clinical services, Tufts Medical School appealed to the trustees, in the name of justice. The Boston University School of Medicine, tainted by a homeopathic past, was less successful in direct requests to the hospital's governing board. But after mayoral intervention from James Michael Curley in 1930, all three schools had medical and surgical teaching services in the hospital.[35]

This manifestation of democracy—the equality of the local medical schools, at least in terms of the favors they could expect from the city government—was made possible by another expression of the same force. The hospital constructed new wards and spawned new services because it was forced to be responsive to demands from potential patients for institutional growth. The medical schools, acting within the democratic system as interest groups marshalling constituencies, were able to channel the public clamor for constant hospital expansion into building programs that fit the needs of medical school imperialism. Ultimately the city hospital reached a capacity of 2,500 beds, with an expensive duplication, and sometimes triplication, of facilities.

We have, in effect, identified the late nineteenth and early twentieth centuries as a "golden age" of sorts for the municipal hospital. This situation resulted from the fact that medical (and social) decisions previously (and in voluntary institutions then still) made by members of a medical and social elite were now made within the context of a political system increasingly responsive to the lower classes. One factor in the legitimation of the hospital as a community institution was the experience of municipal hospitals in undermining the image of hospital patients as a socially marginal, dependent class. This period of institutional development is associated with "machine politics." Political machines still exist; from the point of view of reformers, it is debatable whether municipal governments are any less corrupt now than they were at the beginning of the century. But municipal hospitals have changed. This change should be recognized as resulting, in part, from a metamorphosis in city politics.

Suburbanization, since the 1920s, has removed from the city the descendants of the municipal hospital's turn-of-the century patients. In Boston and Philadelphia, later generations of the immigrant groups to which the city hospital proved such a benefit no longer find the institution geographically convenient. Nor would it be perceived as socially appropriate for the more affluent to use an institution so thoroughly identified with the poor. The contemporary poor do form a substantial patient clientele for the city hospital. Forms of social insurance have enabled—but not forced—the contemporary poor to seek other institutions, particularly voluntary hospitals, for inpatient medical care. The reason that the city hospital has been abandoned, to some measure, by its natural patient constituency is to some degree political.

Suburbanization has had only minimal impact on the city's political leadership; certain ethnic groups may have left, but they have also left behind their leaders to lead others. Entrenched political organizations are much less responsive to Spanish-speaking and black constituencies than they were when more of an ethnic identity prevailed between leaders and electorates. The political organizations which still exist, like the city governments they dominate, have also lost much of their political power to the federal government, since the New Deal. City governments have allowed massive and aging hospital plants, swollen by the demands of medical schools and of patients, to deteriorate. While the costs of maintaining older hospitals have risen, the commitment to provide care has diminished. The failure of political change to keep pace with the changing social composition of the city, or, more accurately, the changing ethnic and racial composition of the classes that need help from the city, has doomed the city hospital. The nature of the institution's commitment to its patients has regressed to about the same point where it was when the patient class originally developed political power, and with it the power to reorient the hospital. Today's answer is to cut services, close wards and, as in the case of Philadelphia, abandon the city's general hospital function altogether.

NOTES

1. Arthur Ames Bliss, *Blockley Days: Memoirs and Impressions of a Resident Physician, 1883–1884* (privately printed, 1916), pp. 14, 59.
2. J. M. Toner, "Statistics of Regular Medical Associations and Hospitals of the United States," *Transactions of the American Medical Association* 24 (1873): 314–33. Toner counted 178 hospitals in his survey in 1873. But at least 58 of these

were insane asylums. Morris J. Vogel, "Patrons, Practitioners, and Patients: The Voluntary Hospital in Mid-Victorian Boston," in *Victorian America*, ed. Daniel Walker Howe (Philadelphia: University of Pennsylvania Press, 1976), pp. 121–38.

3. Charles E. Rosenberg, "Social Class and Medical Care in Nineteenth Century America: The Rise and Fall of the Dispensary," *Journal of the History of Medicine and Allied Sciences* 29 (1974): 40.

4. Erwin H. Ackerknecht, *Medicine at the Paris Hospital, 1794–1848* (Baltimore: Johns Hopkins University Press, 1967); Michel Foucault, *The Birth of the Clinic: An Archaeology of Medical Perception* (New York: Pantheon, 1973).

5. *American Historical Review* 78 (1973): 531–88.

6. Morris J. Vogel, "Boston's Hospitals, 1870–1930: A Social History," (Ph.D. diss., Univ. of Chicago, 1974), pp. 22, 43.

7. See, for example, [William Richards Lawrence], *Medical Relief to the Poor* (Boston: Rockwell and Churchill, 1877); Walker Gill Wylie, *Hospitals: Their History, Organization, and Construction* (New York: D. Appleton and Co., 1877); George S. Hale, "Medical Charities," *Proceedings of the National Conference of Charities and Corrections* 2 (1875): 52–66.

8. *Boston Medical and Surgical Journal* 86 (1872): 81–82.

9. *Boston Evening Transcript*, 21 November 1885.

10. Erving Goffman, *Asylums: Essays on the Social Situations of Mental Patients and Other Inmates* (Garden City, N. Y.: Doubleday Anchor, 1961).

11. Vogel, "Boston's Hospitals," chaps. 3, 4.

12. Charles Perrow, "Goals and Power Structure: A Historical Case Study," in *The Hospital in Modern Society*, ed. Eliot Freidson (New York: Free Press, 1963), pp. 112–46. Perrow dates this period from 1929. This different time sequence is due to his studying a new institution, founded in 1885, whose economic marginality resulted in trustee control into a later period.

13. Thomas C. Amory, Jr., "Address," in *Proceedings at the Dedication of the [Boston] City Hospital* (Boston: J.E. Farwell, 1865), p. 57. Much of the rest of this paper uses Boston as an extended example.

14. Boston, Mass., Boston City Document no. 27, 1880, "Majority and Minority Reports of the Committee on Ordinances on the Order Requesting the Mayor to Petition the Legislature for an Act Incorporating the Trustees of the City Hospital"; Walter Muir Whitehill, *Boston Public Library: A Centennial History* (Cambridge: Harvard University Press, 1956), pp. 107–12, 133; Roger Lane, *Policing the City: Boston, 1822–1885* (New York: Atheneum, 1975), pp. 180–219.

15. By the twentieth century that influence was consolidated, as the political machine was able to control city-wide elections in Boston.

16. See, in this regard, accounts by Martin Lomasney, Councilman Joseph Lomasney, and Alderman Keenan, *Proceedings of the Boston City Council*, 21 June 1888; 18 July 1892; 2 January 1904; 6 December 1909. Settlement workers, aware that the political boss provided some needed services, noted: "he must secure for the sick admission to the hospital." Robert A. Woods, ed., *Americans in Process: A Settlement Study* (Boston: Houghton Mifflin and Co., 1903), p. 174; For requests to excuse payment, Boston City Hospital, Trustees Manuscript Records, 27 October 1897.

17. See, for example, "Reform Needed: What was Shown in Regard to the City Hospital at one of Judge McCafferty's Inquests," *Boston Evening Transcript*, 18 May 1885: "There was evidence that death from the same cause [asphyxiation while unconscious] had occurred on several occasions, and that in such cases as Kelly's the patient would not be received at the City Hospital." Also, *Transcript*, 26 April 1886; 24 September 1889.

18. *Proceedings of the Boston City Council*, 21 and 24 May 1883.

19. Boston City Hospital, *33rd Annual Report, 1896–97*, pp. 19–20; *34th Annual Report, 1897–98*, p. 30; *Boston Medical and Surgical Journal* 139 (1898): 419; Boston City Hospital, Visiting Staff Manuscript Minutes, 9, 19 September, 23 October 1899; Boston City Hospital, Trustees Manuscript Records, 4, 25 October 1899. All Boston City Hospital manuscript records are in the hospital archives, Boston, Mass.

20. Boston City Hospital, *Report of the Trustees of the Boston City Hospital on the Advisability of Establishing Cottage or Branch Hospitals in the Several Wards of the City* (Boston: Rockwell and Churchill, 1893), passim.

21. Boston City Hospital, *39th Annual Report, 1902–03*, p. 25; *44th Annual Report, 1907–08*, pp. 30–31; *45th Annual Report, 1908–09*, p. 25.

22. *Boston Globe*, 20 February 1880.

23. Boston City Hospital, Trustees Manuscript Records, 18 June 1891.

24. Ibid., 22 March 1893.

25. Ibid., 21 February, 22 March, 19 December 1894.

26. Ibid., 29 March 1905.

27. *Proceedings of the Boston City Council* 6 December 1909.

28. Boston City Hospital, *52nd Annual Report, 1915–16*, p. 174.

29. Boston, Mass., Boston City Document no. 27, 1880, p. 96; *Boston Evening Transcript*, 22 February 1879.

30. *Proceedings of the Boston City Council*, 18 November 1880; 9 April 1886; 15 September, 25 October 1902; Boston City Hospital, Trustees Manuscript Records, 18 November 1885; 22 June 1892; 22 February 1893; 17 April 1895; 29 October, 18 November 1896; 25 May, 29 June 1898; 16 June, 27 August, 17 September, 15, 29 October 1902.

31. Boston City Hospital, Trustees Manuscript Records, 6 February 1901; 11 March, 22 April, 13, 27 May 1903; 31 August 1904; 15 March 1909; 26 March 1915.

32. *Boston Medical and Surgical Journal* 148 (1903): 220; *Proceedings of the Boston City Council*, 18 July 1892.

33. See Boston City Hospital, Visiting Staff Manuscript Minutes, 4 April, 11 July 1884; 30 March, 16 November 1896; 25 May 2 June, 1897; 10 January, 31 March, 9 May, 1898; Boston City Hospital, Trustees Manuscript Records, 13 October 1911; 19 March, 8 April 1912.

34. Boston City Hospital, Trustees Manuscript Records, 10 October 1886; Dr. William M. Conant to Dr. Richardson, November 1911, copy in medical education file, Massachusetts General Hospital Archives, Boston, Mass.

35. Boston City Hospital, Trustees Manuscript Records, 17 March 1916; 18 March, 2, 27 May, 21 November 1921; 8 September 1922; 7 December 1923; 15 August 1924; 23 September, 2, 16 December 1927; 2 March, 14 September 1928; 26 April 1929; 28 February 1930.

No third party must be permitted to come between the patient and his physician in any medical matter.

American Medical Association, 1934[1]

8

THE THIRD PARTY: Health Insurance in America

RONALD L. NUMBERS

American medicine, in the nineteenth century, was essentially a two-party system: patients constituted one party, and physicians the other. Medical practice was relatively simple, and doctors, more out of economic necessity than to preserve an intimate physician-patient relationship, personally collected their bills. Most practitioners billed their patients annually, or semi-annually, although those with office practices usually insisted on immediate payment.[2] They were not, however, always free to charge what they pleased. In many communities local medical societies established schedules of minimum fees and instructed members never to undercut their colleagues.[3] There was little objection to providing free care for the poor—or to overcharging the wealthy—but generally the American medical profession preferred fixed fees to the so-called "sliding scale."[4] When hospitals

A slightly different version of this essay appears in *Sickness and Health in America: An Overview,* ed. Judith Waltzer Leavitt and Ronald L. Numbers (Madison: University of Wisconsin Press; © 1978 by the Regents of the University of Wisconsin).

began to proliferate, late in the century, they, too, charged patients directly, according to fixed prices.

But even in the nineteenth century, a small (but undetermined) number of Americans carried some insurance against sickness through an employer, fraternal order, trade union, or commercial insurance company. Most of these early plans, however, were designed primarily to provide income protection, with perhaps a fixed cash benefit for medical expenses; few paid for medical care, and those that did, such as the plans sponsored by remotely located lumber and mining companies, generally contracted with physicians at the lowest possible prices. This type of "contract" practice restricted the patient's choice of physician, allegedly commercialized the practice of medicine, sometimes resulted in shoddy medical care—and always elicited the opposition of organized medicine.[5] During the latter half of the century, the American Medical Association (AMA) repeatedly condemned arrangements that provided unlimited medical service for a fixed yearly sum, and urged the profession to maintain "the old relations of perfect freedom between physicians and patients, with separate compensation for each separate service."[6]

Widespread interest in health insurance did not develop in the United States until the 1910s, and then the issue was compulsory, not voluntary, health insurance. During the late nineteenth and early twentieth centuries, rising costs and increased demands for medical care had prompted many European nations, beginning with Germany, in 1883, to provide industrial workers with compulsory health insurance.[7] Americans, however, paid little attention to these foreign experiments before 1911, when the British parliament passed a National Insurance Act.

Inspired by developments abroad, and by the spirit of Progressivism at home, the reformist American Association for Labor Legislation (AALL), in 1912, created a Committee on Social Insurance to prepare a model bill for introduction in state legislatures.[8] By the fall of 1915, this committee had completed a tentative draft, and was laying plans for an extensive legislative campaign. Its bill required the participation of virtually all manual laborers earning $100 a month or less, provided both income protection and complete medical care, and divided the payment of premiums among the state, the employer, and the employee.[9]

The medical profession's initial response to this proposal bordered on enthusiasm. Three progressive physicians—Alexander Lambert, Isaac M. Rubinow, and S. S. Goldwater—had served on the drafting committee, and for a brief period after the turn of the century, organized medicine was in a reform-minded mood. Upon receiving a copy of the AALL's bill, Frederick R. Green, secretary of the AMA's Council on Health and Public

Instruction, informed the bill's sponsors that their plan for compulsory health insurance was

> exactly in line with the views that I have held for a long time regarding the methods which should be followed in securing public health legislation. . . . Your plans are so entirely in line with our own that I want to be of every possible assistance.

Specifically, Green wanted to give the AALL "the assistance and backing of the American Medical Association in some official way," and he proposed setting up an AMA Committee on Social Insurance to cooperate with the AALL in working out the medical provisions of the bill.[10] As a result of his efforts, the AMA Broad of Trustees, early in 1916, appointed a three-man committee, with Lambert as chairman. He, in turn, hired Rubinow as executive secretary and set up committee headquarters in the same building with the AALL.

The *Journal of the American Medical Association* hailed the appearance of the model bill as "the inauguration of a great movement which ought to result in an improvment in the health of the industrial population and improve the conditions for medical service among the wage earners."[11] In the editor's opinion, "No other social movement in modern economic development is so pregnant with benefit to the public."[12] At the AMA's annual session in June 1916, President Rupert Blue called compulsory health insurance "the next step in social legislation,"[13] and Lambert, as chairman of the Committee on Social Insurance, presented a report that stopped just short of endorsing the measure.[14]

Physician support at the state level was similarly strong. In 1916, the state medical societies of both Pennsylvania and Wisconsin formally approved the principle of compulsory health insurance, and so did the Council of the Medical Society of the State of New York.[15] The reasons for favoring health insurance varied from physician to physician. According to the *Journal of the American Medical Association,* the most convincing argument was "the failure of many persons in this country at present to receive medical care";[16] but the average practitioner, who earned less than $2,000 a year, was probably more impressed by the prospect of a fixed income and no outstanding bills.[17] Besides, the coming of health insurance appeared inevitable, and most doctors preferred cooperating to fighting. "Whether one likes it or not," wrote the editor of the *Medical Record,*

> social health insurance is bound to come sooner or later, and it behooves the medical profession to meet this condition with dignity. . . . Blind condemna-

tion will lead nowhere and may bring about a repetition of the humiliating experiences suffered by the medical profession in some of the European countries.[18]

By early 1917, however, medical opinion was beginning to shift, especially in New York, where the AALL was concentrating its efforts. One after another of the county medical societies voted against compulsory health insurance, until finally the council of the state medical society rescinded its earlier endorsement.[19] Both friends and foes of the proposed legislation agreed on one point: the medical profession's chief objection was monetary in nature. As the exasperated secretary of the AALL saw it, the "crux of the whole problem" was that physicians were constantly hearing the lie that the model bill would limit them to twenty-five cents a visit, or about $1,200 a year.[20] "If you boil this health insurance matter down, it seems to be a question of the remuneration of the doctor," observed one New York physician, who believed that ninety-nine out of one hundred physicians had taken up the practice of medicine primarily "as a means of earning a livelihood."[21] Another New York practitioner, who opposed the AALL's bill, described all other objections besides payment as "merely camouflage for this one crucial thought." Medical opposition would melt away, he predicted, if adequate compensation were guaranteed.[22]

The medical profession was, of course, not alone in opposing compulsory health insurance. Commercial insurance companies, which would have been excluded from any participation, were especially critical; and some labor leaders, like Samuel Gompers, preferred higher wages to paternalistic social legislation.[23]

America's entry into World War I, in April 1917, not only interrupted the campaign for compulsory health insurance, but touched off an epidemic of anti-German hysteria. Patriotic citizens lashed out at anything that smacked of Germany, including health insurance, which was reputed to have been "made in Germany." As the war progressed, Americans in increasing numbers began referring to compulsory health insurance as an "un-American" device that would lead to the "Prussianization of America."[24]

Shortly before the close of the war, California voters, in the only referendum on compulsory health insurance, soundly defeated the measure by a vote of 358,324 to 133,858, and dampened the hopes of insurance advocates.[25] Their spirits revived briefly in the spring of 1919, when the New York State Senate passed a revised version of the model bill, but the bill subsequently died in the Assembly. By 1920, even the AALL was rapidly losing interest in an obviously lost cause.

As the prospects for passage of the model bill declined, the stridency of the doctors who opposed insurance increased. "*Compulsory Health Insur-*

ance," declared one Brooklyn physician, "is an Un-American, Unsafe, Uneconomic, Unscientific, Unfair and Unscrupulous type of Legislation [supported by] Paid Professional Philanthropists, busybody Social Workers, Misguided Clergymen and Hysterical women."[26] In 1919, he and other critics launched a campaign to have the AMA's House of Delegates officially condemn compulsory health insurance. They failed on their first attempt, but the following year the delegates overwhelmingly approved a resolution stating

> that the American Medical Association declares its opposition to the institution of any plan embodying the system of compulsory contributory insurance against illness, or any other plan of compulsory insurance which provides for medical service to be rendered contributors or their dependents, provided, controlled, or regulated by any state or the Federal Government.[27]

This repudiation of compulsory health insurance was not, as one writer has suggested, the result of "an abdication of responsibility by the scientific and academic leaders of American medicine."[28] Nor was it primarily the product of a rank-and-file takeover by conservative physicians disgruntled with liberal leaders.[29] The doctors who rejected health insurance in 1920 were by and large the same ones who had welcomed, or at least accepted it only four years earlier. Frederick Green, the person most responsible for the AMA's early support of compulsory health insurance, was, by 1921, describing it as an "economically, socially and scientifically unsound" proposition, favored only by "radicals," and his experience was not atypical.[30]

No doubt many factors contributed to such changes of heart. Opportunism undoubtedly motivated some, and the political climate surely affected the attitudes of others. But more important, it seems, was the growing conviction that compulsory health insurance would lower the incomes of physicians, rather than raise them, as many practitioners had earlier believed. With each legislative defeat of the model bill, the coming of compulsory health insurance seemed less and less inevitable, and the self-confidence of the profession grew correspondingly. "[T]his Health Insurance agitation has been good for us," concluded one prominent New York physician as the debate drew to a close. "If it goes no farther it will have brought us more firmly together than any other thing which has ever come to us."[31]

An additional factor affecting the medical profession's attitude toward compulsory health insurance was its recent experience with workmen's compensation, which was probably the most common form of health insurance in America from the 1910s to the 1940s. Beginning in 1911, many states passed laws making employers legally responsible for compensating workmen for on-the-job injuries, but few of the early compensation acts provided comprehensive medical benefits. During the war, however, most states added such provisions, or liberalized existing ones, giving American doctors their first taste of social insurance. For many, it was not pleasant. Employers often took out accident insurance with commercial companies, which either contracted with physicians to care for the injured or paid local practitioners according to an arbitrary fee schedule.[32] Neither arrangement pleased the medical profession, which complained that the shoddy treatments resulting from such practices "were akin to mayhem and murder."[33] It was evident from this experience, reported the AMA, that "pus and politics go together."[34]

In 1925, the New York State Medical Society reported that health insurance "is a dead issue in the United States. . . . It is not conceivable that any serious effort will again be made to subsidize medicine as the hand-maiden of the public."[35] The victorious New York physicians had every reason to be confident, but they failed to reckon with economic disaster. The Great Depression invalidated many assumptions about American society and threatened the financial security of both hospitals and physicians. Between 1929 and 1930 hospital receipts, per patient, declined from $236.12 to $59.26, and occupancy rates fell from 71.28 per cent to 64.12 per cent.[36] As the Depression continued, income from endowments and contributions decreased by nearly two-thirds, and the charity load almost quadrupled.[37] Particularly hard hit were the private voluntary hospitals, which had been expanding six times faster than the population.[38] The net income of physicians during the first year of depression dropped 17 per cent, with general practitioners suffering the biggest losses. In some regions, particularly the cotton-growing states, collections from patients fell 50 per cent, and the situation grew worse as the Depression continued.[39]

In response to this disaster, several hospitals began experimenting with insurance. Although not the first, the most influential of these experiments was the Baylor University Hospital plan, often described as the "father" of the Blue Cross movement. In December 1929, Baylor vice-president Justin F. Kimball, former superintendent of the Dallas public schools, enrolled 1,250 public school teachers, who paid fifty cents a month for a maximum of twenty-one days of hospital care, an arrangement consciously modeled after the prepayment plans used in the lumber and railroad industries.[40] The success of single-hospital insurance at Baylor and other places soon led to the development of multiple-hospital plans which included all hospitals in a given area. The first of these appeared in Sacramento, California, in 1932, and by 1937, when the American Hospital Association began approving such programs, there were twenty-six in operation, with 608,365 participating members.[41]

The motives behind these early endeavors are difficult to determine. In two recent studies of Blue Cross, for example, Odin W. Anderson stresses the altruistic spirit of the pioneers, while Sylvia Law emphasizes their economic interests.[42] There is, as one might expect, some evidence for both interpretations. Voluntary hospital insurance, said health-care reformer Michael M. Davis, in 1931, has "the double aim of furnishing a new and broader base of support for hospitals and of helping small income people to meet their big sickness bills."[43] Economic concerns are, however, easier to document than altruism. It is significant that although financially disinterested civic organizations occasionally contributed funds to establish hospital insurance programs, "in most cases the initiative and main drive for the starting of the various plans came from the hospitals of the community —from hospital administrators and trustees."[44] In his 1932 survey of prepayment plans, Pierce Williams concluded that hospitals had promoted insurance primarily "to put their finances on a sound basis."[45]

The reaction of physicians to these early experiments in hospital insurance was mixed. Those affected the most seemed pleased. A physician associated with a Grinnell, Iowa, plan described the attitude of local practitioners as "very cordial,"[46] and Kimball reported that Dallas doctors appreciated both the increased availability of hospital care for their patients and the fact that insurance got "the patient's hospital bill out of the way of the doctor's personal collections."[47] The AMA, however, was openly antagonistic, characterizing prepayment plans "as being economically unsound, unethical and inimical to the public interests."[48] According to the director of the association's Bureau of Medical Economics, such schemes were largely "a result of 'tactics of desperation,' in which hard-pressed hospitals are seeking 'any port in a storm.' "[49] The AMA's solution to the problem of financing health care was to urge people "to save for sickness."[50]

Despite these negative pronouncements, health insurance continued to grow—especially after the publication in 1932 of the final report of the Committee on the Costs of Medical Care. This group of between forty-five and fifty prominent Americans drawn from the fields of medicine, public health, and the social sciences set out in 1927 to ascertain the medical needs of the American people and the resources available to meet them. Ray Lyman Wilbur, a former president of the AMA, served as chairman, and over half of the members were physicians. At the end of five years of exhaustive study, funded by several philanthropic organizations, a majority of the committee, including the chairman, modestly recommended the adoption of group practice and voluntary health insurance as the best means of solving the nation's health care problems.[51]

But even this was too radical for eight of the physicians on the committee, who, with one other member, prepared a minority report denouncing "the thoroughly discredited method of voluntary insurance" as being more objectionable than compulsory health insurance. Health insurance, said the minority, would inevitably lead to the

> solicitation of patients, destructive competition among professional groups, inferior medical service, loss of personal relationship of patient and physician, and demoralization of the profession. It is clear that all such schemes are contrary to sound policy and that the shortest road to the commercialization of the practice of medicine is through the supposedly rosy path of insurance.

The dissenting doctors did, however, favor action to alleviate the financial plight of the medical profession, which was caused, in part, they felt, by the obligation to provide free care to the poor. Thus they recommended that the government relieve physicians of this unfair "burden" by assuming financial responsibility for the care of the indigent. The results of such a plan, they said, "would be far reaching." In particular, the income of physicians would increase, and young doctors would find it easier to begin the practice of medicine.[52]

Although some state medical societies (including those in Alabama and Massachusetts) endorsed the majority report,[53] and although more of the physicians on the committee had voted with the majority than with the minority, the AMA's House of Delegates declared, in 1933, that the minority report represented "the collective opinion of the medical profession." Group practice and health insurance, said the delegates, "would be inimical to the best interests of all concerned."[54] Morris Fishbein, the outspoken editor of the association's *Journal,* characteristically reduced the issue to "Americanism versus sovietism for the American people."[55] "The alinement is clear," he wrote:

> on the one side the forces representing the great foundations, public health officialdom, social theory—even socialism and communism—inciting to revolution; on the other side, the organized medical profession of this country urging an orderly evolution guided by controlled experimentation.[56]

The alignment may have seemed clear in 1932, but a revival of public interest in compulsory health insurance soon blurred it. In 1934, President Franklin D. Roosevelt appointed a Committee on Economic Security to draft legislation for a social security program, which, everyone assumed, would include health insurance. Pressure from organized medicine, however, forced the president to drop health care from the bill that he sent to Congress in 1935. Undaunted, progressive members of his administration continued to agitate for compulsory health insurance, and in 1938 they sponsored a National Health Conference in Washington. This event aroused great popular interest in a government-sponsored health program, resulting, the next year, in Senator Robert F. Wagner's unsuccessful bill to provide medical assistance for the poor, primarily through federal grants to the states.[57]

In view of these developments, the AMA reversed its position on voluntary health insurance, hoping that such action would quiet demands for a compulsory system. In 1937, the House of Delegates approved group hospitalization plans that confined "their benefits strictly to the facilities ordinarily provided by hospitals; viz., hospital room, bed, board, nursing, routine drugs."[58] A short time later the association began taking credit for promoting the growth of hospitalization insurance, which it had so bitterly opposed only a few years before.[59]

At the same time that it was giving its blessing to hospitalization insurance, the AMA was working out a physician-controlled plan to provide medical care insurance. In 1934, the House of Delegates took a tentative step in that direction by agreeing on ten principles to govern "the conduct of any social experiments." These included complete physician control of medical services, free choice of physician, the inclusion of all qualified practitioners, and the exclusion of persons living above the "comfort level." The delegates stopped short of endorsing health insurance and made a point of emphasizing the traditional view that medical costs "should be borne by the patient if able to pay at the time the service is rendered."[60]

In February 1935, shortly after the Committee on Economic Security reported to the president, the AMA House of Delegates met in special session—the first since World War I—to reaffirm its opposition to "all forms of compulsory sickness insurance." Recognizing the need to offer an alternative to government-sponsored insurance, the delegates encouraged "local medical organizations to establish plans for the provision of adequate medical service for all of the people . . . by voluntary budgeting to meet the costs of illness."[61] The language was vague, but the intention was clearly to foster the creation of medical insurance plans which would be controlled by medical societies.

In the aftermath of the National Health Conference of 1938, the AMA called a second special session on insurance. This time the House of Delegates approved the development of "cash indemnity insurance plans" for low-income groups, controlled by local medical societies.[62] By offering cash benefits instead of service benefits, physicians hoped to retain their freedom to charge fees higher than the insurance benefits, whenever it seemed appropriate.[63] In 1942, to meet competition from commercial insurance companies, the AMA took the final step of approving medical service plans.[64]

By the late 1930s, a number of local medical societies, particularly in the Northwest, had already organized "medical service bureaus," offering medical care for a fixed amount per year.[65] In 1939, the California Medical Association, in an effort to stave off compulsory state health insurance, established the first statewide medical service plan.[66] Seven years later, when the AMA created Associated Medical Care Plans, the precursor of Blue Shield, there were forty-three medical-society plans with a combined enrollment of three million members.[67] In most places, coverage was limited to low-income families, who would otherwise have been among those least able to pay physicians' fees.

The threat of "socialized medicine" was no doubt the most compelling reason why organized medicine decided to embrace health insurance. As the demand for compulsory health insurance grew, more and more physicians came to see voluntary plans as their "only telling answer to federalization and regimentation."[68] "[I]t is better to inaugurate a voluntary payment plan," advised the secretary of the State Medical Society of Wisconsin, "rather than wait for a state controlled compulsory plan."[69]

But fear of compulsory health insurance was not the only reason why the medical profession changed its mind. By the late 1930s, many physicians were also discerning potential benefits in health insurance.[70] A 1938 Gallup poll showed that nearly three-fourths of American doctors favored voluntary medical insurance, and over half were confident that it would increase their incomes.[71] Health insurance, predicted one Milwaukee physician, "would do away with the uncollectible accounts. . . . It would offer to the physician an opportunity of earning a living commensurate with the value of the service that he performs."[72] Furthermore, by paying for expensive services like X rays and laboratory tests, it would, physicians believed, enable them to practice a better quality of medicine.[73]

Once the profession recognized these possible benefits, it sought absolute control over medical service plans. In many states, physicians won the right to monopolize medical care insurance through special enabling acts, which critics ironically regarded as "un-American."[74] In other places, organized medicine tried to discourage physicians from participating in plans not sponsored by medical societies by threatening them with expulsion and denial of hospital privileges. In 1938, such heavy-handed tactics brought the AMA a federal indictment (and eventual conviction) for violation of antitrust laws.[75]

Despite a genuine concern for the welfare of their patients, doctors did not embrace health insurance primarily to assist the public in obtaining better medical care. In fact, throughout the 1930s, spokesmen for organized medicine repeatedly denied that health care in America was inadequate and attributed the good health of Americans to "the present system of medical practice," that is, to the traditional two-party system.[76] The physicians of Massachusetts may, as they claimed, have supported a medical service plan in recognition of "a problem in the distribution of the cost of decent medical care." But even in that progressive state, competition from consumer cooperatives was just as important.[77]

Proudly displaying the medical profession's stamp of approval, health insurance entered a period of unprecedented growth (see figure 1). By 1952, over half of all Americans had purchased some health insurance, and prepayment plans were being described as "the medical success story of the past 15 years."[78] Behind this growth was consumer demand, especially from labor unions; after World War II, the unions began bargaining for health insurance to meet rapidly rising medical costs that were making the prospect of sickness the "principal worry" of industrial workers. Following a 1948 Supreme Court ruling that health insurance benefits could be included in collective bargaining, "the engine of the voluntary health insurance movement," to use Raymond Munts' metaphor, moved out under a full head of steam. Within a period of three months, the steel industry alone signed 236 contracts for group health insurance, and auto workers were not far behind.[79]

Growth statistics, however, do not tell the whole story. Although most Americans did have some health insurance by mid-century, coverage remained spotty. In 1952, insurance benefits paid only 15 per cent of all private expenditures for health care (see figure 2). Besides, the persons most likely to be insured were employed workers living in urban, industrial areas, while the unemployed, the poor, the rural, the aged, and the chronically ill—those who needed it the most—often went uninsured.[80]

With voluntary plans failing to protect so many Americans, the perennial debate over compulsory health insurance flared up again. Encouraged by organized labor, the Social Security Board, in 1943, drafted a bill (named after its congressional sponsors, Senators Robert Wagner and James Murray and Representative John Dingell) providing health insurance to all persons paying social security taxes, as well as to their families. The time, however, was inauspicious. The Second World War was diverting the

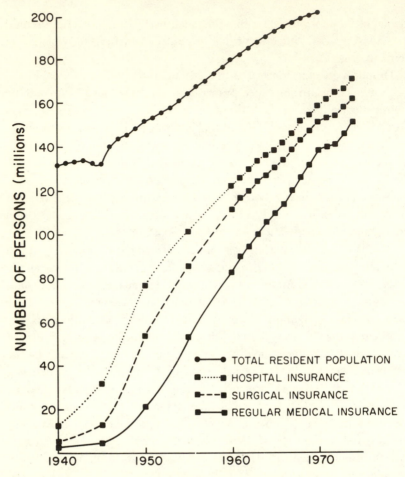

Figure 1. The growth in health insurance from 1940–1976.
Source: *Source Book of Health Insurance Data, 1975–76* (New York: Health Insurance Institute, 1976), p. 22; U.S. Bureau of the Census, *Historical Statistics of the United States: Colonial Times to 1970* (Washington: Government Printing Office, 1975), part 1, p. 8.

nation's attention to other issues, and without the president's active support, the bill died quietly in committee.[81]

Two years later, with the war over and Harry S. Truman in the White House, prospects for passage appeared much brighter. Since his days as a county judge in Missouri, Truman had been concerned about the health needs of the poor, and within a few weeks of assuming the presidency he decided to lend his support to the health insurance campaign. Following a strategy session with the president, Wagner, Murray, and Dingell reintroduced their bill, this time adding dental and nursing care to the proposed benefits.[82]

These developments terrified the AMA, which viewed the Wagner-Murray-Dingell bill as the first step toward a totalitarian state, where American doctors would become "clock watchers and slaves of a system."[83] To head off passage of such legislation, the AMA, in 1946, began backing a substitute bill, sponsored by Senator Robert A. Taft, which authorized federal grants to the states to subsidize private health insurance for the indigent.[84]

The basic problem, as the association's spokesman Morris Fishbein defined it, was one of "public relations." The medical profession had "to convince the American people that a voluntary sickness insurance system . . . is better for the American people than a federally controlled compulsory sickness insurance system."[85] Actually, most Americans needed little convincing. A 1946 Gallup poll showed that only 12 per cent of the public favored extending Social Security to include health insurance, and more individuals thought the Wagner-Murray-Dingell proposal would have a negative effect on health care than believed that it would be beneficial.[86]

Truman's surprise victory in 1948, at the close of a campaign that featured health insurance as a major issue, convinced the AMA that it was

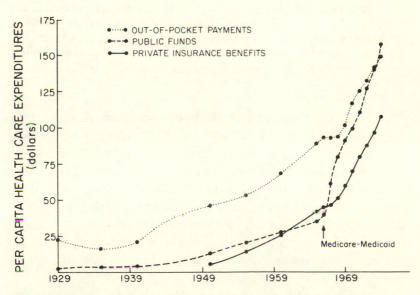

Figure 2. Sources of per capita health care expenditures, 1929–74. Source: Nancy L. Worthington, "National Health Expenditures, 1929–74," *Social Security Bulletin* 38 (February 1975): 16.

time to declare all-out war. Shortly after the election returns were in, the House of Delegates voted to assess each member twenty-five dollars to raise a war chest for combatting "socialized medicine," which was defined as "a system of medical administration by which the government promises or attempts to provide for the medical needs of the entire population or a large part thereof."[87] Within a year $2,250,000 had been raised, and the public relations firm of Whitaker and Baxter was putting it to effective use in an effort to "educate" the American people. The showdown came in 1950, when organized medicine won a stunning victory in the off-year elections, forcing many candidates to renounce their earlier support of compulsory health insurance and defeating "nearly 90 percent" of those who refused to back down.[89]

Throughout this controversy, representatives of organized medicine insisted that the country did not need compulsory health insurance, just as they had insisted in the early 1930s that voluntary insurance was unnecessary. "There is no health emergency in this country," said a complacent AMA president in 1952. "The health of the American people has never been better."[90] If some individuals could not afford proper medical care, it was probably the result of self-indulgence, rather than genuine need:

> Since one out of every four persons in the United States has a motor car, one out of two a radio, and since our people find funds available for such substances as liquors and tobacco in amounts almost as great as the total bill for medical care, one cannot but refer to the priorities and to the lack of suitable education which makes people choose to spend their money for such items rather than for the securing of medical care.[91]

What Americans needed, said the doctors, was more voluntary insurance, which had worked out so well that most physicians, by the early 1950s, no longer thought coverage should be restricted to low-income groups.[92] The financial and political benefits of this kind of health insurance were so great that the medical profession jealously protected it. When rumors began circulating that some surgeons were doubling their fees to insured patients, the AMA called for an immediate crackdown. "Voluntary prepayment plans are the medical profession's greatest bulwark against the socialization of medicine," said one official. "This program must not be jeopardized by avaricious physicians."[93]

The election of a Republican administration, in 1952, effectively ended the debate over compulsory health insurance, and organized medicine breathed a sigh of relief. "As far as the medical profession is concerned," wrote the AMA president, "there is general agreement that we are in less danger of socialization than for a number of years. . . . We have been given the opportunity to solve the problems of health in a truly American way."[94] The "American way," it went without saying, was the way of voluntary health insurance.

The Eisenhower years indeed proved to be tranquil ones for the medical profession. Encouraged by their physicians and by the constantly rising costs of medical care, an increasing number of Americans purchased health insurance, until by the early 1960s nearly three-fourths of all American families had some coverage (see figure 1). Still, this paid for only 27 per cent of their medical bills, and many citizens, especially the poor and the elderly, had no protection at all.[95]

This problem led Representative Aime Forand, in the late 1960s, to reopen the debate over compulsory health insurance with a proposal for a program limiting coverage to Social Security beneficiaries. In 1960, Senator John F. Kennedy introduced a similar measure in the Senate.[96] To organized medicine, even such restricted coverage amounted to "creeping socialism,"[97] and the AMA would have none of it. The association's "strongest objection" continued to be that "it is unnecessary and would lower the quality of care rendered"—the same argument it had been using since the 1910s. Its only concession was to approve a government plan providing assistance to "the indigent or near indigent," which would benefit physicians as much as the poor.[98] Thus in 1960, Congress, with AMA approval, passed the Kerr-Mills amendment to the Social Security Act granting federal assistance to the states to meet the health needs of the indigent and the elderly who qualified as "medically indigent."

If the medical profession hoped to forestall the coming of compulsory health insurance by this small compromise, Senator Kennedy's election to the presidency that fall soon convinced them otherwise. Upon occupying the White House, he immediately began laying plans to extend health-insurance protection to all persons on Social Security, whether "medically indigent" or not. The AMA denounced his plans as a "cruel hoax" that would disrupt the doctor-patient relationship, interfere with the free choice of physician, impose centralized control, and—worst of all—undermine the financial incentive to practice medicine. National health insurance would not only endanger the quality of medical care, but would discourage the best young people from entering medicine.[99] Despite these ominous predictions, Congress, in 1965, voted to include health insurance as a Social Security benefit (Medicare) and to provide for the indigent through grants to the states (Medicaid). Thus, after fifty years of debate, compulsory health insurance finally came to America.

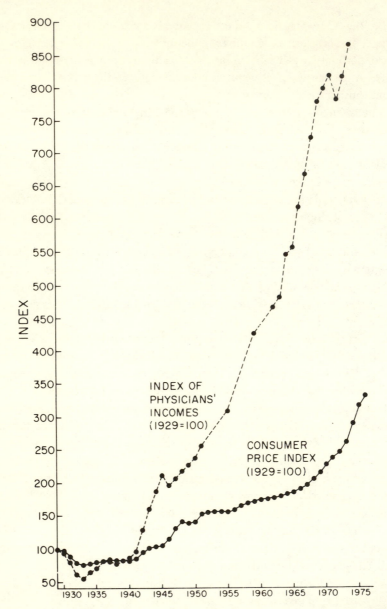

Figure 3. Comparison of physicians' incomes with the consumer price index, 1929–75.

Source: *Historical Statistics of the United States: Colonial Times to 1970* (Washington: Government Printing Office, 1975), 1: 175–76, 210–11; *Statistical Abstract of the United States: 1975* (Washington: Government Printing Office, 1975), p. 77; *Medical Economics* 37 (24 October 1960): 40, and 52 (10 November 1975): 184; U.S. Bureau of Labor Statistics, *Consumer Price Index, 1971–76.* Graph prepared by Lawrence D. Lynch.

In 1967, just two years after the passage of the Medicare bill, third parties, for the first time, paid more than half of the nation's medical bills.[100] Many Americans continued to be without health insurance coverage, but seldom by choice.[101] Although critics frequently attacked the health-insurance industry, no one advocated returning to a two-party system. In the opinion of one observer, the acceptance of health insurance was a phenomenon "without parallel in contemporary American life."[102] Prepayment plans benefited both providers and consumers of medical care —but especially the providers.

Hospitals, the pioneers of voluntary health insurance, profited from the start. In 1947, Louis Reed reported that hospital administrators agreed unanimously that insurance plans had reduced their volume of free care and had increased revenues.[103] In the years between 1939 and 1951, the amount of charity care provided by Philadelphia hospitals, for example, fell from 60 per cent to 24 per cent.[104] Later, in the 1960s and 1970s, the windfall from Medicare and Medicaid enabled many hospitals to improve —or at least to expand—their facilities.

Health insurance also proved advantageous to physicians, especially in financial terms. In the period following the development of medical service plans, their incomes climbed dramatically (see figure 3); and, according to some analysts, the "most significant factor" contributing to this increase was third-party payments, which rose from 15.5 per cent to nearly 50 per cent of physicians' incomes in the two decades between 1950 and 1969.[105] Proving a cause-and-effect relationship is difficult, but the testimony of physicians themselves supports this view. In 1957, for example, over half of the doctors in Michigan reported increased incomes as a result of prepaid medical care, with small town physicians and general practitioners registering the greatest gains. The most frequently cited explanations were that the programs provided better bill collecting and attracted more patients.[106]

Certainly there can be little doubt that Medicare and Medicaid benefited the medical profession handsomely. In fact, Robert and Rosemary Stevens concluded that "it seemed to be the physicians who gained the most."[107] After complaining for years that compulsory health insurance would beggar the profession and reduce the financial incentive to practice medicine, physicians discovered the results to be just the opposite. In the first year under Medicare the rate of increase in physician fees more than doubled (from 3.8 per cent to 7.8 per cent), while the rate of increase of the Consumer Price Index rose only from 2.0 per cent to 3.3 per cent.[108] A 1970 Senate Finance Committee investigation turned up at least 4,300 individual physicians who had received $25,000 or more from Medicare in 1968, and 68 of these had gotten over $100,000 each. Although most of this money was earned fairly, reports of questionable practices abounded. Some physicians allegedly saw patients more often than necessary, billed for care never given, and, on occasion, even resorted to the notorious "gang visit," charging $300 or $400 for one cursory sweep through a hospital ward or nursing home.[109] Such flagrant abuses prompted the president of one local medical society to warn his colleagues "to quit strangling the goose that can lay those golden eggs."[110]

Compared with the relatively tangible benefits of health insurance for hospitals and physicians, those to patients are more difficult to calculate. Prepayment plans undeniably gave Americans greater access to medical care than ever before, eased the financial strain of paying medical bills, and brought peace of mind to millions of policyholders. A grateful public showed its appreciation by buying increasingly comprehensive coverage. But it is not certain that the policyholders enjoyed better health for it. On the one hand, there are studies showing that "those who were eligible for Medicaid were likely to have better health than similar groups who were not."[111] But other studies indicate that although Medicare apparently encouraged more expensive types of treatment, like surgery, rather than radiation, for breast cancer, recovery rates remained roughly the same.[112]

Under health insurance from 1941 to 1970, life expectancy at birth in America did increase from 64.8 years to 70.9 years.[113] But again, it is hard to determine how much, if any, of this should be credited to improved medical care, much less to the way in which it was financed. By the early 1970s, even organized medicine was downplaying the ability of the medical profession to prolong life and preserve health. As Max H. Parrott, of the AMA testified in 1971, choice of lifestyle had become as important as medical care in determining the nation's health: "No matter how drastic a change is made in our medical care system, no matter how massive a program of national health insurance is undertaken, no matter what sort of system evolves, many of the really significant, underlying causes of ill health will remain largely unaffected."[114] In a society in which heart disease, cancer, accidents, and cirrhosis of the liver all ranked among the top ten killers,[115] it was indeed unrealistic to expect health insurance to cure the nation's ills.

NOTES

1. Minutes of the Eighty-Fifth Annual Session, 11–15 June, 1934, *Journal of the American Medical Association* 102 (1934): 2200.

2. D. W. Cathell, *The Physician Himself and What He Should Add to His Scientific Acquirements,* 3d ed. (Baltimore: Cushings and Bailey, 1883), pp. 16, 175–76; Charles Rosenberg, "The Practice of Medicine in New York a Century Ago," *Bulletin of the History of Medicine* 41 (1967): 229–30.

3. George Rosen, *Fees and Fee Bills: Some Economic Aspects of Medical Practice in Nineteenth Century America,* Supplement No. 6, *Bulletin of the History of Medicine* (Baltimore: John Hopkins Press, 1946).

4. Jeffrey Lionel Berlant, *Profession and Monopoly: A Study of Medicine in the United States and Great Britain* (Berkeley: University of California Press, 1975), pp. 101–2.

5. Pierce Williams, *The Purchase of Medical Care through Fixed Periodic Payment* (New York: National Bureau of Economic Research, 1932); Jerome L. Schwartz, "Early History of Prepaid Medical Care Plans," *Bulletin of the History of Medicine* 39 (1965): 450–75.

6. *1846–1958 Digest of Official Actions: American Medical Association* (Chicago: American Medical Association, 1959), pp. 121–22.

7. For a summary of the European experience, see Richard Harrison Shryock, *The Development of Modern Medicine* (New York: Hafner Publishing Co., 1969), pp. 381–402.

8. This account of the first American debate over compulsory health insurance is based on my *Almost Persuaded: American Physicians and Compulsory Health Insurance, 1912–1920* (Baltimore: John Hopkins University Press, 1978).

9. *Health Insurance: Standards and Tentative Draft of an Act* (New York: American Association for Labor Legislation, 1916).

10. Green to J. B. Andrews, 11 November 1915, American Association for Labor Legislation Papers, Cornell University, Ithaca, N.Y.

11. "Industrial Insurance," *Journal of the American Medical Association* 66 (1916): 433.

12. "Cooperation in Social Insurance Investigation," ibid., pp. 1469–70.

13. Rupert Blue, "Some of the Larger Problems of the Medical Profession," ibid., p. 1901.

14. Report of the Committee on Social Insurance, ibid., pp. 1951–85.

15. Proceedings of the Medical Society of the State of Pennsylvania, 18–21 September 1916, *Pennsylvania Medical Journal* 20 (1916): 135, 143; Proceedings of the House of Delegates, State Medical Society of Wisconsin, 5 October 1916, *Wisconsin Medical Journal* 15 (1916): 288; Minutes of the Council, Medical Society of the State of New York, 9 December 1916, *New York State Medical Journal* 17 (1917): 47–48.

16. "Social Insurance in California," *Journal of the American Medical Association* 65 (1915): 1560.

17. Income statistics are scarce for this period, but a 1915 survey of physicians and surgeons in Richmond, Virginia, showed that "the very large proportion of physicians were earning less than $2,000," and income tax records for Wisconsin, in 1914, indicate that the average income of taxed physicians was $1,488. Committee on Social Insurance, *Statistics Regarding the Medical Profession,* Social Insurance Series Pamphlet No. 7 (Chicago: American Medical Association, n.d.), pp. 81, 87.

18. "Opposition to the Health Insurance Bill," *Medical Record* 89 (1916): 424.

19. Report of the Committee on Legislation, *New York State Journal of Medicine* 17 (1917): 234.

20. J. B. Andrews to New York members of the AALL, 3 November 1919, AALL Papers.

21. "A Symposium on Compulsory Health Insurance Presented before the Medical Society of the County of Kings, Oct. 21, 1919," *Long Island Medical Journal* 13 (1919): 434. George W. Kosmak made the statement.

22. M. Schulman to J. B. Andrews, 22 February 1919, AALL Papers.

23. See Gompers's testimony before the *Commission to Study Social Insurance and Unemployment: Hearings before the Committee on Labor, House of Representatives, 64th Congress, First Session, on H.J. Res. 159, April 6 and 11, 1916* (Washington: Government Printing Office, 1918), p. 129.

24. See Roy Lubove, *The Struggle for Social Security, 1900–1935* (Cambridge: Harvard University Press, 1968), pp. 66–90.

25. On the California debate, see Arthur J. Viseltear, "Compulsory Health Insurance in California, 1915–18," *Journal of the History of Medicine and Allied Sciences* 24 (1969): 151–82.

26. "A Symposium on Compulsory Health Insurance . . . ," p. 445. John J. A. O'Reilly made the statement.

27. Minutes of the House of Delegates, *Journal of the American Medical Association* 74 (1920): 1319.

28. John Gordon Freymann, "Leadership in American Medicine: A Matter of Personal Responsibility," *New England Journal of Medicine* 270 (1964): 710–15.

29. Elton Rayack, *Professional Power and American Medicine: The Economics of the American Medical Association* (Cleveland: World Publishing Co., 1967), pp. 143–46. For a similar view, see Carleton B. Chapman and John M. Talmadge, "The Evolution of the Right to Health Concept in the United States," *Pharos* 34 (1971): 39.

30. Green, "The Social Responsibilities of Modern Medicine," *Transactions of the Medical Society of the State of North Carolina,* 1921, pp. 401–3.

31. Henry Lyle Winter, "Social Insurance," *New York State Journal of Medicine* 20 (1920): 20.

32. On the early history of workmen's compensation in America, see Harry Weiss, "The Development of Workmen's Compensation Legislation in the United States" (Ph.D. diss., University of Wisconsin, 1933); and Lubove, *The Struggle for Social Security,* pp. 45–65.

33. Bureau of Medical Economics, *An Introduction to Medical Economics* (Chicago: American Medical Association, 1935), p. 80.

34. Committee on Social Insurance, *Workmen's Compensation Laws,* Social Insurance Series Pamphlet No. 1 (Chicago: American Medical Association, [1915]), p. 60.

35. Report of the Committee on Medical Economics, *New York State Journal of Medicine* 25 (1925): 789.

36. Sylvia A. Law, *Blue Cross: What Went Wrong?* 2d ed. (New Haven: Yale University Press, 1976), p. 6. According to the *Journal of the American Medical Association,* the percentage of occupied beds in nongovernmental hospitals declined from 64.6 per cent to 63.2 per cent between 1929 and 1930: "Hospital Service in the United States," the *Journal of the American Medical Association* 100 (1933): 892.

37. J. T. Richardson, *The Origin and Development of Group Hospitalization in the United States, 1890–1940,* University of Missouri Studies, vol. 20, no. 3 (Columbia: University of Missouri, 1945), p. 12.

38. "Hospital Service in the United States," pp. 892–94.

39. Maurice Leven, *The Incomes of Physicians: An Economic and Statistical Analysis,* Committee on the Costs of Medical Care, Publication No. 24 (Chicago: University of Chicago Press, 1932), pp. 76–81. The fraction of California doctors earning less than $6,000 a year rose from approximately one-half, in 1929, to three-fourths, in 1933; Arthur J. Viseltear, "Compulsory Health Insurance in

California, 1934–1935," *American Journal of Public Health* 61 (1971): 2117.

40. J. F. Kimball, "Group Hospitalization," *Transactions of the American Hospital Association* 33 (1931): 667–68; J. F. Kimball, "Prepayment Plan of Hospital Care," *Bulletin of the American Hospital Association* 8 (1934): 42–47; Odin W. Anderson, *Blue Cross Since 1929: Accountability and the Public Trust* (Cambridge, Mass.: Ballinger Publishing Co., 1975), pp. 18–19.

41. Louis S. Reed, *Blue Cross and Medical Service Plans* (Washington: Government Printing Office, 1947), pp. 10–12.

42. Anderson, *Blue Cross Since 1929*, pp. 29–44; Law, *Blue Cross*, pp. 6–8. Anderson quotes one pioneer, J. Douglas Colman, as saying that "all this notion that it was going to solve the financial problems of hospitals was farthest from their [the Blue Cross founders'] minds." But Colman himself became involved with prepayment plans because hospitals might have to close without them: "An Interview with J. Douglas Colman," *Hospitals* 39 (1965): 45–46.

43. Michael M. Davis, "Effects of Health Insurance on Hospitals Abroad," *Transactions of the American Hospital Association* 33 (1931): 585. At the same meeting where Davis read this paper, the president of the AHA called for insurance as a partial answer to the problem of decreasing occupancy rates; idem., pp. 195–97.

44. Reed, *Blue Cross*, pp. 13–14.

45. Williams, *The Purchase of Medical Care*, p. 219.

46. Letter from E. E. Harris, 10 December 1930, quoted ibid., p. 238.

47. Kimball, "Prepayment Plan of Hospital Care," p. 45.

48. *1846–1958 Digest*, p. 313.

49. R. G. Leland, "Prepayment Plans for Hospital Care," *Journal of the American Medical Association* 100 (1933): 871. For similar expressions, see the address of president-elect Dean Lewis, Minutes of the Eighty-Fourth Annual Session, 12–16 June 1933, idem., p. 2021, and the editorial "Hospital Insurance and Medical Care," idem., p. 973.

50. *1846–1958 Digest*, p. 313.

51. *Medical Care for the American People: The Final Report of the Committee on the Costs of Medical Care*, Committee on the Costs of Medical Care, Publication No. 28 (Chicago: University of Chicago Press, 1932), pp. v–viii, 120.

52. Ibid., pp. 164–65, 171–72. The committee's study of the incomes of physicians revealed that "the average volume of free work furnished by physicians throughout the country is only 5 per cent of the total." Leven, *The Incomes of Physicians*, p. 66.

53. Oliver Garceau, *The Political Life of the American Medical Association* (Hamden, Conn.: Archon Books, 1961), p. 138.

54. Minutes of the Eighty-Fourth Session, 12–16 June 1933, *Journal of the American Medical Association* 100 (1933): 48.

55. "The Report of the Committee on the Costs of Medical Care," ibid., 99 (1932): 2035.

56. "The Committee on the Costs of Medical Care," ibid., p. 1952.

57. The fullest account of this second debate over compulsory health insurance is Daniel S. Hirshfield, *The Lost Reform: The Campaign for Compulsory Health Insurance in the United States from 1932 to 1943* (Cambridge: Harvard University Press, 1970). But see also Roy Lubove, "The New Deal and National Health," *Current History* 45 (August 1963): 77–86, 117; Edwin E. Witte, *The Development of the Social Security Act* (Madison: University of Wisconsin Press, 1962); Arthur J. Altmeyer, *The Formative Years of Social Security* (Madison: University of Wisconsin Press, 1966); and James G. Burrow, *AMA: Voice of American Medicine* (Baltimore: Johns Hopkins Press, 1963), pp. 185–252.

58. Minutes of the Eighty-Eighth Annual Session, 7–11 June 1937, *Journal of the American Medical Association*, 108 (1937): 2219.

59. Minutes of the Special Session, 16–17 September 1938, ibid. 111 (1938): 1193.

60. Minutes of the Eighty-Fifth Annual Session, 11–15 June 1934, ibid. 102 (1934): 2199–2201.

61. Minutes of the Special Session, 15–16 February 1935, ibid. 104 (1935): 751.

62. Minutes of the Special Session, 16–17 September 1938, ibid. 111 (1938): 1216; *1846–1958 Digest*, pp. 321–22. At this session black physicians representing the National Medical Association pledged to join the struggle against compulsory health insurance, even though it might not be in the best interest of their race. *Journal of the American Medical Association* 111 (1938): 1211–12.

63. Nathan Sinai, Odin W. Anderson, and Melvin L. Dollar, *Health Insurance in the United States* (New York: Commonwealth Fund, 1946), pp. 64–65.

64. Minutes of the Ninety-Third Annual Session, 8–12 June 1942, *Journal of the American Medical Association* 119 (1942): 728.

65. Reed, *Blue Cross*, pp. 136–46.

66. Viseltear, "Compulsory Health Insurance," pp. 2115–26; Arthur J. Viseltear, "The California Medical-Economic Survey: Paul A. Dodd versus the California Medical Association," *Bulletin of the History of Medicine* 44 (1970): 151. Although the second debate over compulsory health insurance took place primarily on the national level, many compulsory health insurance bills were also introduced in state legislatures. See Carl W. Strow and Gerhard Hirschfeld, "Health Insurance," *Journal of the American Medical Association* 128 (1945): 871.

67. Anderson, *Blue Cross Since 1929*, p. 54.

68. R. L. Novy, "In Retrospect: Changing Attitude of the Medical Profession," *Journal of the Michigan State Medical Society* 49 (1950): 708. See also George Farrell, "Development of Voluntary Nonprofit Medical Care Insurance Plans," *New York State Journal of Medicine* 57 (1957): 560–64.

69. J. G. Crownhart, "The Economic Status of Medicine," *Wisconsin Medical Journal* 33 (1934): 230. I wish to thank Jennifer Latham for her assistance in locating this, and other documents relating to health insurance in Wisconsin.

70. E. Minihan and T. Levi, of the University of Wisconsin, develop this point in their unpublished paper, "The Political Economy of Health Care Financing: The Foundation for Medical Care in Wisconsin" (April 1975), pp. 22–23.

71. George H. Gallup, *The Gallup Poll: Public Opinion, 1935–1971*, 3 vols. (New York: Random House, 1972), 1: 107.

72. James C. Sargent, "Shall Medicine Be Socialized?" *Wisconsin Medical Journal* 32 (1933): 562. See also Donald K. Freedman and Elinor B. Harvey, "Development of Voluntary Health Insurance in the United States," *New York State Journal of Medicine* 40 (1940): 1704.

73. Reed, *Blue Cross*, p. 230.

74. "Wisconsin Cooperative Association Assails State Medical Society," *Wisconsin Medical Journal* 45 (1946): 3.

75. *The United States of America, Appellants, vs. The American Medical Association . . . Appellees* (Chicago: American Medical Association, 1941).

76. Minutes of the Ninetieth Annual Session, 15–19 May 1939, *Journal of the American Medical Association* 112 (1939): 2295–96. See also the comments of president-elect J. H. J. Upham, Minutes of the Eighty-Eighth Annual Session, 7–11 June 1937, idem., 108 (1937): 2132.

77. James C. McCann, "Medical Service Plans," ibid. 120 (1942): 1318.

78. President's Commission on the Health Needs of the Nation, *Building America's Health*, 5 vols. (Washington: Government Printing Office, [1952]), 1: 43; 2: 257.

79. Raymond Munts, *Bargaining for Health: Labor Unions, Health Insurance,*

and Medical Care (Madison: University of Wisconsin Press, 1967), pp. 10–12, 49, 250. See also Frank G. Dickinson, "The Trend Toward Labor Health and Welfare Programs," *Journal of the American Medical Association* 133 (1947): 1285–86.

80. President's Commission on the Health Needs of the Nation, *Building America's Health,* 1: 43; 2: 253–54; Reed, *Blue Cross,* pp. 28, 119; Sinai, Anderson, and Dollar, *Health Insurance,* pp. 57–58, 73; Odin W. Anderson and Jacob J. Feldman, *Family Medical Costs and Voluntary Health Insurance: A Nationwide Survey* (New York: McGraw-Hill, 1956), pp. 14–20.

81. Altmeyer, *The Formative Years,* p. 146; Peter A. Corning, *The Evolution of Medicare: From Idea to Law* (Washington: Government Printing Office, 1969), pp. 53–55.

82. Monte Mac Poen, "The Truman Administration and National Health Insurance" (Ph.D. diss., University of Missouri, 1967), pp. 54–63.

83. "The President's National Health Program and the New Wagner Bill," *Journal of the American Medical Association* 129 (1945): 950–53. See also "Senator Wagner's Comments," idem, 128 (1945): 667–68.

84. Burrow, *AMA,* p. 347.

85. Fishbein, "The Public Relations of American Medicine," *Journal of the American Medical Association* 130 (1946): 511.

86. Gallup, *The Gallup Poll,* 1: 578; see also, 2: 801–4, 862–63, 886.

87. *1846–1958 Digest,* p. 331; Minutes of the Interim Session, 30 November– 1 December 1948, *Journal of the American Medical Association* 138 (1948): 1241; "A Call to Action against Nationalization of Medicine," idem., pp. 1098–99; "Reply by Officers and Trustees," idem. 139 (1949): 532. AMA officers later referred to this action as "American Medicine's Declaration of Independence"; Report of Coordinating Committee, idem. 147 (1951): 1692.

88. Burrow, *AMA,* pp. 361–64.

89. R. Cragin Lewis, "New Power at the Polls," *Medical Economics* 28 (January 1951): 76.

90. John W. Cline, "The President's Page: A Special Message," *Journal of the American Medical Association* 148 (1952): 208.

91. "A Call to Action against Nationalization of Medicine," ibid. 138 (1948): 1098. This comment was made in response to the Federal Security Administrator's statement that millions of Americans could not afford proper medical care. See Oscar R. Ewing, *The Nation's Health: A Report to the President* (September 1948).

92. Odin W. Anderson, *The Uneasy Equilibrium: Private and Public Financing of Health Services in the United States, 1875–1965* (New Haven: College and University Press, 1968), p. 140.

93. John W. Cline, "The President's Page: A Special Message," *Journal of the American Medical Association* 148 (1952): 1036.

94. Louis H. Bauer, "The President's Page," ibid. 150 (1952): 1675.

95. Ronald Andersen and Odin W. Anderson, *A Decade of Health Services: Social Survey Trends in Use and Expenditure* (Chicago: University of Chicago Press, 1967), pp. 75, 109, 153. See also Ethel Shanas, *The Health of Older People: A Social Survey* (Cambridge: Harvard University Press, 1962).

96. On the events leading up to Medicare, see Max J. Skidmore, *Medicare and the American Rhetoric of Reconciliation* (University, Ala.: University of Alabama Press, 1970), pp. 75–95.

97. J. H. Houghton, "President's Message to the House of Delegates," *Wisconsin Medical Journal* 64 (1965): 208.

98. "New Drive for Compulsory Health Insurance," *Journal of the American Medical Association* 172 (1960): 344–45. See also Edward R. Annis, "House of Delegates Report," idem. 185 (1963): 202.

99. Donovan F. Ward, "Are 200,000 Doctors Wrong?" ibid. 191 (1965):

661–63; *The Case against the King-Anderson Bill (H.R. 3820)* (Chicago: American Medical Association, 1963), pp. 17, 118–19.

100. Nancy L. Worthington, "National Health Expenditures, 1929–74," *Social Security Bulletin* 38 (February 1975): 13–14.

101. Estimates of the number of uninsured in the early 1970s varied between 17 and 41 million; see Marjorie Smith Mueller, "Private Health Insurance in 1973: A Review of Coverage, Enrollment, and Financial Experience," *Social Security Bulletin* 38 (February 1975): 21. The liklihood of a family's having health insurance corresponded directly with income. Over 90 per cent of families earning above $10,000 in 1970 carried hospital insurance, for example, while less than 40 per cent of families with incomes under $3,000 had it. Cambridge Research Institute, *Trends Affecting the U.S. Health Care System* (Department of Health, Education, and Welfare Publication No. HRA 76–14503; Washington: Government Printing Office, 1976), p. 188.

102. President's Commission on the Health Needs of the Nation, *Building America's Health* 4: 43.

103. Reed, *Blue Cross*, p. 230.

104. President's Commission on the Health Needs of the Nation, *Building America's Health*, 5: 390–91.

105. John Krizay and Andrew Wilson, *The Patient as Consumer: Health Care Financing in the United States* (Lexington, Mass.: Lexington Books, 1974), p. 111. During the 1960s, physicians' incomes increased faster than those of other professionals, including chief accountants, attorneys, chemists, and engineers; idem., p. 109.

106. *An Opinion Study of Prepaid Medical Care Coverage in Michigan* (Michigan State Medical Society, 1957), p. 140.

107. Robert Stevens and Rosemary Stevens, *Welfare Medicine in America: A Case Study of Medicaid* (New York: The Free Press, 1974), p. 191. "One unforeseen result of Medicare and Medicaid," say the Stevenses (p. 194), "was that in formalizing the system of doctors' charges by developing profiles of the 'usual and customary' fees prevailing in each area, some physicians became aware of what others were charging. Quite clearly, there was some 'standardizing-up'. . . ."

108. Theodore R. Marmor, *The Politics of Medicare* (London: Routledge and Kegan Paul, 1970), p. 89.

109. *Medicare and Medicaid: Problems, Issues, and Alternatives,* Report of the Staff to the Committee on Finance, U.S. Senate (Washington: Government Printing Office, 1970), pp. 9–10, 13.

110. Quoted in Stevens and Stevens, *Welfare Medicine in America*, p. 197.

111. Ibid., p. 202.

112. Victor R. Fuchs, *Who Shall Live: Health, Economics, and Social Change* (New York: Basic Books, 1974), pp. 94–95.

113. U.S. Bureau of the Census, *Historical Statistics of the United States: Colonial Times to 1970*, 2 vols. (Washington: Government Printing Office, 1975), 1: 55. The great gains came before the 1960s; between 1961 and 1970, life expectancy increased only from 70.2 to 70.9, and actually decreased slightly for black males.

114. *National Health Insurance Proposals: Hearings before the Committee on Ways and Means, House of Representatives, Ninety-Second Congress, First Session on the Subject of National Health Insurance Proposals, Oct.–Nov., 1971* (Washington: Government Printing Office, 1972), p. 1950.

115. Monroe Lerner and Odin W. Anderson, *Health Progress in the United States, 1900–1960* (Chicago: University of Chicago Press, 1963), p. 16.

9
ISABEL HAMPTON AND THE PROFESSIONALIZATION OF NURSING IN THE 1890s

JANET WILSON JAMES

In the fall of 1889 a young woman in Chicago and another in Baltimore took up jobs which were to have a major impact in the interlocking worlds of social welfare and health care, as well as on the status of women. Jane Addams opened the doors of Hull House; Isabel Hampton took charge of the new school for nurses at the Johns Hopkins Hospital, which had opened the previous spring. At the time, Miss Hampton and her training school were more in the public eye. The Johns Hopkins Hospital, sixteen years in the planning and building, was widely expected to inaugurate a new era in medical research and education, as well as in hospital construction, administration, and patient care. Miss Addams and her project for a social settlement had become somewhat familiar to Chicagoans but were unknown outside the city. Time was to reverse the spotlight. Today Jane Addams is a historical figure of the first rank, while Isabel Hampton, who led the movement that still continues for the professional independence of a major occupation for women, is buried in seldom-read histories of nursing to be found only in nursing school libraries.

Hampton's relative obscurity owes something to the fact that her effort took place within a social structure over which she had little control, and hence was only partly successful. Jane Addams, on the other hand, was an entrepreneur in what her contemporaries called philanthropy, who independently fashioned an institution. Yet the two had much in common. Both were feminists of a nondoctrinaire sort, who, in their girlhood of the 1870s, had absorbed some sense of the opportunities appearing in the world outside the confines of the Victorian home. Evading marriage, each cast about for wider spheres of influence. Industrial society at the time was beginning to institutionalize women's traditional domestic functions, both economic and nurturing. Without much risk of criticism, women willing to try something new in an urban setting could be guardians of culture in libraries, uplift the poor in charity organizations and settlement houses, or nurse sick paupers in hospitals that were being made safe and respectable through sanitary reform. Jane Addams determined to "study medicine and 'live with the poor,' "[1] but lost her enthusiasm for science in medical school and found another way to benefit the lowly. The less affluent Isabel Hampton fled from teaching district school into nursing and discovered a struggling new women's field without standards or leadership.

The Johns Hopkins Hospital Training School for Nurses was Hampton's opportunity. In the hospital, professionalization was in the air, and feminism was politely knocking at the gate. A group of well-to-do Quaker women in Baltimore, several of them daughters of the trustees, had enlisted friends in other eastern cities together with a number of well-known female physicians in an ambitious effort to secure funds for establishing the long-awaited Johns Hopkins University School of Medicine. The ladies attached two conditions: that entrance standards be raised, above those in existence anywhere else, and that admission be open to women. The conditions were not so welcome as the money. The first caused the medical staff a moment of panic. Yet the central purpose of the Hopkins plan had always been to raise the standards of the medical profession and medical care through the striking example of a hospital which should function as a laboratory for teaching and research; it was not hard for them to raise their sights a bit higher. The second condition occasioned more misgivings, for they had not envisioned women as part of the select company who would lead the way into modern medicine.[2]

After the fund had reached the $100,000 mark, the hospital trustees gave a luncheon for the donors. The speaker was Dr. Mary Putnam Jacobi of New York, whose professional attainments surpassed those of all other medical women and most medical men of her day. Dr. Jacobi declared that two ruling ideas animated her group—one, that medical education was "an intellectual matter," and the profession "not a mere trade, to be practiced for pecuniary profit"; the other, that "women are to participate to the full in this intellectual aspect of medicine."[3] The luncheon was held at the Nurses' Home at the hospital, where everyone met on common ground, so to speak, for on the propriety of training women as nurses, all were agreed.[4] A training school had been a feature of the farsighted plans for the hospital from the beginning, at a time when no such schools existed in the United States except in a few women's hospitals staffed by women physicians. Such a school, constituting a skilled labor force of apprentices directed by experienced head nurses and a woman superintendent, was an essential part of the concept of the modern hospital as defined by Florence Nightingale, along with pavilion-style wards, and elaborate provision for hygiene, through sanitation and ventilation. A model of hospital design, the Johns Hopkins was prepared to set the pace for the training of nurses, also.

This intention was clear at the ceremony inaugurating the training school in October 1889. "A large and distinguished audience" was on hand, including the mayor of Baltimore, James Cardinal Gibbons (archbishop of this oldest American diocese), President Daniel Coit Gilman of the Johns Hopkins University and Mrs. Gilman, hospital trustees and medical staff, several superintendents of nursing schools from Philadelphia hospitals, and the Sister Superior of Baltimore's Mount Hope Retreat, together with about a hundred interested local ladies. Isabel Hampton hailed the progress of nursing ("of the various professions opened to women during the past few years, none have made more sure and rapid growth nor met with greater public favor than that of the Trained Nurse"). She pointed out that the Hopkins school had already attracted women of "superior attainments," and promised that "as the University and Hospital are looked to from all quarters for what is best in science, so . . . this School may be looked to for what is best in nursing." The hospital's superintendent, Dr. Henry M. Hurd, assured the gathering that in this training school, "service in the Accident Department and in the Dispensary; in the Medical, Surgical, Gynaecological and Pay Wards" would be accompanied by "carefully devised courses of study and systematic mental training. . . . In the eyes of the Trustees," he added, "nursing the sick is not to be considered a trade but a learned profession."[5]

The speakers' emphasis on the word "profession" is striking, since the question of whether nursing is a profession in any strict sense of the word is still moot today. It is true that the term, then as now, was commonly applied to vocations which, if less exacting and autonomous than medicine, for example, could be considered equally altruistic. Hurd and Hampton could simply have been indulging in rhetoric intended to enhance the status of nursing. Nor did the term, in 1889, have today's sociological denotations; medicine itself had not become a profession in the full modern sense.

On the other hand, the speakers had the confident air of heralds of progress, and the place and the company gathered there were significant. At Johns Hopkins, President Gilman had created the American prototype of the modern university, with its research orientation and its facilities for graduate training. Thus he was already a prime mover in shaping modern professional standards and distinctions. At the request of the hospital trustees, the majority of whom also served as trustees of the university, Gilman had personally set up the hospital's administration and sought out its key personnel, including Dr. Hurd and Miss Hampton. Furthermore, if the female fund-raisers for the prospective medical school succeeded with their plan, the school's entrance requirements would set new standards for the medical profession. At the same time, admission of women medical students would be a striking advance for their sex.

Looking back at that day from the viewpoint of our own, one may wonder why there was no thought at Johns Hopkins of bringing the training of nurses into the university structure at some level. The social psychologist Anselm Strauss calls this "a curious paradox," although he correctly observes that not even Isabel Hampton envisioned such a connection for nursing.[6] To imply, however, that the group at Hopkins refused to seize a genuine opportunity for the advancement of nursing and women is to raise a false issue and one that distracts attention from the real significance of the plans for the training school. College education for nurses (as for 95 per cent of the American population) was not a social necessity in 1889, any more than it was for teachers, who constitute a more appropriate reference group than physicians. The training school was and would remain a part of the hospital, not of the university. But the Johns Hopkins was to be a new kind of hospital, in which patient care would be closely related to medical teaching and research. The nurses would be part of a community of science, and the elaborate ceremony opening the school signified a deep interest in and high expectations for this important department of the new institution. The talk of professionalism was not idle. The major impetus for the professionalization of nursing in the United States was to come, in the decade of the 1890s, from the Johns Hopkins training school and its successive women administrators, with some assistance from their male associates.

Lavinia Dock, who was Isabel Hampton's assistant superintendent of nurses at Johns Hopkins, learned from hard experience, and from the example of British nurses of her generation, the peculiar problems of professionalization in her field. Dock's nursing career made her a feminist, and the themes of independence, autonomy, and self-determination resound through her account of what the historian today might call the "modernization" of nursing.[7] She knew well the tension, classic in the modern history of health care, between efforts to raise standards of education and practice on the one hand, and, on the other, the controls exerted over women by society in general, and over nurses by the medical and hospital professions. In the early years at Johns Hopkins this tension had somewhat abated, and the atmosphere was unusually favorable to professional growth. We must begin, therefore, by separating out the historical elements in that atmosphere.

The hospital and the school had their roots in Baltimore's Quaker community, and its traditions of humanitarianism and the equality of the sexes. Both the founder, Johns Hopkins, and Francis T. King, president of the board of trustees, had a lifetime interest in medical charities. Hopkins, a survivor of the cholera epidemic of 1832, had retained from that experience a shocked memory of the dearth of medical and nursing care and hospital facilities. For many years he and King served on the board of the Maryland Hospital in Baltimore. They were therefore acquainted with the state of such institutions in mid-century America: charitable shelters for the sick poor, where "nursing" was a low-paid, low-status job for laboring class women, who, over a twelve-hour day, attended to the physical needs of the patients while doing the heavy domestic work on the wards. In 1867 Hopkins, King, and the other board members reported that the hired nurses at the Maryland Hospital lacked "method, order, invention, or energy" and were not "sufficient in number or intelligence to perform their duties." That was the year when Hopkins secured an act incorporating a new hospital and set up its board of trustees, with King at the head. To found this institution and a university, he left his fortune of $7 million, the largest sum any American had yet bequeathed for philanthropic purposes. In his final letter of instructions, written in March 1873, Hopkins made it clear that a "training school for female nurses" was to be established "in connection with" the hospital, a facility intended, in his sober words, to "compare favorably" with the best in Europe or America.[8]

Behind the specifications of Hopkins's letter lay not only his own experience as a local hospital trustee but some lessons of recent history. The mortality from disease among soldiers in the Crimean War and the American Civil War had drawn public attention both to glaring deficiencies in army hospital and medical care and to the capabilities of women in organizing at least partial remedies—from the towering figure of Florence Nightingale to America's lesser heroines in hospital service and in the work of the Sanitary Commission. It seems likely, from his choice of words, that Hopkins had in mind the model training school for nurses which Miss Nightingale had established in 1860 at St. Thomas's Hospital in London. The school had certain feminist aspects. Except for orders regarding the care of patients, the Nightingale plan rejected medical administration of nursing services in favor of an independent, women's nursing organization, the training school, "connected with" the hospital but having its own funds, a separate nurses' home, and a lady superintendent. The Nightingale model thus in a sense restored to women, in a secular framework, a measure of the autonomy they had lost in Protestant countries with the decline of the religious nursing orders.[9] In response, nursing in England had begun to regain status and to attract more intelligent and dedicated women. One may surmise that this reform made a strong appeal to Hopkins and King. After Hopkins's death, King journeyed to England in 1875 to see the Nightingale school at first hand. He had "lengthy interviews" with Miss Nightingale and after his return sat "night after night" (as his daughter recalled) talking about her work.[10]

Meanwhile other Americans in large cities, activated by the same concerns, and led by women veterans of wartime volunteerism, had also been studying the training school at St. Thomas's. In 1873, the first three American "Nightingale schools" for nurses opened in connection with hospitals in New York, Boston, and New Haven. As King and his fellow trustees (the majority of them also Quakers) carefully proceeded with the planning and construction of the Johns Hopkins Hospital over a period of fifteen years, they were able to observe the progress of these pioneering experiments.

At Bellevue in New York, for instance, "pupil nurses" replaced the "hired nurse" of a former day. These trainees, recruited from "a better class of women" and working under the direction of a woman superintendent, did give the patients more humane and conscientious care, and introduced cleanliness and order into institutions where these had been lacking. Nevertheless, the long hours, heavy work, and working class image hung on. The "training" was mostly hard experience under scanty supervision by the superintendent and by head nurses who were themselves only second-year students. Once a week, in the evening, after twelve hours or longer on the wards, the nurses were exposed to an elementary lecture by a physician; as a young lecturer at the Bellevue Medical School, Dr. William H. Welch, who would become chief of pathology at Hopkins, had delivered such talks to classes of weary young women hardly able to keep awake. In the second year of training school, "pupils" were sent out to nurse in private homes, their pay going into the school or hospital treasury. At the end of the two-year course they "graduated" and left the hospital for a career of live-in private duty nursing, caring mostly for obstetrical or "fever" (typhoid or pneumonia) cases in the homes of those sufficiently well-to-do to afford such a luxury.

The Bellevue training school produced most of the nursing leaders of the next generation, including Hampton and Dock; it also inspired them to strenuous efforts toward more radical improvements. The school's founders had done their best, but even the combined resources of this group of aristocratic women, most of them veterans of war relief work who had turned to reforming public charities in New York, could raise standards no further. Municipal officials and the medical staff were satisfied with things as they were. The pupils, receiving room and board and a meager wage called an "allowance" for personal expenses, provided nursing service at low cost. The more visible abuses of the old system had been removed, and the quality of nursing service was adequate, especially for a patient population whose medical care was an act of charity. The greater respectability of the pupil nurses, and the glamor shed upon nursing by Florence Nightingale, concealed from the public, from hospital administrators, and from the pupils themselves the fact that they were as much an exploited female labor force as the old hired nurses had been.

In planning the nursing for the Johns Hopkins Hospital, its trustees began afresh, rethinking nursing in the context of a new kind of institution. As their chief medical adviser they chose John Shaw Billings, of the United States Army Medical Corps. Essentially a sanitarian of the Nightingale era, Dr. Billings was convinced that buildings were the key to the problem. Not only would correctly designed structures eliminate contagion and cross-infection, but in a hospital intended "to assist in educating physicians, in training nurses, in promoting discoveries in medicine," they would also attract "proper and suitable persons to be the soul and motive power of the institution" by providing a favorable environment for growth.[11]

As an admirer of Miss Nightingale's principles of hospital design, Billings had supposed that her training school for nurses would also provide the model for the school at Hopkins. But a tour of hospitals all over Europe, followed by an inspection of the American schools and a study of the literature on the subject (almost all of it "favorable to . . . the Nightingale system"), completely changed his mind. The essentially feminist plan of the Nightingale school he found personally exasperating and administratively unsound. He could not advise the trustees "to establish an independent female hierarchy, which will consider from the very commencement, that one of its main objects is to endeavor to be independent of all males, who are to be considered as the natural enemies of the organization." The superintendent of nurses would have her hands full "teaching the women how to nurse"; she should report to the hospital authorities.[12]

As an army man Billings was accustomed to nursing by hospital orderlies; he was reluctant to see nursing become an entirely female occupation and would have liked the trustees to "try the experiment of training a few, say half a dozen male nurses."[13] Nevertheless he agreed that in general women made better nurses and had no doubt that "an educated, properly trained female nurse," in many cases "as important to the success of treatment as a competent doctor," was essential "in a properly conducted hospital ward."[14] On this ground all could agree.

One problem remained, and Billings, not given to beating around the bush, approached it directly. Promiscuous sex had been part of the folklore surrounding the hired nurse, but Florence Nightingale and the women advocates of trained nursing believed that the superior character of the trained nurse would banish immorality from the wards. Billings, remarkably free of the conventional Victorian assumptions about female sexuality, was skeptical. "If a female nurse is a properly organized and healthy woman," he declared, "she will certainly at times be subject to strong temptation under which occasionally one will fall, and this occurs in all hospitals in which women are employed without any exception whatever."[15]

Billings now returned to the drawing board. To "remove opportunities" for temptation as much as was practicable, the nurses' quarters would be located not in the hospital but, as Miss Nightingale advised, in a separate home, though on the hospital grounds. Francis King was insistent that the home be "a model of excellence and of sanitary perfection." Billings exerted himself and produced "a large and handsome building," as he described it at the hospital's opening exercises, "separated from the others, and exclusively appropriated to the female nurses, where each can have her comfortable room," along with "a common parlor, library, dining-room, bath-rooms, and, in short, the arrangements of a first-class hotel. . . . The intention is that when the nurse has finished her . . . tour of duty with the sick, she shall come quite away from the ward and all that pertains to it, and take her rest and recreation in a totally different atmosphere."[16]

Such surroundings could be expected to attract women qualified to be nurses not only for the new medicine but for an expanded patient population. It was already evident that with increased powers of healing, hospitals in the future would no longer be merely charitable shelters for the sick poor but centers of scientific care for all. Voluntary hospitals had always made some provision for the upper classes—travelers, for instance, who might fall ill in a strange city. Following Johns Hopkins's wish, Dr. Billings included "special accommodations" for "pay and private patients" in his earliest plans. Fourteen years later, when the hospital opened, he took pains to assure the well-to-do "that when they are afflicted with certain forms of disease or injury they can be better treated in a properly appointed hospital than they can be in their own homes, no matter how costly or luxurious these may be."[17]

Though Billings's rejection of independent status may have been a loss for the training school, Daniel Coit Gilman's plan for the administration of the hospital proved a gain. As Dr. William Osler told the story, the manager of the Fifth Avenue Hotel in New York, a friend of Gilman's, gave him a tour of its operations, from which he emerged with the idea of organizing the hospital "in departments, with responsible heads, and over all a director," each unit being "the exact counterpart of one of the sub-divisions of any great hotel or department-store."[18] The training school thus acquired an equal standing among components of the hospital that served to enhance the superintendent's authority.

There remained the major administrative appointments, for the head of the training school and the director of the hospital. Gilman's choice for the latter post, Dr. Henry M. Hurd, was an experienced administrator of asylums for the insane. Dr. Hurd cared about the quality of hospital life. Though he was in agreement with Billings on the importance of "strict accountability for the performance or neglect of duty," he had a distaste for the stiff military approach. To Hurd the prime consideration was "the development of kindly instincts and humane methods of thought among all employés." Discipline ought to be "sustaining in its nature and calculated to develop the individual." Far from a mere "avocation, a trade, a preparation for getting a living," the nursing of the sick should be infused with "sympathy, kindly feeling, enthusiasm and personal interest," the nurse "happy and contented in her chosen calling."[19]

As a man of science, however, Hurd saw other aspects of the nurse's role besides nurturing. He had realized from the beginning that the school "must inevitably feel the influence of the great University to which the Hospital is so nearly allied."[20] Soon after his appointment, the trustees despatched him on a tour of training schools in Boston, New York, New Haven, and Philadelphia. He returned with the recommendation "that careful attention should be given to the more purely intellectual part of the nurse's training," with studies "systematized and extended beyond what is at present attempted in any existing school."[21] Sympathetic from the beginning to nurses' aspirations, Dr. Hurd became a willing speaker at training schools graduation exercises, on which occasions he was wont to assay the professional status of nursing and urge a forward step. His description at the opening of the Hopkins school of "the hands of the nurse" as "a physician's hands *lengthened out* to minister to the sick" was to become a favorite quotation of Isabel Hampton's when explaining her profession to the public.

For the post of superintendent of the training school there had been "scores of applicants," including the heads of most of the major existing

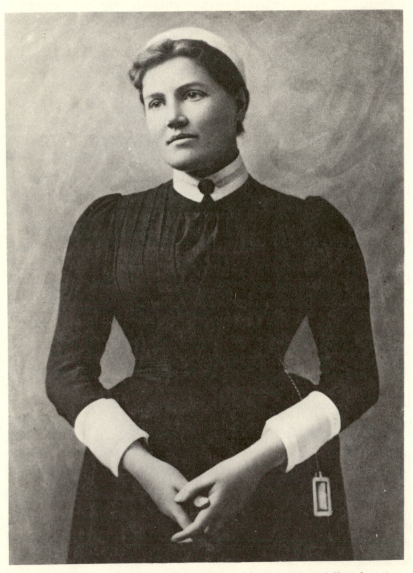

Isabel Hampton Robb. Portrait by William Sergeant Kendall, Administration Building, The Johns Hopkins Hospital.

training schools.[22] King, Dr. Billings, Gilman, and Dr. Osler, hospital physician-in-chief, interviewed the four leading candidates. Osler recalled later that "as Miss Isabel Hampton left the room, Mr. King looked approvingly at Mr. Gilman, who smiled assent at Dr. Billings. I whistled gently the first two bars of the tune of *'Conquering kings their titles take—from the foes they captive make';* as it was quite plain that a commanding figure, a sweet face, and a sweeter voice had in the short space of fifteen minutes settled the election of the Head of The Training school." Osler did add that "of course, the fact of two years experience at Chicago was taken into consideration."[23]

The four men had interviewed a young woman of twenty-nine, unusually tall at five feet ten inches, with fair hair, high coloring, blue eyes, and an ample figure, in the Lillian Russell style of the day. Her feminine attractions and air of authority may have swept the field, but the interviewers also sensed other qualities that fitted her to play a key role in their undertaking. Francis King, his daughter remembered, came home that day and said, "I have found an administrator." Like the staff physicians, Hampton had gone beyond a mastery of the existing knowledge and skills in her field to conceive broad and ambitious plans for its future, with which she had identified her own career. Like them, she had a strong physique and a vivid personality—in her case, a combination of dignity, charm, and enthusiasm and a maternal sense that evoked a strong positive response from patients, colleagues, and students alike.[24]

At New York's Bellevue Hospital she had seen the best and worst of hospital nursing in the 1880s. Some fellow pupils later remembered her as something of a nuisance, determinedly precise and methodical, despite the pressure of work in the busy wards, and constantly asking questions. Others, who, like her, were dissatisfied with their scanty instruction, met in her room in the evenings after the long working day to study anatomy and physiology out of medical books they bought themselves. When *Century* magazine in 1882 published a major article on the "new profession for women," it was illustrated by a sketch of first-year pupil Isabel Hampton measuring out medicines in a Bellevue ward.[25]

After graduation came two years of nursing at an Episcopal home in Rome for sick English and American travelers. There she gained social experience, a love for Italy and the arts, and a cosmopolitan outlook unknown in the small Canadian town of Welland, Ontario, where she had grown up. She came to Hopkins from three years (Osler's memory erred) as Superintendent of Nurses at the Illinois Training School in Chicago, whose pupils staffed wards in the Cook County Hospital. There she had worked well with the women's board of the school, won over hostile doctors to cooperation, and even, by "judicious engineering," induced the commissioners to make "long-needed improvements" in the hospital.[26]

Within the Illinois school, Hampton extended the instruction, meager though it was, into the second year, introducing for the first time in a training school something like a graded course of study. In addition, she abolished the practice of sending senior pupils out to work in private homes, and arranged an affiliation with the private Presbyterian Hospital where they might have supervised experience in the care of private patients.[27] Already her determination to eradicate the old image of the nurse was evident. A former pupil of this era later recalled that as Miss Hampton made rounds with the pupil head nurses, she gave little talks impressing "the fact that nursing is womanly work and we need lose no refinement in doing it. That one who became coarsened and hardened by her experience must blame herself, not the work. And in a last talk she expressed the hope that her pupils might marry and have homes and children."[28]

Hampton's ideal was to produce nurses who would meet the best British Victorian standards of womanhood. Perhaps even more than the moderately feminist American-born leaders of her generation, she took seriously the religious, moral, and cultural responsibilities assigned to her sex. She saw in nursing an opportunity for individual development and social service. Only a slight shift from the domestic scene would be required. Nurses, whether pupils or graduates, caring for rich or poor in home or hospital, were performing a nurturing function essential to human welfare. At the same time, modern medicine, hygiene, and dietetics were opening up new vistas of health. In her position close to the family, the nurse could exert enormous influence. As Lavinia Dock later recalled, Hampton held "the highest belief in the mission of women as the superior moral force, and in the possibility of universal happiness."[29]

Ontario, in the 1880s, had provided no outlet for her energy and ambition. A static provincial economy, her sex, and her social position as the daughter of a tradesman barred the way upward. Adelaide Nutting, her successor at Hopkins, who worked with her longer than anyone else, reflected at Hampton's death in 1910 that "had she been a man and in the business world, nothing could have kept her from an active and controlling share in some of the great organizations and combinations of which the world now hears so much."[30] In the United States, she saw an opportunity to improve society and make a career for herself by expanding woman's influence through a role already prescribed for her—to make nursing work "second to none done by women" through what has since come to be called professionalization.[31]

By the time Miss Hampton took up her job in Baltimore, the reputation of the Johns Hopkins Hospital, already widespread even before its opening, had attracted inquiries about the training school from a group of young women of strong educational background and social position. A comparison with the first and second generations of pupil nurses at the Boston Training School (one of the schools of the Nightingale model founded in 1873), who staffed the Massachusetts General Hospital, shows a marked difference.

In the records of the 181 candidates admitted to the Boston Training School in the decade of the 1870s, birthplaces were recorded in 119 cases. Only 14 of the candidates were natives of Boston; most of the others came from rural Massachusetts and other New England states (53), or from the Maritime Provinces of Canada (28). Of the 120 whose religion was recorded, 109 were Protestants. Previous occupations were noted, but only the paid ones. Eight pupils had been teachers, ten domestics, one a hospital attendant (hired nurse), five seamstresses, two machine operators, and one a clerk; the others must have been accustomed to hard work in small town or rural households.[32]

Fifteen years later, in 1889, the year the Johns Hopkins Hospital opened, the committee managing the Boston Training School assured the public that "the quality of the nurses" had improved, with "every effort" being made "to maintain and elevate the standard of teaching and requirements." Applicants now filled out a form with personal information and were required to furnish a reference from "some responsible person as to their moral character."[33] Between 1888 and 1891, 125 women entered training at the Massachusetts General. In some cases brief notes on education, intelligence, and "refinement" were entered in the ledgers that came to be known as enrollment books. In the 96 instances where previous education was evaluated, 50 were "poor" or "fair" and 46 "good." Judgments on intelligence, not surprisingly, corresponded with the educational ratings. Thirty-four women were considered "refined," 8 were judged to be lacking in refinement. Notes on the records of the latter make such comments as "liked by patients, good-natured, loud, flirtatious," "noisy, lacked attention to detail," and "talked too much."

The Boston Training School records show that the school in the years between 1888 and 1891 was drawing from the same largely rural and northern areas; only four pupils were from Boston. Twenty-eight had come from elsewhere in Massachusetts; twenty-five from Maine, New Hampshire, and Vermont; and thirty-four from Canada (almost all from the Maritimes). Southern New England contributed four, New York and New Jersey, twelve, and the Midwest, five.

At Johns Hopkins, Isabel Hampton began by setting up a records system later described as "the most perfect of its kind in any school" of the day;[34] this included complete duty records for both pupils and head nurses as well as correspondence with those applicants whom she accepted.[35] She herself made the admissions decisions; her authority in training school affairs is indicated by the reported experience of Dr. Hurd, who in her absence once wished to admit a Baltimore girl whom he knew, but with some irritation had to accept the reminder of assistant superintendent Lavinia Dock that the decision must await Miss Hampton's return.[36] She based her judgments on a letter from the candidate, including specified information about education, health, and freedom from home responsibility, plus recommendations from a physician and a clergyman. The level of personal cultivation revealed in the candidate's letter weighed heavily.

The application records reveal a great deal about the candidates' backgrounds and motivations. The records of 105 pupils admitted in the school's first four years (September, 1889 through August, 1893) show that the would-be Hopkins nurses, like those at the Boston Training School, came mainly from regions close to the school and from Canada: 24 from Baltimore and elsewhere in Maryland, 12 from other states in the upper South and the District of Columbia, 10 from Pennsylvania, 8 from New York and New England, and 23 from Canada, virtually all from the province of Ontario. The letters, however, portray a middle to upper-middle-class group, drawn from the larger towns and cities rather than from rural areas. A large majority of the young women, moreover, had completed a good secondary education at a local seminary. In church membership they were heavily Episcopalian (53) and Presbyterian (14). Their physicians and clergymen were family friends who had known "Bessie" or "Effie" from girlhood and usually emphasized the family's elite social standing, as well as, on occasion, the writer's bias regarding work for women. Thus Susie Carroll of Little Rock, Arkansas, age twenty-five, was "a lady by heredity, breeding and culture and qualified by education and natural endowment to learn any vocation appropriate for her sex." Agnes Lease, twenty-eight, of Mt. Pleasant, Maryland, would be leaving "a happy and comfortable home in order to engage in labor in a harder field, is educated and intelligent beyond the average of your applicants as you will find. She is perfectly proper and refined in all her tastes."

Only a few of the applicants to the Johns Hopkins Training School were dependent on themselves for support. Most were simply restless, tired of the domestic responsibilities of the unmarried daughter or sister in the family, and eager for an absorbing occupation out in the world. The price of separation was often a painful conflict with parents who felt that woman's place was in the home and also, in many cases, that nursing was

too hard and socially demeaning. Mary Heriot of Charleston, South Carolina, having at age thirty won such a battle, wrote "I am single, and my
life is my own, to do as I please with, from now on." Mary Collins,
twenty-three, daughter of a Washington, D. C., physician, had studied
abroad and was accomplished in organ, piano, French, and German but had
"no special occupations except home duties." According to her pastor,
"Maidie" waged her campaign with "great fortitude and patience"; her
father finally took her side against her mother and wrote Miss Hampton
himself: "As her desire, for years, has been to prepare herself for a career
of usefulness as a trained nurse, she now leaves home with my full consent
and blessing. Her mother very naturally, under the circumstances, raises
some objections. . . ."

Those few who had been employed had worked mostly in such genteel
occupations as teaching and giving lessons in music and languages, or
serving as companions and housekeepers to the aged. Two who entered in
1892 had had business experience: Harriet Carr, educated at a Sacred Heart
convent, who had connected herself with a new industry employing women
and was assistant secretary at "the telephone company head office" in
Hamilton, Ontario; and Julia Feeley of Pittsfield, Massachusetts, a graduate
of Miss Salisbury's School for Young Ladies, who at thirty-three had been
for six years "cashier in a large dry goods house in this city." Evvy Smith
of St. Catharines, Ontario, had been keeping house for her father since her
mother's death; with a second marriage he had acquired stepchildren to
support, and her way was now clear to "earning an independent living."

Even after a student had arrived in Baltimore and was enrolled in the
school, family claims had priority. The monthly reports of the training
school record a number of incidents where students or even head nurses
were called home by family illness. In September, 1896, Kate Galloway, a
senior (second-year) student, had to give up training and go home at her
sister's sudden death to take charge of the latter's small children. In March,
1892, two pupils were even "called home by the illness of friends." In 1891,
one pupil's mother came and took her away after she had been in school
for a month; "objected to her being a nurse" was Dock's note.

The large number of Canadian women in American nursing schools and
leadership posts in these early generations has often been noted. The
Canadians were breaking loose from a domestic setting which, because of
class traditions, was even more strictly bounded than that of the American
girl. In British Canadian families of the middle and upper-middle class, no
occupation other than teaching was permissible; to be sure, few others were
available. Better economic opportunities, moreover, were drawing many
young men west to make their fortunes, creating a surplus of women with

few alternatives to marriage. Isabel Hampton had been able to enroll at Bellevue (in 1881) only because teaching primary school had made her independent at twenty-one; a friend who had been admitted at the same time, but who was still living at home, was not permitted to go by her parents. Adelaide Nutting, a Canadian woman of strong intellect who was to follow Isabel Hampton as the preeminent leader in American nursing, was thirty when she joined the first class at Johns Hopkins; Adelaide and her mother, who came of a "good" family, had struggled for years, despite meager resources, to keep up appearances so that the girl could "circulate" on the fringes of Ottawa society; her mother was dead and hope of marriage gone before she left home.[37] Ida McArthur, twenty-five, of Bowmanville, Ontario, who had had three years of schooling in Toronto, finally won her parents' consent to apply at Hopkins when her father lost his money. ("Though not accustomed to very hard work," she wrote Hampton, "I feel sure I should be able to do all that you desire.")

The applicants showed a striking eagerness for new experience, making touching efforts to convince Hampton of their suitability for nursing. Alice Preston of Troy, New York, had helped with the nursing in two fatal illnesses in her family. ("The undertaker didn't have to do a thing except carry the casket downstairs the day of the funeral. The nurse and I did everything for Miss Mollie even to the measuring for the casket. . . . Words cannot express my longing to become a nurse as soon as possible.") Katharine Laing of Philadelphia, thirty-two, earnestly "hope[d] that you will be able to accept me and let me begin as soon as possible. I have been waiting for this day, so many years, that now I feel, I do not want to lose a moment." Applications came also from several upwardly mobile nurses trained at other schools. Hannah Neill, thirty-three, wished to have a better training "and nice associates at the same time. . . . I have a horror of entering some of the Schools here who admit any class of pupils. . . . I am perfectly willing to unlearn everything not approved and to begin as a new beginner."

Some of the young women persisted despite considerable anxiety over their physical capacity to endure the training, not surprising in a day when many doctors felt that women lacked the stamina even for college study. As Lucy Sharp, twenty-eight, of North Carolina wrote, "I know of no particular way to guage [*sic*] my strength don't think I can lift much more than fifty lbs. without feeling it"; furthermore, she was "liable to suffer a good deal of pain every month when unwell am often obliged to lay quiet one day and sometimes even two."

Though they may have known little of medical science, the successful candidates, each through her own break with the past and her venture into an unfamiliar world, had prepared themselves for membership in the Hopkins community; in the 1890s, women as well as medicine were exploring the unknown. The remarkable spirit of unity, almost comradeship, that was shared by the people working in the hospital grew, in part, at least, out of a common past experience.

For the members of the first pupil class, their initial months of training were both exhilarating and confusing. Miss Hampton gave all the nursing instruction. Only one text had been written, Clara S. Weeks's *A Text-book of Nursing* (1885), which the author herself described as a mere compendium; "all the rest of our study," one of the pupils recalled, "and all our materia medica we got from notes which Miss Hampton had written herself for us to copy and study." The methods Hampton taught, however, were often not followed by the head nurses on the wards, who came from a variety of different training schools in the United States and England: each thought "her own . . . the only correct way." For the moment, however, there was time to feel a sense of participating in an historic undertaking. Everything was new, and as Lavinia Dock remembered, "a fresh and inspiring atmosphere did indeed permeate the whole place. . . . When I think of the hospital now," she mused in 1910, "it is always this picture that I see:—the nurses in their blue dresses streaming down the corridor, the green lawn, and young trees outside in the sunshine . . . ; and Miss Hampton's caryatid-like figure, clad either in white or black, [her eyes] . . . radiant with pride and joy in her flock."[38]

Determined to give the school a clear identity as an educational institution, Hampton began by assuming a new title, Principal of the Training School, in addition to the standard Superintendent of Nurses. Her innovations in Chicago furnished a starting point for arranging the instruction. The central problem was to manage admissions and graduations of students, and to maintain a regular schedule of graded classwork, without disrupting the nursing service at the hospital. Hampton compromised. New pupils at Hopkins entered the hospital during three-month periods in the spring and fall and began their classes with the next term.[39] The twelve-hour day on the wards was eased to permit two hours off duty in the afternoon and one free afternoon a week. This made time for a few regular weekly classes: two a week, in nursing, by Miss Hampton for first-year students, and one for seniors. The staff physicians gave a weekly lecture to each group in the evening.

An expert teacher, Hampton emphasized the use of visual aids (what she called "object-teaching"). She equipped the classroom with a skeleton, a mannikin to demonstrate "visceral anatomy," charts, specimens, and pictures, and enlisted the doctors' aid in securing other material for "demonstrations." A collection of about twenty medical texts and other works in medicine and nursing made up a good working library. As at most of the better training schools, notes taken in class had to be carefully written out in ink and handed in to be corrected and preserved for future reference. Hampton required written as well as oral examinations and gave the seniors extra practice in writing through dictation, quizzes corrected and criticized in class, and the preparation of short papers on such subjects as the more important drugs, observations of symptoms, and treatment in emergencies.[40]

She also set the pace in introducing new subject matter in nursing. Other training schools had given pupils lectures on, or lessons in cooking, but Hampton, aware of new research in foods and nutrition, secured a resident "Diet School Teacher," a graduate of the Boston Cooking School, who not only taught cooking for invalids but also gave some elementary instruction in food chemistry. A course in Swedish massage, eight demonstration lectures by Miss Hampton herself, also offered a precedent for other schools.[41]

Even thus augmented, formal instruction could hardly be more than incidental to the strenuous on-the-job vocational training. This, in turn, was outstanding at Hopkins, not only because of the special quality of the hospital and its medical staff but because of the supervision given the pupils as they rotated on a fairly regular schedule through the wards, the operating room, and the dispensary. Hopkins wards were headed by graduate nurses, rather than by the second-year pupils found in such positions at most nursing schools, and Miss Hampton herself spent much time in supervision and ward teaching. Pupils soon were impressed with her governing concepts: a humanitarian sympathy for all sufferers; the importance of "thoroughly clean surroundings and pure air" as "conditions absolutely necessary to the recovery of patients"; and her insistence that "system and method prevail throughout . . . ; the work is not done haphazard."[42] One student retained a vivid memory of her "taking me, a raw probationer, into an isolation backroom to nurse a baby with virulent gonorrheal conjunctivitis. She did not need to touch it; in clear words she explained the technique minutely, the danger to be incurred, and my responsibility to myself as well as to the child, and after assuring herself that I understood the significance of each act she watched me do the first dressing. I listened to her talking to the baby's mother, and I realized for the first time I had seen the ideal of a trained nurse."[43]

With such inspiration, morale was high.[44] In February, 1891, Dr. Hurd, submitting his first report as hospital superintendent, listed the work of the training school at the head of the achievements that had already given the hospital "an acknowledged position in the medical work of the country as a growing center of instruction and usefulness." In Baltimore the school, the city's first, had become the object of considerable pride and interest. Young women of good family were entering this "new field of usefulness," and Miss Hampton, introduced to local society by Francis King, found time for an occasional luncheon, tea, or concert, joined the Women's Fund Committee for the medical school, and "became well known as a delightful representative of the great Hospital and of a new profession for women." President and Mrs. Gilman gave pictures to decorate the Nurses' Home, and Miss Mary Garrett, a leader and chief donor of the Women's Fund Committee, supplied books for its library. When the first class graduated in June, 1891, the occasion was made a special ceremony. Francis King and Miss Hampton spoke briefly; Dr. Osler gave the main address and provided bouquets of roses, which Mrs. Gilman presented as each of the eighteen young women received her diploma from Dr. Hurd.[45]

Osler's address, entitled "Doctor and Nurse," and the courtly gesture of the roses hinted at a certain ambivalence on the doctors' part toward the women who had been trained to be their skilled assistants. For the nurses, the physicians were their superiors, their judges within the hospital and before the public, and their professional role models; they were also men, whom most of the young women were conditioned to regard as authority figures. To a large extent dependent upon these men for their own image of themselves, they received mixed signals.

Each of the famed Hopkins doctors had his own dramatic personal style, but in their official pronouncements and perhaps also their conscious minds they were united in hailing the trained nurse as an ally (as Osler put it) in "lessening the sad sum of human misery and pain by spreading . . . knowledge of . . . [the] grand laws of health." The chiefs of services enjoyed their association with Miss Hampton and then with her successor Adelaide Nutting, a more reserved personality, but a woman of breeding and intellect. They were also greatly interested in all the teaching that went on in the hospital, including the training school. Dr. Osler and Dr. Howard A. Kelly, however, never allowed the nurses to forget their lowly professional origins and the weaknesses which they, as women, were heir to. Dr. Kelly, for instance, reminded the second graduating class of their "inestimable privilege to have elevated the class you represent, from that of self-taught, selfish hired attendants." Democracy and enlightenment had created "a new and beautiful ministry," physicians and nurses joining with pastors in devoted and self-abnegating service to humankind. "I need not add," he continued, "that nurses dominated by this spirit do not everywhere fill the rank and file of the profession." Osler, on his part, was addicted to stereotypes of garrulous nurses babbling of patients' private affairs and "things medical and gruesome."[46]

It is hard to believe that Isabel Hampton's carefully selected candidates stood in need of these admonitions, yet considering them as women fresh from a domestic world of close personal relationships and informal, spontaneous sociability, with an education that at best had provided more cultivation than intellectual discipline, one can conceive that they may have had some difficulty in adjusting to a more formal, institutional setting.

The problem of professional relationships prompted the writing of *Nursing Ethics* (1900), Hampton's second book, which created and named a subject that still lingers in nursing school curricula. Like much else, the concept was borrowed from the doctors and then devalued. "Ethics," for nurses, turned out to be essentially a code of etiquette. Like most etiquette books, it was designed to enable the reader to acquire the standards of a higher social class. The complex history of nursing, however, imparted to the code a distinctive emphasis on stringent discipline.

Historically, this element was in part a legacy from the military, religious, and nursing orders going back to the Middle Ages, with their traditions of obedience, subordination, and self-abnegation. Imbibing these through her training and experience, Florence Nightingale transmitted them to the secular, progress-minded nineteenth century. The standards of behavior they set were useful in the difficult task of upgrading the nursing service, and, fitting in with the British class structure, tolerable to English nurses of the new breed. The few American training schools of the first generation had not attempted this degree of control, but by the 1890s, circumstances were changing. One has only to read the directions, in Hampton's earlier textbook (*Nursing: Its Principles and Practice*, 1893), for cleaning the ward or preparing a patient for surgery to visualize the strenuous and unremitting activity of the daily twelve-hour war against germs, with no other weapons than cleanliness. To carry this enormous workload, pupil nurses, no matter what their standing in the loosely defined American middle class, had to be habituated to organization and discipline.

Few American girls had disciplined work habits, those from more affluent families being perhaps the least accustomed to constraint. And as was not the case in the other professions into which women above the working class were moving, such as teaching, librarianship, and social work, the pupil nurses were coming into contact, and working closely with not only other women, children, and families, but with men, ranging from the patients at the bottom of the social scale to the Johns Hopkins doctors at the top. Isabel Hampton, with her Canadian background and a mother who, as Adelaide Nutting remarked in several biographical reminiscences, was "a great believer in law and order and government, and a staunch upholder of British ideals in discipline,"[47] clearly found the old military tradition congenial. She also thought discipline essential, for if women were to win acceptance and status as nurses, to earn a good living, and, as she dreamed, to play their part in social reform, they must demonstrate their usefulness, and first of all convince their superior officers, the doctors.

Nursing ethics offered the key to success. Hampton and her successors in the genre identified three problem areas: manners, work habits, and sex, and laid down rules designed to transform the girlish chatterbox into a dignified and discreet nurse able to pick her way in a complex world of work where middle class women were new and conspicuous.

In the early days at Hopkins, in the relatively relaxed atmosphere of the new hospital, Hampton, in her textbook, had attempted to define for her pupil nurses a manner both professional and womanly. On the ward, the nurse should "extend the same courtesy that she would show to visitors in her own home," rising to greet "the medical officers connected with the ward, the superintendent of the hospital, superintendent of nurses, and strangers." By 1900, working in the now renowned Hopkins or any other crowded, busy hospital, the gracious hostess had become a member of a platoon. "The head nurse and her staff should stand to receive the visiting physician, and from the moment of his entrance until his departure, the attending nurses should show themselves alert, attentive, courteous, like soldiers on duty."[48]

The proper attitude toward the patient underwent a similar change. According to the textbook of 1893, the nurse "should always make the patients feel that they are her first consideration, and that to do anything for their comfort is her greatest pleasure." She was adjured to be "particularly attentive and kind to a new patient: the dread of entering a hospital is bad enough, but much of the gloom can be removed by the bright, cheerful greeting of the nurse. . . ." The patient's friends, acknowledged to be "often the greatest trials that a nurse has to contend with," were likewise to be treated with patience. By 1900 this positive approach had given way to a warning that the pupil must be "very circumspect in her own language, and encourage nothing from patients, or their friends, that borders on familiarity, vulgarity, or frivolity."[49]

Home training, it appeared, was no longer sufficient. The ebullient young woman sometimes adjusted with difficulty to hospital routine. The probationer had to be warned that "unnecessary questions, talking and noise, are absolutely prohibited during the rounds of the medical staff," the junior pupil reminded that "the desire to talk incessantly, or to make unnecessary comments, should always be controlled," and the senior pupil admonished that "the operating room is no place for indulging in talking or frivolity of any kind." It was not permitted when off duty to "go into the hospital to visit"; similarly, having friends from outside the hospital "to visit one in the ward is quite out of place."[50]

Relationships with both sexes were hedged about with cautionary advice. Toward each other, pupils should show "nothing in the way of personal feeling," equally avoiding on the one hand "personal jealousy, discord, and faultfinding," and, on the other, "sentimental, intense personal friendships."[51]

Relationships with the opposite sex presented dangers which, though only obliquely referred to, had been, as we have seen, a source of serious concern since the beginning of hospital reform. Furthermore, the spinsterhood of nurses summoned up images of females desperate to secure a mate. Dr. Osler was prone to fantasies about the "gradually accumulating surplus of women who will not or cannot fulfil the highest duties for which nature designed them," whom he regarded as "a dangerous element."[52]

Since male folklore made woman the aggressor, nursing ethics, like the society at large, assigned her the responsibility for chastity, with careful explanations. "The ordinary little attentions and social privileges" that the pupil nurse "may have been accustomed to in the small social circle at home" could not be allowed in "the large wards of a hospital." Encounters with internes or resident physicians during the solitary hours of night duty were a subject of particular concern. The nurse must "emphatically" discourage "any disposition on the part of the doctor to stop for a friendly chat," or prolong his stay. ("If she is the only woman in a ward full of men," she risked losing their respect, thus lowering "the professional dignity of the entire nursing staff.") Should the doctor have to be called several times during the night, she must resist the temptation of giving him "any refreshment from provisions belonging to the ward."[53]

Other admonitions completed the restraint of impulse and the cultivation of caution: gossip was repeatedly condemned in every possible context; sympathy and sentiment were given limits; above all, the nurse must take care "not to make in any direction any unnecessary advances."[54] Middle class habits of neatness, punctuality, truthfulness, study, method and order, personal hygiene, and table manners were inculcated as fundamentals. Finally, the military and religious traditions were explicitly invoked. "Above all, let her remember what she is told to do, and no more. . . ." And, amid injunctions to patience, gentleness, cheerfulness, and good temper, "the nurse's work is a ministry; it should represent a consecrated service, performed in the spirit of Christ, who made himself of no account but went about doing good."[55]

Isabel Hampton's working relationships with the Hopkins doctors were the subject of considerable gossip. At times, in the hospital, their interests clashed. Hampton's rotation of pupils from one service to another disrupted continuity in the wards, and her insistence on her authority to appoint head nurses, because of their teaching function, brought her to an impasse with surgeon William S. Halsted, who understandably wished to choose and retain his own operating team.[56] There was also some clash of wills with Dr. Hurd, a strong administrator, reserved, meticulous, and frugal; but though he does not seem to have been a popular figure with the nurses, he believed in the improvement of nursing, and not only because, as he said of Hampton after her death and his own retirement, he had "rarely, if ever, seen a woman with a more winning presence."[57]

The work of Dr. William H. Welch, the hospital's pathologist, did not bring him in contact with the nurses, but in after years he, too, faithfully seconded their efforts to improve their professional standing. Dr. Osler, Henry Hurd remarked tactfully after his death, "seemed always appreciative and helpful while at the same time he had an air of detachment as one who was endeavoring to see where the movement for the education of nurses would ultimately lead." Hampton, like Adelaide Nutting, was doubtless aware that Osler "liked certain nurses because he liked them as women."[58] The unfailing support of Francis T. King resolved many issues in Hampton's favor through the trustees' power of the purse. King's daughter recalled of Hampton that it was one of her father's "greatest pleasures to confer with her, and to listen to and encourage her admirable plans"; Miss Hampton nursed him herself in his last illness.[59]

The doctors' influence on the training school and the development of nursing went far beyond nursing ethics. Hampton worked with them at a time when the medical profession itself was reaching for a higher status in society, on the basis of its new powers of healing, and the men at Hopkins were in the forefront of this effort. As they built a new clinical base for medical education and research by redefining the functions of the hospital, they were also influencing the profession at large. Each in his own way, they cultivated a wide acquaintance, took an active part in professional associations, selected and trained younger men and placed them in important posts, conducted research and published it, founded new journals, and delved into medical history for past glories with which to identify. William Osler, the professor of medicine, gentleman scholar, embodiment of masculine charm and wit, served as a role model to a profession moving upward. Shining in medicine's reflected light, caught by the magnetism of the doctors' personalities and their confident sense of mission, the nurses imitated their professional structures.

Among the many ways in which the Hopkins doctors' example left its mark was the use of history to establish a sense of professionalism. One of the medical staff's Monday evening clubs devoted itself to historical studies; Osler and Kelly collected books on the history of medicine. Kelly, the leading gynecologist of his day, built up a library on the history of women, and his assistant, Dr. Hunter Robb, gave a series of papers at Historical Club meetings on noted French and German midwives of the past, whose work he extolled as professional in many respects.[60] It was during these years that Adelaide Nutting began her collection of books relating to the history of nursing, and she and Lavinia Dock conceived the idea of writing a book to celebrate the ancient antecedents of their profession and its progress to their own day. In the twentieth century, medical history was to thrive, as the prestige of the profession grew; attracting able, trained historians with or without medical degrees, it became a distinguished sub-field within the historical profession. Nursing history, lacking these vital transfusions, was kept alive in nursing school curricula by faithful followers of Lavinia Dock but finally fell into a state of inanition.

In June, 1894, Isabel Hampton resigned her post at the Johns Hopkins Hospital to marry Dr. Hunter Robb and move with him to Cleveland. In keeping with nursing ethics, their courtship had been discreetly conducted outside the hospital, causing no gossip except among the doctors.[61] She had organized the school and administered it for nearly five years, choosing as assistants two of the ablest women of her generation, Lavinia Dock and Adelaide Nutting. Within the hospital she had achieved the best training program of the day and a clearly defined professional standard of nursing service: by 1894, every nursing post on the staff was held by one of her graduates. She had written, in the late afternoons of those early years, in her office, after the day's work was over, *Nursing: Its Principles and Practice*, a detailed, 480-page text that would be standard in nursing courses for more than a generation.[62] Dr. Billings, in a review, remarked that the book was of interest to doctors as well as to nurses, "indicating what a trained nurse of the present day may be expected to know and to be able to do."[63]

Hampton had also readied a plan for a major new advance in the training of nurses that would shift the balance from service to education by extending the course to three years, reducing the workday to eight hours, and eliminating the money payment to pupils. In addition, she had laid the groundwork for the remainder of her career, which was to be devoted to organizing and upgrading the profession as a whole, and presenting to the nurses and to the public her conception of the nurse's role in the contemporary movement for social reform.

Her plans for professional organization, specifically for a national association of nurses, and an advanced training course for teachers and administrators, had been at least partly formulated by the time she came to Johns Hopkins. Lavinia Dock, who remembered enthusiastic conversations about "nursing growth, organisation and activities" over leisurely Sunday morning breakfasts in the alcove of the nurses' dining room, had no doubt that these ideas had originated with Hampton.[64] The systematized program of training and practice at Hopkins was intended to be an example that would inspire efforts for uniform standards everywhere; the group loyalty Hampton strove to instill was intended as a base for a larger "sisterhood."[65] Her efforts to extend the pupils' outlook beyond the confines of the hospital would build an awareness of social issues and thus provide worthy goals for united effort.

Some of the Hopkins pupils, before entering nursing, had been active in their churches, and hence may have had some experience in group work with other women, but there is no evidence of this in the application letters. The first step in building loyalty was to reconcile the pupils to working with others "with whom in every-day life one would have little in common." Nursing ethics, mindful of women's proverbial lack of loyalty to other women, next required them to refrain from disparaging other pupils "either to friends in the city or to doctors."[66] Graduates grew accustomed to working together, and strengthened their loyalty to the school in an alumnae association, founded in 1892, only the third to be organized in a nursing school (after Bellevue and the Illinois Training School), and the first to which all graduates of the school were admitted.[67]

Loyalty to the school, carried to an extreme, however, could be counterproductive. Pupils were admonished that "a nurse can give no stronger evidence of ignorance or narrow-mindedness than by behaving as if she considered herself, her school and her hospital better than any other."[68] From opening day, when nursing superintendents from Philadelphia were invited to the ceremony, Isabel Hampton's cordiality worked to break down the isolation of schools. Starting with her Canadian friends in nursing, a stream of training-school superintendents came to Baltimore to visit the hospital, the beginning of a communications network.[69] Lucy Walker, the English-trained superintendent of Philadelphia's Presbyterian Hospital school, timidly ventured to Baltimore in 1893, hoping to learn something about the new system which she had heard of for training nurses in the preparation of diets for the sick. Having no letter of introduction, she was amazed to be "at once received" by Hampton, who spent the day with her, invited her to lunch, and "explained her kitchen to the minutest detail."[70]

To open up some views of the world outside to pupils and nursing staff, Hampton took a leaf from the Journal Club which had been formed by the Hopkins doctors for discussion of current medical literature, and whose meetings she and Dock sometimes attended. A Nurses' Journal Club, founded in 1891, met for an hour every other Monday evening, officially "to keep in touch with what is being done in other schools and hospitals," but unofficially, also, to give the nurses practice in expressing themselves and to introduce them to important issues in nursing. Most of the participants read aloud from articles in medical or nursing journals; a few short original papers of a very informal sort were produced each year, on subjects like "Loyalty among Nurses," or "The Care of Children." Lavinia Dock may have been responsible for inserting in the program occasional articles from current magazines of opinion touching on subjects like capital punishment, the Negro nursing school at Hampton Institute, and Hull House (Jane Addams's first published account). In May, 1892, Father James O. S. Huntington, the reform-minded Episcopal priest, gave a short talk. A meeting in Miss Hampton's last year at Hopkins was devoted to "The Unregarded Causes of Ill Health in American Women."[71]

As she prepared her students and staff for participation in a profession, the growing reputation of the hospital and the training school brought Hampton opportunities to present her concepts of nursing and its goals to the public. She took full advantage of these, beginning with her address at the school's opening exercises.[72] On each occasion, varying the approach and emphasis with the audience, she pictured the new nurse, educated and idealistic, fitted to bring skilled care to all classes of society, whether in the hospital or at home. She then deplored the lack of uniform standards of training. A principal target was the small hospitals which conducted "schools" without the resources to offer a rounded nursing experience, throwing on the market poorly trained nurses who gave the profession a bad name.[73]

The new nurse described in these speeches tended to separate into two very different identities. In her hospital role, the nurse was the physician's obedient and loyal assistant, but the district nurse, bringing to the sick poor, in their homes, skilled care and instruction in the laws of sanitation, was an independent figure. In the latter role, the nurse occupies center stage, her medical supervisor somewhere in a shadowy background. She is an expert in household economy, versed in bacteriology, a woman of refinement and tact, who can convert her patients to "a healthier, better way of living" without arousing antagonism. The nurse could thus join the ranks of the progressive citizens of the day, bringing her own answer to the question, "What is to be done with the lower social conditions of life?"[74]

With her usual quickness and perceptiveness, Isabel Hampton had recognized the potentialities of a new kind of work which would both fulfill woman's mission of social uplift and enhance the status of nurses. District nursing, first developed in England, had been introduced in several American cities in the late 1880s by women who founded charitable associations to direct and finance the program. Chicago ladies had established such an organization during Isabel Hampton's last year at the Illinois Training School.[75]

Hampton carried with her to Baltimore the hope of introducing district nursing into the instruction and practice of the pupil nurses at Johns Hopkins, an advanced idea that was not to be realized to any extent in nursing education until the 1930s.[76] The Hopkins doctors were much attracted to this concept of social reform through the medium of medicine and hygiene.[77] But even the Johns Hopkins Hospital's funds were not bottomless, and as its work swiftly expanded, the pupil nurses could not be spared for an expensive experiment.

In interpreting nursing outside the hospital, however, Hampton continued to present the district nursing dimension. In May, 1890, when the National Conference of Charities and Correction held its annual meeting in Baltimore, in order to inspect the innovative facilities of the Johns Hopkins Hospital, she became the first nurse to address this influential group. Her report emphasized nursing's role in both scientific medicine and the contemporary vision of scientific charity, and the necessity of "exceptional women and training" to perform this work. She described the plight of a worthy profession without professional organization or any fixed standards of practice.[78]

That summer, on vacation in England, she visited one of the district nursing branches in London; the following spring, on a trip to Boston, she studied the operations of the Instructive District Nursing Association, considered the best in the United States. With this background she appealed to the Charity Organization Society of Baltimore later that year for a combined effort on the part of doctors, clergy, religious sisterhoods, nurses, and businessmen to establish district nursing in the city, pointing out that dispensaries could not reach "mothers of families, . . . chronic patients, and those who still retain their old prejudice against hospitals."[79] A few years later Lillian Wald, in New York, would invent the term *public health nurse* and capture nationwide interest by combining district nursing with a new kind of charitable institution called the *social settlement.* Isabel Hampton had done much to pave the way.

Hampton's efforts to define the status and role of nursing crystallized in the International Congress of Charities, Correction and Philanthropy that was held in Chicago as part of the Columbian Exposition of 1893. Hopkins-connected medical men dominated the Congress special section on hospitals; Hampton's Hopkins position gave her a leading role in planning the meetings devoted to nursing, and a platform for her views.

The range of papers showed not only Hampton's wide knowledge of the field and the people in it but also her excellent political sense.[80] Dock recalled later that "Miss Hampton really went through a mental process of construction of the entire subsequent evolution of the nursing profession. She placed the papers so that certain ideas should be worked out, and waited almost breathlessly for the results. . . ."[81] The most crucial, the papers on the history and organization of American training schools, the importance of training school alumnae groups, and the need for an all-inclusive nurses' association went to her fellow Canadians, the superintendents with whom she had often talked about their common problems.

Meanwhile Dr. Billings and Dr. Hurd had arranged for the superintendent and the assistant superintendent of the Johns Hopkins Hospital Training School to speak at the two most prominent meetings. The congress convened in mid-June. Early in the week, when one session considered major aspects of hospital administration, Lavinia Dock, appearing with Dr. Hurd, Dr. Edward Cowles of Boston, a German hospital director, and a Philadelphia hospital trustee, discussed "The Relation of Training Schools to Hospitals." In midweek came a presentation before the entire congress, when Isabel Hampton, sharing the platform with Dr. Billings and the English hospital authority Henry Burdett, delivered her carefully prepared paper on "Educational Standards for Nurses."

The two women knew hospital nursing in institutions ranging all the way from city or county hospitals, "where local politics grow at the expense of the neglected sick poor, . . . hating to be interfered with," to the munificently endowed Johns Hopkins, where hospital and school enjoyed "identity of interest and aims; a sense of mutual obligation; a reciprocal feeling of personal pride, admiration and attachment." Most hospital-school relationships, they knew, fell somewhere in between, characterized by "a formlessness, a lack of tradition, an adoption of hasty and tentative methods, and an acceptance of imperfect results." For all this the public blamed the nurses, "though much of the fault lies with the hospital."[82]

Dock reminded her audience of hospital leaders that trained nursing, interacting with "a dawning rationalism in medicine, antisepsis in surgery, [and] a growing intelligence of public opinion," had done much to bring hospitals into their present high esteem, and that it alone was responsible for the improved moral atmosphere of "the once foul old hospitals." Admittedly the new nursing system was more expensive than the old, yet the schools, by promising an education, insured "a steady supply of intelligent women," who, under school discipline, performed "an amount and quality of work which the hospitals could not possibly secure if they had to pay for it." In addition, many hospitals still made the pupil nurses support the school as well, by sending them outside on private duty.[83]

What the training offered by a hospital school should be was the topic of Hampton's paper, which she regarded as "the culmination of her teaching work."[84] In it she served notice that the achievements of the pioneer generation of schools were no longer good enough. Although virtually all hospital nursing was now done by training-school pupils, so widely did the schools vary in their requirements that the term "trained nurse" could mean "anything, everything, or next to nothing." She spoke plainly for the first time of the hospitals' responsibility to provide a real education in return for the nursing service, rendered for less than the pay of a ward maid. Hampton called for a spirit of unity and cooperation among the superintendents to determine upon a uniform system of instruction and work toward it, and proposed her plan of a three-year course with an eight-hour day of "practical work." In conclusion, she described the ideal background for a trained nurse: an education equal to that of the best high schools, and, to instill habits of throughness and system, home training in household economy, "a branch of woman's work . . . neglected or superficially understood by so many women in all ranks of life."[85]

In public meetings before an international audience of leaders in hospital work, Hampton and Dock had frankly discussed the basic, interlocking problems of nursing: the variability in training-school standards and hospital support. The dilemma, in somewhat altered form, would still be dogging the profession seventy-five years later.

There remained the question of what nurses themselves could do to raise their professional sights and standards. Hampton, in her address, had called for cooperation among the superintendents; Dock, in another portion of hers, although not mentioning Florence Nightingale by name, had advocated a return to the Nightingale system of a clear separation of the areas of medical and nursing authority. "The organization of a training school is and must be military," she declared, with "absolute and unquestioning obedience," and a chain of command leading to the head of the school. In the direct care of the sick the doctors gave the orders; in the internal affairs of the school, including teaching and discipline, the superintendent's authority should be absolute.[86] These themes would be picked up by the succeeding papers given before the nursing subsection,[87] whose meetings many of the hospital administrators also attended, since the schedules of the two subsections had been planned not to overlap.

Dock's paper provoked an interesting discussion from the audience. The speakers, nurses and hospital men, agreed on the necessity of full authority for the training-school superintendent, though Dr. Billings argued that women able to exercise such power were "extremely rare, just as men who are qualified to take charge of and command a big establishment are extremely rare." The real difficulty, he thought, would come over a question of disciplining "some nurse who is perhaps attractive in manner and ways," and "particularly satisfactory" to some trustee or member of the medical staff. But even in these cases, he concluded, "the rule of the superintendent of the training school goes with me." Dr. Hurd added his earnest conviction that there was a unity of interest between hospital and school.[88]

Hampton and Dock were disappointed at the timidity of the other nursing papers, especially that of Edith Draper, superintendent of the Illinois Training School, on "The Necessity for an American Nurses' Association."[89] The formidable presence of Henry Burdett, arch-foe of the British organization of a similar name, may have been intimidating, as was the paper sent to the congress by Florence Nightingale, who denounced the modern tendency to make nursing a profession, instead of a calling, and dismissed "examinations, public registration, graduation" as affording no proof of the dedicated character necessary for the true nurse. Miss Draper referred only vaguely to "a system of registering" to be administered by the association, without mentioning legislation, and Irene Sutliffe of the New York Hospital School, clinging to the Nightingale image, offered as justification for "a well-regulated association of nurses" its aid in the restoration of such ideals as "the beauty of self-sacrifice."[90]

The conflict in the nurses' minds between, on the one hand, the ideals according to which trained nursing had been founded and on which it had depended to create a new image, and, on the other, the realities of a modern profession, surfaced in a discussion following the paper by Louise Darche, superintendent of the New York City Training School at the pauper hospital on Blackwell's Island. Darche had described a school registry as one of the American alterations in the Nightingale plan. The nurses present seized upon this opportunity to discuss "prices," despite a clearly uneasy fear that such concern might be considered mercenary. The custom of having fees fixed by the registry was defended as preventing any unpleasantness with private employers, and the nurse's right to give her services for nothing was anxiously reserved. Lilla Lett, of St. Luke's Hospital in Chicago, offered as a possible model the plan in effect at her registry, where by agreement her graduate nurses worked without pay on cases in poor families for two weeks out of the year. But Lillian Wald, who had just begun her work among immigrant families in New York, struck a vigorous modern note: the nurse "should have the privilege of setting her own price. It is as much professional work as that of the physician."[91]

Hampton had known at least half of the superintendents attending the meetings for several years, through Canadian or Bellevue connections, but many of the other women later remembered that the chief event of the congress had been getting acquainted, and then suddenly realizing that "the deficiencies and difficulties of their work were peculiar to the whole nursing profession, and not to one school or hospital."[92] Hampton herself made essential contacts at the congress with the leaders from the Massachusetts General and Boston City hospital schools.

In one of the discussions about nurses' associations, she had laid down professional priorities. A national superintendents' association should come first; later the alumnae associations in the individual schools, of which only a few had yet been founded, could form the base for an association of all nurses. Following her suggestion that the superintendents should meet to discuss organizing, a few of the leaders conferred in Lilla Lett's sitting room at St. Luke's and determined to call a meeting after the session. "About eighteen" stayed to form the American Society of Superintendents of Training Schools in the United States and Canada. The name would carry no aggressive connotations or overtones of British militancy, and the election of officers brought into the movement the essential New England contingent. The two vice-presidents were veteran graduates of the Boston Training School, associated with the Massachusetts General Hospital: Mary E. P. Davis, superintendent of the University of Pennsylvania Hospital and its training school, and Sophia Palmer, founder and superintendent of the school at the Garfield Memorial Hospital in Washington, D.C. Lucy Drown, of the Boston City Hospital, was made treasurer. Anna Alston, of New York's Mount Sinai Hospital, became the first president; Isabel Hampton's old friend Louise Darche, secretary.

With the perspective of after years, Lavinia Dock could smile at the "awful solemnity" with which this nucleus of a profession took its first combined step. So conscious of standards was the new body that it excluded superintendents of small hospital training schools even when their own training had been unexceptionable, and she marveled that those present who fell under this decree made not a murmur of protest.[93]

It is worth noting that the members of the new society must have been aware of other women's recent activity in forming organizations. National women's suffrage and temperance organizations were now some twenty years old; the rising women's colleges had associations of alumnae, whose nomenclature the training schools borrowed for their own organizations of graduates; the proliferating women's clubs had recently founded a General Federation. A month earlier the fair had seen a much-publicized gathering of delegates from women's organizations, the World's Congress of Representative Women; daily, in the Woman's Building, a continuous Congress of Women was meeting with presentation of papers by or about women that eventually filled a thick volume.[94] A society of nurses would be something different, organized from the top down, because of the hospital authority structure, yet potentially more widely inclusive than any of the strongly middle class women's organizations of that day. And, conscious of a history of their own whose great leaders were still alive, the founder generation of nurses had its special, if only partly conscious, feminism. As Louise Darche had said in ending her paper, "From its nature nursing is peculiarly a woman's work; a woman originated the training-school system in England, women started it in this country, women have brought it to its present stage of development, and it is to women we must look for its future advancement."[95]

Looking back at the congress after the passage of eighty-five years, one can see that in a sense the nursing papers which Isabel Hampton arranged constituted the first of a series of investigative reports which, once every generation, would diagnose and prescribe for the ills of this indispensable but floundering profession.[96] Like the later reports, the World's Fair program singled out nursing education as the key problem; like them, also, it estimated society's needs for nursing more accurately than society's readiness to pay the cost. In contrast to the others, the program was almost entirely the work of the nursing leadership, particularly Hampton and Dock, prepared for this role by their participation in the remarkably open community that launched the Johns Hopkins Hospital.

The Society of Superintendents proceeded briskly with its organization. With Dr. Billings's aid, Miss Darche rounded up the names of seventy-one superintendents to approach, and when the group met again in January, 1894, in New York, there were thirty new members. The forty-four superintendents present adopted a constitution defining the object of the society: "to further the best interests of the nursing profession by establishing and maintaining a universal standard of training and by promoting fellowship among its members. . . ."[97] Succeeding annual meetings debated the central concerns that had emerged at the World's Fair: the raising of standards of training along the lines Hampton had laid down; the operation of registries—bread and butter to the private duty nurse; the nurse's obligation of moral and social uplift; and the organization of an all-inclusive association.

In the society's discussions, hope mingled with hesitation and doubt. Hampton took a leading part in the proceedings and kept her key projects alive by securing the appointment of sympathetic committees. Lavinia Dock submitted comprehensive and astute reports on the registry problem, and explained the operations of other national professional associations, especially the American Medical Association. Everyone could agree that pupil nurses should not be sent out on private duty (a resolution to this effect was passed in 1896) and that training-school alumnae associations should be encouraged. The idea of a three-year course made headway, and by 1900 many schools were changing over. But the eight-hour day seemed only remotely possible; it would not become standard for nurses until the New Deal in the 1930s made it standard for everyone. The nonpayment plan, Hampton's idea for financing "a really liberal education as an equivalent for the three years' service,"[98] was adopted only by the few schools like Johns Hopkins that could attract young women of some means. Most superintendents were sure that without the cash allowance, worthy candidates would be unable to enter nursing, and the society finally refused even to endorse nonpayment.[99]

As Adelaide Nutting, who became head of the training school at Hopkins in 1894, took up the leadership of the superintendents' effort to raise standards of training, Hampton concentrated on the remaining goals of her long-cherished plan for the nursing profession. Lavinia Dock's study having prepared the way, a national organization of nurses came into being at a small meeting of superintendents and representatives of training-school alumnae associations at Manhattan Beach, New York, in September, 1896. Hampton, absent from meetings that year for the birth of her first child, returned, to be triumphantly elected the first president of the Nurses' Associated Alumnae of the United States and Canada.[100] Within three years a professional journal was in publication.

Hampton then found the capstone for her structure and set it in place. A debate at the Society of Superintendents' meeting in 1898 over qualifications for membership enabled her to initiate a discussion of training for superintendents, and to propose replacing the hard school of experience with a formal course such as normal schools provided for teachers. The duly appointed study committee returned the next year with a fait accompli. Proceeding alone, after the committee as a whole had been unable to settle on a common meeting date, Hampton and Nutting had arranged with

Dean James E. Russell, of the newly founded Teachers College at Columbia University, for a year's course in "hospital economics" for graduate nurses, to begin that fall,[101] the origin of the department of nursing education which would train most of the leaders in the profession for the next forty years.

The decade of the 1890s had seen professionalization advance from little more than an idea in Isabel Hampton's head to seeming completion. And yet as the decade, and the century, ended, a feeling of frustration set in among the superintendents, as if their goal had somehow eluded their grasp. The Spanish-American War publicly demonstrated the lack of public influence of the Associated Alumnae, whose offer to recruit nurses was totally ignored by the government. Instead, women of social position and influence won the ear of the Surgeon-General, and volunteers were selected by Dr. Anita McGee, under the sponsorship of the Daughters of the American Revolution.[102]

By 1898, too, the superintendents were uncomfortably aware of widespread public criticism of trained nurses, particularly of that great majority of graduates who earned their living caring for cases in private homes. For the most part, it was not the nurse's skill or knowledge that was questioned, but her personal conduct: she was said to be too talkative or too arbitrary, she was wasteful of household supplies. One may surmise that families under strain of serious illness had difficulty adjusting to the constant presence of a stranger with ill-defined status and authority, a normal share of human failings, and usually some ignorance of upper class mores. The superintendents responded to this criticism with a stepped-up effort (reflected in Hampton's *Nursing Ethics* of 1900) to stiffen the morals and conduct of the pupil nurses. Superintendents' control of admission and expulsion must be absolute; candidates younger than twenty-five, not yet past the "silly age," should be rejected. As for carelessness and extravagance, the fault, of course, lay in the pupil's upbringing, but it was nevertheless the superintendent's duty "by precept and example and continued watchfulness during the two or three years we have them with us in training" to reform the character and send out "examples of economy as well as angels of mercy."[103]

Had they known it, the superintendents, in their renewed affirmation of Victorian middle class standards of female behavior, were binding nursing to a code that was obsolescent and already being challenged by a rising current of feminism. They were also flying in the face of demographic change. The last great wave of immigration was adding millions each year to the population, at the same time that city life and the prestige of modern medicine began to draw not only the ailing poor but the middle classes into the hospital. New institutions had to be built, and the small hospital (Hampton's bête noir) suddenly multiplied, as the upper levels of society, shrinking at first from the general hospital with its pauper associations, patronized proprietary institutions established by enterprising doctors. To assure themselves cheap labor, these proprietary hospitals opened so-called training schools, without assuming the obligations of such schools, as Hampton and the society conceived them.[104] After a decade of exciting challenge and dedicated work, Hampton and her small corps of superintendents, with their weak educational system and fledgling professional institutions, saw the private-duty market flooded with a new multitude of "trained nurses" from "schools" indifferent or oblivious to "professional" standards or refined demeanor. The employer, already disappointed in his expectations of gentle womanly nurture and economical use of linens, neither a virtue imparted in the rugged ordeal of hospital training, now was further put off by such poorly trained personnel.

Even in the 1890s, Hampton and the other superintendents of the best hospital schools had at times been forced to accept students whom they considered unqualified, simply to meet the needs for nursing service. From 1900 on, as hospitals multiplied and other occupations less demanding and isolating opened up to women, even the good schools had to dip down into the labor pool and admit ever more youthful and more poorly prepared students. By 1912, more than 55 per cent of pupil nurses were only twenty years old, or younger. The supply of middle and upper-middle-class girls with good educational backgrounds dwindled further, as many who might have entered nursing in the 1890s elected to go to college. Of the 303 students in seven New York City training schools in 1910 (most of the seven among the best in the country) more than half had had less than four years of high school.[105]

In 1890, with 35 training schools in operation, and something under 500 graduate nurses in the United States, Isabel Hampton's long-range plans had seemed practicable. But even in 1893 her new Society of Superintendents did not represent the majority of existing schools and nurses. By 1900 there were 432 schools; in 1909 they numbered 1096.[106] Only a minority of their superintendents belonged to the society, and only a minority of graduates joined their school alumnae associations (and through them, the Associated Alumnae), or subscribed to the struggling *American Journal of Nursing,* which for years lacked money for an office outside the editor's home. The Hospital Economics course at Teachers College attracted a bare handful of students in its first half-dozen years, and was kept alive only by contributions of money and teaching services from Hampton, Nutting, and a few others.[107]

Hampton's remedy for the dilution of standards by small training schools was still the idea of a central school offering a rounded experience in several small hospitals with different medical specialties. By 1905 she had broadened this concept to advocate a coordinating central institution in each state.[108] But the bigger version, like the smaller one, failed to come to grips with the basic problem of securing adequate financial support.

Of Hampton's proposed instructional reforms, the three-year course, by reducing turnover, worked to the hospitals' benefit and was generally adopted, but only a few institutions enriched the educational program as she had expected; elsewhere the old two-year curriculum was just spread thinner. She had triumphantly abolished the practice of sending senior students out to duty in private homes, but now some schools were making money by assigning seniors to special duty with private patients in the hospital for long periods. She had introduced graduate head nurses at Hopkins; now many hospitals put senior pupils back in charge, under the direction of a graduate nurse supervisor.[109]

As nurses actually lost ground in their efforts to establish standards, their counterparts, the doctors, were well on the way to bringing their sprawling profession under control. The American Medical Association was reorganized in 1901, and in 1904 it began the process of inspection and grading of medical schools which, culminating in the Flexner report of 1910, forced dozens of inadequate schools to close.

Within the profession which she loved with a possessive affection, Hampton's leadership was inevitably challenged. The two stalwart leaders of the Massachusetts General Hospital contingent, Sophia Palmer and Mary E. P. Davis, old friends and classmates and shrewd businesswomen, quickly made themselves felt in the Society of Superintendents. Palmer had taken the lead at the Manhattan Beach meeting which founded the Associated Alumnae, and in 1900, Palmer and Davis, to Hampton's exasperation, single-handedly launched the *American Journal of Nursing,* much in the fashion that Hampton and Nutting had produced the course at Teachers College. Relations were further strained when Palmer criticized the management of the course. With the Hopkins group, of course, Hampton's ties were strong, but even her long, affectionate friendship with Adelaide Nutting cooled as Nutting's strong intellect and will carried her to the forefront of organized nursing and, in 1907, to a professorship at Teachers College.[110]

Meanwhile Lavinia Dock moved into a different world, Lillian Wald's Nurses' Settlement on Henry Street in New York. Isabel Hampton had been the earliest public champion of district nursing, which she correctly perceived to be a field that nursing could develop for its own, a role that could attain a distinct social importance. Now, however, while private-duty nursing became the weary target of public criticism, the public lavished appreciation and support on Lillian Wald and her visiting nurses. The organizations which Hampton had brought into being struggled with internal problems, while more broadly based activity by women in movements for health, education, and recreation receded from their view. Miss Wald allied herself not with the medical profession but with the growing public health movement, secured the endowment which finally put the Teachers College course on its feet, and eventually took a leading part in forming a separate professional body, the National Organization for Public Health Nursing. And all the while, Henry Street was becoming the center of a circle of brilliant women social reformers and feminists in which Lavinia Dock found herself completely at home.[111]

To Isabel Hampton, life in Cleveland as Mrs. Hunter Robb also brought some measure of disappointment. True, she enjoyed the social prestige awarded the wife of one of the city's leading physicians, and found time for local nursing affairs, serving on the executive committee of the Visiting Nurse Association from its founding in 1901, and as chairman of the training-school committee of the Lakeside Hospital. Looking back on those years, Clevelanders felt that she had created a strongly supportive atmosphere for the profession there. Considerable evidence survives to indicate that her marriage was less than happy, however, though Dr. Robb does not seem to have interfered with his wife's professional work in any way. Household duties did sometimes interfere, and irked her generally. She loved her two sons, but reportedly overindulged them; after the birth of the second, in 1902, when she was forty-two, she became less active professionally. In June 1910, at the age of fifty, Isabel Hampton Robb was killed in a streetcar accident in Cleveland.[112]

As Adelaide Nutting reflected after Hampton's death, she had had, at Johns Hopkins, an opportunity to "create standard, precedent, and tradition at will, under conditions which were at that time little less than ideal."[113] Trained nursing was just emerging from its pioneer stage. At Johns Hopkins, thanks in part to Hampton's leadership and magnetism, it received recognition as an essential auxiliary of modern medicine, and a good measure of encouragement to keep pace with medicine and share in its rising status. The Hopkins experience encouraged Hampton's attempts to make nursing an organized, self-regulating profession for women; the World's Fair provided a highly visible public debut, and, under Hampton's spell, the impetus for the rapid formation of professional nursing organizations.

But the Hopkins experience of the early 1890s was a unique historical moment, and the Hopkins ambience did not prove reproducible elsewhere. Within the expanding hospital world of the new century, competition for funds intensified, and the nurses and their training schools inevitably emerged a poor second to the staff physicians. Caught in a vicious circle of public criticism, they clung to outworn notions of female gentility that frowned upon aggressiveness. Isolated and overworked in the hospital and on private duty, they were separated from the vital branch of their profession which engaged in active combat with social problems in the outer world, and sought to raise the status of women. The leadership at the top of what came to be the nursing establishment, encumbered by middle class prejudice (in the guise of idealism), continued to call for higher standards, with little response from the general public or a major part of their own constituency. The status quo would be accepted as woman's place for a generation or more to come.

NOTES

1. *Twenty Years at Hull-House* (New York: Macmillan, 1910), p. 61.

2. In their tentative acceptance of the women's committee's proposal, the trustees carefully defined the sphere of women doctors. "This board is satisfied that in hospital practice among women, in penal institutions in which women are cared for, and in private life where women are to be attended, there is a need and place for learned and capable women physicians." "Medical School Fund," *Johns Hopkins Hospital Bulletin* 1 (November 1890): 103.

3. Ibid., p. 104.

4. Ibid. Both the women's committee and the trustees prefaced their remarks on the admission of women as medical students by strong statements on the importance of training women as nurses.

5. Ibid., 1 (December 1889): 6–8.

6. "The Structure and Ideology of American Nursing," in *The Nursing Profession*, ed. Fred Davis (New York: John Wiley and Sons, 1966), p. 69.

7. M. Adelaide Nutting and Lavinia L. Dock, *A History of Nursing*, vols. 1 and 2 (New York: G. P. Putnam's Sons, 1907); Dock, *A History of Nursing*, vols. 3 and 4 (New York: G. P. Putnam's Sons, 1912). Many times revised by Dock and Isabel M. Stewart, and finally by Stewart and Anne L. Austin, this classic work reached its 5th edition in 1962. Other authoritative surveys by nursing leaders are Mary M. Roberts, *American Nursing* (New York: Macmillan, 1954), and Isabel M. Stewart, *The Education of Nurses* (New York: Macmillan, 1943). Richard H. Shryock, *The History of Nursing: An Interpretation of the Social and Medical Factors Involved* (Philadelphia: W. B. Saunders, 1959), is an excellent survey by a distinguished historian of medicine; see also his "Nursing Emerges as a Profession: The American Experience," *Clio Medica* 3 (1968): 131–47. For sociological treatments see Davis, *Nursing Profession*, and Amitai Etzioni, *The Semi-Professions and Their Organization: Teachers, Nurses, Social Workers* (New York: Free Press, 1969).

8. Ada M. Carr, "The Early History of the Hospital and the Training School," *Johns Hopkins Nurses Alumnae Magazine* 8 (June 1909): 54–75; John S. Billings

et al., Hospital Plans (New York: W. Wood, 1875); Donald Fleming, *William H. Welch and the Rise of Modern Medicine* (Boston: Little Brown, 1954). For the history of hospitals, see W. Gill Wylie, *Hospitals: Their History, Organization, and Construction* (New York: Appleton, 1877); Henry C. Burdett, *Hospitals and Asylums of the World*, 4 vols. (London: J. and A. Churchill, 1893), vol. 3; Commission on Hospital Care, *Hospital Care in the United States* (New York: Commonwealth Fund, 1947), chaps. 30–33; Morris J. Vogel, "Boston's Hospitals, 1870–1930: A Social History" (Ph.D. diss., University of Chicago, 1974); Charles E. Rosenberg, "And Heal the Sick: The Hospital and the Patient in the 19th Century America," *Journal of Social History* 10 (Summer 1977): 428–47.

9. See Shryock, *History of Nursing*, pp. 278–81.

10. Elizabeth King Ellicott, address to the Maryland State Association of Graduate Nurses in 1900, quoted in Ethel Johns and Blanche Pfefferkorn, *The Johns Hopkins Hospital School of Nursing, 1889–1949* (Baltimore: Johns Hopkins University Press, 1954), p. 22.

11. Johns Hopkins Hospital, *Reports and Papers Relating to Construction and Organization*, no. 1 (1876), pp. 6–8.

12. Ibid., no. 3 (1877), pp. 8–10.

13. Ibid., p. 11.

14. "The Plans and Purposes of the Johns Hopkins Hospital," *Addresses at the Opening of the Hospital, May 7, 1889* (Baltimore: J. Murphy and Co., 1889), p. 29.

15. Johns Hopkins Hospital, *Reports and Papers*, no. 3, p. 11.

16. Ibid.; Henry M. Hurd, address at 25th anniversary of the Johns Hopkins Hospital, 1914, typescript in William H. Welch Papers, Welch Medical Library, Johns Hopkins Medical School, Baltimore, Md.; Billings, "Plans and Purposes," p. 30.

17. Billings *et al., Hospital Plans*, p. 9; Billings, "Plans and Purposes," p. 19.

18. Harvey Cushing, *The Life of Sir William Osler*, 2 vols. (Oxford: Clarendon Press, 1925), 1: 303.

19. "Hospital Organization and Management" (1897), quoted in Thomas S. Cullen, *Henry Mills Hurd* (Baltimore: Johns Hopkins University Press, 1920), p. 76; "The Relation of the Training School for Nurses to the Johns Hopkins Hospital," *Johns Hopkins Hospital Bulletin* 1 (December 1889): 7. Mrs. Hurd was an active member of the Women's Fund Committee for the medical school.

20. "Relation of Training School to Hospital," p. 8.

21. Hurd to King, 4 Sept. 1889, typed copy in Nightingale Collection, Welch Medical Library, Johns Hopkins Medical School, Baltimore, Md.

22. William Osler, "The Inner History of the Johns Hopkins Hospital," *Johns Hopkins Medical Journal* 125 (October 1969): 187; Dock, *History*, 3: 122; Carr, "Early History of the Hospital," p. 65.

23. Osler, "Inner History," pp. 187–88.

24. Among the many glowing descriptions of her, see Lavinia L. Dock and Henry M. Hurd in "The Isabel Hampton Robb Memorial Fund," *Johns Hopkins Nurses Alumnae Magazine* 11 (April 1912): 6, 16. Also Elizabeth King Ellicott, in "Memorial Services for Isabel Hampton Robb," *Johns Hopkins Hospital Bulletin* 21 (August 1910): 11. For her maternal sense see, for instance, Edith W. Ware, interview with Grace Baxter, n.d., typed summary, Department of Nursing Education Archives, Teachers College, Columbia University (hereafter cited as Dept. Nurs. Ed. Archives, TC).

25. M. E. Cameron, "Isabel Hampton—Pupil Nurse in the Bellevue Training School for Nurses, 1881–1883," *American Journal of Nursing* 11 (October 1910): 10–13; Lavinia L. Dock, in "Memorial Fund," p. 7; M. Adelaide Nutting, in

"Memorial Services for Isabel Hampton Robb," *Johns Hopkins Hospital Bulletin* 21 (August 1910): 6.

26. Hampton to Elizabeth Birdseye, 11 July 1886, Nightingale Collection; Edith A. Draper, "Isabel Hampton Robb," *American Journal of Nursing* 2 (January 1902): 244.

27. Lavinia Dock in "Memorial Fund," p. 7; Isabel McIsaac, "Should Undergraduates Be Sent Out to Private Duty," Society of Superintendents, *Third Annual Report* (1896) p. 67.

28. Cora Overholt as quoted in "Memorial Services," *American Journal of Nursing* 11 (October 1910): 32.

29. Dock, *History*, 3: 124.

30. "Isabel Hampton Robb—Her Work in Organization and Education," *American Journal of Nursing* 11 (October 1910): 19.

31. Isabel Hampton Robb, "An International Educational Standard for Nursing," reprint from *New York Medical Journal*, 15 January 1910, p. 7, in nursing history files, Office of Director, Massachusetts General Hospital School of Nursing (hereafter cited as MGHSN), Boston, Mass.

32. These and the following data on pupils of the Boston Training School come from the manuscript enrollment books, Office of Director, MGHSN.

33. *Report of the Directors of the Boston Training School for Nurses Attached to the Massachusetts General Hospital*, 1889, pp. 4, 6.

34. Carr, "Early History," p. 70.

35. The monthly records of the nursing department and the files of letters from applicants accepted are preserved in the Welch Medical Library at the Johns Hopkins Medical School. Unless otherwise noted, they are the source for this and the next seven paragraphs.

36. Lavinia Dock's note on the application of Wilhelmina Wade, September 1891, records that Dr. Hurd was "displeased."

37. See family correspondence in Nutting Papers, Dept. Nurs. Ed. Archives, TC.

38. Georgia Nevins and Adelaide Nutting in "Memorial Services," *American Journal of Nursing* 11 (October 1910): 39, 28; Nutting in "Memorial Services for Isabel Hampton Robb," *Johns Hopkins Hospital Bulletin* 21 (August 1910): 8; Carr, "Early History," p. 73; Dock, "Recollections of Miss Hampton at the Johns Hopkins," *American Journal of Nursing* 11 (October 1910): 16–17. Since in the first years there were no medical students at the hospital, the nurses, as the only young people, may have enjoyed a special place in the sun. This could (in part, at least) account for the idyllic memories of Carr, Dock, and others.

39. Hampton described this solution in her textbook, *Nursing: Its Principles and Practice* (Philadelphia: W. B. Saunders, 1894). The admission records confirm that she used such a system at Hopkins.

40. Hampton, *Nursing*, pp. 19–20, 33, 34.

41. Hampton, "Practical and Scientific Instruction in Invalid Cooking," *Johns Hopkins Hospital Bulletin* 1 (December 1890): 108; Henry M. Hurd, in "Robb Memorial Fund," p. 18; Carr, "Early History," p. 71; Hampton, *Nursing*, p. 40.

42. Hampton, *Nursing*, pp. 56, 42, 17. " 'The comfort of the patient' was the keynote of all our practical instruction," an early pupil recalled. Georgia Nevins, in "Memorial Services," *American Journal of Nursing* 11 (October 1910): 29.

43. Grace Baxter to Adelaide Nutting, n.d. [probably about 1940], incomplete typed copy, Dept. Nurs. Ed. Archives, TC.

44. "She filled us with great pride in our work," Adelaide Nutting later wrote. "It seemed to us better worth doing than any other work in the world." "Memorial Services," *Johns Hopkins Hospital Bulletin* 21 (August 1910): 9.

45. *Second Report of the Superintendent of the Johns Hopkins Hospital, January 31, 1891*, pp. 32–33; Edith Ware, typed notes on two interviews with Adelaide Nutting, one undated, the other 31 June 1939, Dept. Nurs. Ed. Archives, TC; Johns and Pfefferkorn, *Johns Hopkins Hospital School of Nursing*, pp. 80–83; *Johns Hopkins Hospital Bulletin* 2 (July 1891): 95.

46. Osler, "Medicine and Nursing," in *Essays on Vocation* ed. Basil Mathews (London: Oxford University Press, 1919), p. 9; Kelly, *The Ministry of Nursing* (Baltimore: Griffen, Curley, 1892), pp. 5–8; C. N. B. Camac, comp., *Counsels and Ideals, from the Writings of William Osler* (Boston: Houghton Mifflin, 1905), pp. 94, 121.

47. Nutting, "Isabel Hampton Robb," *American Journal of Nursing* 11 (October 1910): 19–20; "Memorial Services," *Johns Hopkins Hospital Bulletin* 21 (August 1910): 9.

48. *Nursing*, p. 55; *Nursing Ethics* (Cleveland: E.C. Koeckert, 1900), p. 173.

49. *Nursing*, pp. 56–57; *Nursing Ethics*, p. 79.

50. *Nursing Ethics*, pp. 65, 78, 52, 61.

51. *Nursing*, p. 57; *Nursing Ethics*, pp. 139–40.

52. William Osler, "Nurse and Patient," in *Aequanimitas* (Philadelphia: P. Blakiston's Sons and Co., 1905), p. 164.

53. *Nursing Ethics*, pp. 64, 132, 85.

54. Ibid., p. 63.

55. Ibid., pp. 57, 38.

56. Edith Ware, interviews with Ida Carr, 13 June 1940; Dr. J. M. T. Finney, 10 June 1940; Adelaide Nutting, December 1940; Dr. William T. Howard, 13 June 1940; typed notes in Dept. Nurs. Ed. Archives, TC.

57. Hurd, "Robb Memorial Fund," p. 16. On Hurd and the nurses, see, e.g., Edith Ware interview with [Ruth B.?] Sherman, 8 June 1940, typed notes in Dept. Nurs. Ed. Archives, TC.

58. Hurd, in *Sir William Osler, Bart.: Brief Tributes to His Personality, Influence and Public Service* (Baltimore: Johns Hopkins University Press, 1920), pp. 105–6; Edith Ware, interview with Isabel M. Stewart (Nutting's friend and successor at Teachers College), November 1940, typed notes in Dept. Nurs. Ed. Archives, TC. The highly articulate Osler often expressed (sometimes under heavy veils of literary allusion) the medical profession's perception of nurses and nursing as a threat. See, for instance, "The Hospital as a College," an address given in 1903, arguing for increased clinical teaching of medical students: "I envy for our medical students the advantages enjoyed by the nurses, who live in daily contact with the sick, and who have, in this country at least, supplanted the former in the affections of the hospital trustees." *Aequanimitas*, p. 333.

59. Elizabeth King Ellicott, in *Johns Hopkins Hospital Bulletin* 21 (August 1910): 11–12; Carr, "Early History," p. 71.

60. William Sydney Thayer, "Reminiscences of Osler," *Osler and Other Papers* (Baltimore: Johns Hopkins University Press, 1931), pp. 30, 37; for Robb's papers, see the following issues of the *Johns Hopkins Hospital Bulletin:* 2 (December 1891); 4 (September 1893); and 5 (January–February 1894). See also Kelly's review of John A. Ouchterlony, *Pioneer Medical Men and Times in Kentucky*, in *Johns Hopkins Hospital Bulletin* 3 (April 1892), which lauds the work of Mrs. Frances Coomes, "a surgeon, physician and obstetrician." Kelly's library on women's history forms part of the Nightingale Collection at the Welch Medical Library.

61. Osler, "Inner History of the Hospital," p. 188.

62. Lavinia Dock, "Recollections," p. 18. "Her power of concentration," Dock said, "was admirable, and she had a tranquil poise, not easily disturbed even by

interruption. After coming in from last rounds I would sit down and hear the newest pages. Dr. Robb used also to wander in and help with suggestions as to phrasing." On the longevity of the textbook see Dr. Hurd's comment in "Memorial Fund," p. 18.

63. *Johns Hopkins Hospital Bulletin* 5 (April 1894): 55.

64. "Recollections," p. 17; Dock, *History*, 3: 123–24; Isabel M. Stewart and Anne L. Austin, *A History of Nursing* (New York: G. P. Putnam's Sons, 1962), p. 199.

65. She used this term in *Nursing*, p. 58.

66. *Nursing*, p. 58, and *Nursing Ethics*, p. 139.

67. Dock, *History*, 3: 124–25.

68. Hampton, *Nursing Ethics*, pp. 258–59.

69. Adelaide Nutting later wrote that Hampton and Dock, at this time, also "studied progress made in other training schools and in other branches of education." "The Work of the Johns Hopkins School for Nurses," *Johns Hopkins Hospital Bulletin* 25 (December 1914): 5.

70. Lucy Walker-Donnell to Nutting, 25 May 1940, Dept. Nurs. Ed. Archives, TC; Nutting, "Work of the Johns Hopkins School," p. 5.

71. A notice of the club's establishment was carried in the 23 May 1891 issue of *The Nightingale*, one of the short-lived nursing periodicals of the day. The *Johns Hopkins Hospital Bulletin* printed its annual reports; see 2 (April 1891): 65–66; 3 (June 1892): 79–80; 4 (October 1893): 100. The report for 1893–94, printed in leaflet form, is in the Nightingale Collection as are typed copies of some of the original papers.

72. The other addresses were "Training Schools for Nurses," at the National Conference of Charities and Correction in 1890, "District Nursing," at the annual meeting of Baltimore's Charity Organization Society in 1891, and "Educational Standards for Nurses," at the Chicago World's Fair in 1893; all are cited below.

73. As an alternative, she proposed a central school connected with a group of small institutions which could provide training comparable to that of a large general hospital. Stepping carefully, she did not emphasize the opportunities for self-determination which such a school would afford, run by nurses, and with nurses on its board together with representatives of the hospitals and the medical profession.

74. "Training Schools for Nurses," *Proceedings of the National Conference of Charities and Correction* (1890), pp. 145–46; "District Nursing," in Hampton, *Educational Standards for Nurses* (Cleveland: E. C. Koeckert, 1907), pp. 52–53.

75. District nursing had been pioneered in the United States in 1877, as a charitable effort, under the nonsectarian Protestant auspices of the New York City Mission and Tract Society, with Mrs. William H. Osborn, board chairman of the Bellevue Training School, paying for the services of a Bellevue graduate. For the historical background, see Annie M. Brainard, *The Evolution of Public Health Nursing* (Philadelphia: W. B. Saunders, 1922).

76. The Johns Hopkins School of Nursing added public health nursing to the curriculum in 1933, the Massachusetts General Hospital School in 1938. See Sylvia Perkins, *A Centennial Review: The Massachusetts General Hospital School of Nursing, 1873–1973* (n.p.: [Massachusetts General Hospital] School of Nursing, Nurses Alumnae Association, 1975).

77. Dr. Hurd, in his annual reports, repeatedly called attention to the need for a system of district nursing in Baltimore, to "lighten the heavy burden of poverty and preventable disease" (*Second Report of the Superintendent*, p. 31). Dr. Kelly, an exponent of the social gospel, who had begun his medical practice in a mill town outside of Philadelphia, pressed the trustees to introduce such a system, in his

address to the training-school graduates in 1892 (*The Ministry of Nursing,* pp. 10–13). Dr. Osler, deeply interested in containing the spread of tuberculosis, is reported to have told Miss Nutting, in a burst of enthusiasm, that if he had not been a physician he would have wanted to be a district nurse. (Edith Ware, interview with Isabel Stewart, November 1940, typed notes in Dept. Nurs. Ed. Archives, TC).

78. "Training Schools," p. 145 and passim.

79. "District Nursing," pp. 46ff.

80. The papers were originally published in John S. Billings and Henry M. Hurd, eds., *Hospitals, Dispensaries and Nursing: Papers and Discussions in the International Congress of Charities, Correction and Philanthropy, Section III, Chicago, June 12th to 17th, 1893* (Baltimore: 1894). The papers on nursing were reprinted in *Nursing of the Sick, 1893* (New York: McGraw-Hill, 1949).

81. Dock, "Recollections," p. 18.

82. Dock, "The Relation of Training Schools to Hospitals," in *Nursing of the Sick,* pp. 14, 13.

83. Ibid., pp. 18, 21, 19, 20.

84. Dock, *History,* 3: 126.

85. Hampton, "Educational Standards for Nurses," in *Nursing of the Sick,* pp. 5, 7, 8, 11.

86. Dock, "The Relation of Training Schools to Hospitals," pp. 16–17.

87. See especially Louise Darche, "Proper Organization of Training Schools in America," in *Nursing of the Sick,* pp. 101–3.

88. Dock, "The Relation of Training Schools to Hospitals," pp. 23–24.

89. Dock, *History,* 3: 126.

90. Nightingale, "Sick Nursing and Health Nursing," *Nursing of the Sick,* p. 36; Draper, "Necessity of an American Nurses' Association," idem., p. 151; Sutliffe, "History of American Training Schools," idem., p. 92.

91. Darche, "Proper Organization," pp. 104–6.

92. Isabel McIsaac, presidential address to International Council of Nurses, Buffalo, New York, September 1901, in *American Journal of Nursing* 2 (October 1901): 2.

93. Dock, *History,* 3: 127; Society of Superintendents, *First and Second Annual Reports,* 1895, p. 3 (hereafter SS, *First Report,* etc.).

94. May Wright Sewall, ed., *The World's Congress of Representative Women,* 2 vols. (Chicago: Rand McNally, 1894); Mary K. O. Eagle, ed., *The Congress of Women* (Chicago: International Publishing Co., 1894).

95. Darche, "Proper Organization," p. 103.

96. Later reports are: Committee for the Study of Nursing Education, *Nursing and Nursing Education in the United States* [the Goldmark Report] (New York: Macmillan, 1923); Esther Lucile Brown, *Nursing for the Future* (New York: Russell Sage Foundation, 1948); and Jerome P. Lysaught, *An Abstract for Action* (New York: McGraw-Hill, 1970).

97. SS, *First and Second Reports,* pp. 8, 10. (The third and subsequent *Annual Reports* were published individually.)

98. SS, *Second Report,* p. 37.

99. SS, *First Report,* p. 16; *Seventh Report,* p. 29.

100. Dock, *History,* 3: 128–29; *The Trained Nurse* 16 (October 1896): 534. A scattering of the early records of this organization, now the American Nurses Association, may be found in the Nursing History Archives, Boston University.

101. SS, *Fifth Report,* pp. 66–70; *Sixth Report,* pp. 61–64. On the germina-

tion of the idea, see Dock, *History*, 3: 131–33; Dock, in "Memorial Fund," pp. 9–10; Nurses' Alumnae Association, Proceedings of the 12th Convention, in *American Journal of Nursing* 9 (September 1909): 955.

102. Hampton, "Some of the Lessons of the Late War and Their Bearing upon Trained Nursing," in her *Educational Standards for Nurses;* Sophia Palmer, "Women in the War," SS, *Sixth Report,* p. 69.

103. For a sample of the criticisms of private duty nurses and the superintendents' reaction, see, in SS, *Fifth Report:* Mary Agnes Snively, presidential address, p. 8; Eva Allerton, "How Far Are Training Schools Responsible for Lack of Ethics among Nurses" (and discussion following), pp. 45ff.; Linda Richards, "The Superintendent of the Training School," p. 52; in SS, *Sixth Report,* Alice I. Twitchell, "The Tendency of Trained Nurses to Extravagance" and discussion, pp. 38ff.; editorial, *American Journal of Nursing,* 9 (October 1908): 5.

104. Isabel M. Stewart, *The Education of Nurses,* p. 140.

105. Ibid., p. 153.

106. Ibid., p. 128, 130, 139.

107. In 1910, for instance, the Society of Superintendents had 360 members. (Adelaide Nutting in "Memorial Services," *Johns Hopkins Hospital Bulletin* 21 [August 1910]: 10.) In the same period less than half the graduates of the Massachusetts General Hospital training school belonged to their alumnae association. (Perkins, *Centennial Review,* p. 67.) Nurse historians have understandably glossed over the low participation in professional organizations, though Mary Roberts refers to it (*American Nursing,* p. 46). The difficulties of the early years of the Teachers College course are documented in Teresa E. Christy, *Cornerstone for Nursing Education* (New York: Teachers College Press, 1969), chaps. 2 and 3.

108. Stewart, *Education of Nurses,* pp. 173–74.

109. Ibid., pp. 155–56.

110. On the Manhattan Beach meeting, see Dock, *History,* 3: 129. Hampton's reactions to Palmer and Davis's entrepreneurship with the *American Journal of Nursing* are evident in her letters to Nutting, in Dept. Nurs. Ed. Archives, TC. See also, on her relationship with Palmer, Edith Ware, notes on interview with Harriet Fulmer, 14 November 1940. The cooling of the Hampton-Nutting friendship can be inferred from such letters as Hampton to Nutting, 28 December [1907], and Ware, notes on interview with Mrs. Lord, 12 June 1940, all in Dept. Nurs. Ed. Archives. On Palmer's criticisms of the Teachers College course, see Christy, *Cornerstone for Nursing Education,* pp. 23ff.

111. Hampton must also have found disheartening the rise of medical social work in hospitals, its early divorce from nursing, and its quick professionalization on an independent basis.

112. This account of Hampton's life in Cleveland is based on a skeptical reading of Edith Ware's notes (Dept. Nurs. Ed. Archives, TC) on the gossipy reminiscences given her thirty years after Hampton's death. See, for instance, Dr. Lewellys F. Barker and Mrs. Lord (a former pupil), 12 June 1940; Dr. Howard A. Kelly and Dr. William T. Howard, 13 June 1940; Isabel Stewart, November 1940; Mrs. John H. Lowman, Annie Brainard, and Elizabeth M. Folchemer, 18 November 1940; Marian G. Howell and Mrs. Charles F. Hoover, 19 November 1940; Helena McMillan, 16 November 1940; Louise Muller and Mrs. A. R. Colvin [Sadie Tarleton], 15 November 1940.

113. "Isabel Hampton Robb," *American Journal of Nursing* 11 (October 1910): 22.

10 *THE SOCIOCULTURAL IMPACT OF TWENTIETH-CENTURY THERAPEUTICS*

EDMUND D. PELLEGRINO

INTRODUCTION

Nothing more clearly sets contemporary medicine apart from its antecedents than its remarkable therapeutic effectiveness. Physicians now routinely intervene, specifically and radically, in the natural history of previously fatal diseases. No disorder, however complex or intractable, is beyond the possibility of conquest. Man's Promethean hope of removing the restraints of disease on history seem less illusory than ever before.

Medicine's capabilities are felt far beyond the immediacies of the patient-physician encounter. By curing, eradicating, or controlling so many devastating diseases, medicine now shapes the economic, demographic, and social structure of human populations. Its newer, as yet incompletely exploited capabilities in genetics and behavioral modification promise to shape the future of human nature itself.

Equally powerful, though more subtly expressed, are the sociocultural influences of twentieth-century therapeutics. Medicine is now a paradigm of the mixed blessings of technology. Therapeutics is as awesome as nuclear power or space travel but, for most people, far more immediate and urgent. The physician is our Merlin, at once beneficent and threatening, able to overwhelm as well as enhance human existence. Public admiration is mixed with suspicion, as expenditures and expectations rise, simultaneously with calls for regulation and accountability.

Despite these ambivalencies—or perhaps because of them—medicine is emerging as a prime shaper of cultural values. It no longer reflects faithfully a dominant and homogeneous value system, as in the past. Instead, by offering so many possibilities for controlling human destiny, it more often challenges or contravenes traditional value systems. Each new medical possibility forces a redefinition of the good life, the nature of man, and the purposes of his existence. It is what we believe about these matters that ultimately must direct how we will use medical technology.

In a pluralistic society, in which traditional values are eroded, what medicine *can* do easily becomes what medicine *should* do. Medicine itself can become a sort of salvation theme, justified by its own powers, rather than by the ends it serves. Man's sense of the fragility of human existence can thus be reduced to a hope in immortality through pharmacology, or genetic engineering, or making the "new man" by electrochemical control of human behavior.

This essay traces the historical and cultural influence of modern medicine, as exemplified in the power of its therapeutics. Two unifying themes are used—the concepts of disease localization and the design of specific therapeutic agents to act at the locus of disease. These two concepts are distinctive of contemporary medicine. The history of their origins, and their impact on the intellectual history of the profession as well as on society's view of that profession, lead to our concern for the future impact of medicine on our culture.

ORIGINS OF TWENTIETH-CENTURY THERAPEUTICS

Professor Charles Rosenberg's paper, "The Therapeutic Revolution" (chapter 1 of this volume), provides a thoughtful analysis of the transition in the sociocultural character of therapeutics in the nineteenth century.[1] As he shows, at the beginning of that century, therapeutics was fixed in a notion of health and illness held in common by physicians and their patients. On this view, illness was an imbalance in the economy of the whole body, expressed in a disturbance in the relationships of input or output of food, sweat, secretions, urine, phlegm, and the like. Treatment was aimed at restoring harmony and balance between environment and constitution. This was best accomplished not by specific attack on some symptoms of disease, but by inducing a physiological effect—sweating, febrilysis, diuresis, vomiting—which helped the body to recover its internal and external balance.

The nineteenth-century notion of health as balance is a very old one. It appears as the harmony of body and soul in Alcmaeon, Hippocrates, Plato, and Aristotle, and is variously termed *isonomia, eukrasia,* or *sophrosyne*[2]. This view of health persists in our own times and is enjoying a recrudescence today in the movement towards holistic, wholistic, or psychosomatic medicine—all of which emphasize treatment of the "whole person" and not the part alone. These modern versions, however, usually accept the value of specific therapy and disease localization but emphasize their employment in a context of care for the whole person. While in this essay we shall place emphasis on localization, and reductionism, they cannot be said to have entirely replaced holistic theories of therapeutics and the notion of health as harmony.

As the nineteenth century advanced, the integrated view of illness and therapeutics was increasingly challenged by the growing idea of diseases as discrete clinical entities, with inherent "natural" histories perhaps less susceptible to intervention by holistic therapy than had been supposed. Therapeutic nihilism, or at least therapeutic parsimony, came to be espoused by some eminent clinical teachers, and as vehemently denounced by others. Most physicians persisted in the old ideas, although gradually skepticism took hold. In the last third of the century, doses were less heroic, bleeding disappeared. Purges, emetics, and diuretics remained popular, however.

At the close of the nineteenth century, physicians were understandably ambivalent about accepting the new conception of a type of therapeutics specifically tailored to particular disease entities which had slowly been emerging during the course of the century. The agents so classified were few but undeniably impressive (table 1). The rationalism of Claude Bernard's plea for scientific, experimental medicine promised more. Yet it was difficult, as always, to give up long held theories about the nature of disease and how it should be treated. The burgeoning achievements of pharmaceutical chemistry, anesthesia, and surgery in the early twentieth century, however, finally compromised the older theories. While the tensions between holistic and discrete explanatory systems continues, the balance, today, has been tipped heavily in favor of the discrete and the radical in therapeutics.

While the concepts which underlie contemporary therapeutics were growing in the nineteenth century, we can trace their origins in the medical thought of the sixteenth and seventeenth centuries.[3] It is surely naive to select any single theoretical innovation as the origin of a scientific or cultural idea. Characteristically, such ideas appear recurrently in incomplete, ill-defined, and often unpopular forms before they become part of the professional or cultural apparatus. Nonetheless, a few innovative thinkers appear to have been especially influential in developing the modern ideas of specificity and discreteness which form the conceptual basis for twentieth-century medicine and therapeutics (figure 1).

Perhaps the first real challenge to the idea of illness as a whole-body phenomenon came with Thomas Sydenham's plea for a nosology of disease

Table 1

Chronology of Specificity in Therapeutics

	Agent	*Use*
1753	lime juice	scurvey
1785	digitalis	heart failure
1806	morphine isolated	pain
1818	transfusion	blood loss
1819	colchicine	gout
1820	quinine isolated	malaria
1831	chloroform synthesized	anesthesia
1832	atropine isolated	anti-spasmodic
1862	chloral hydrate	somnifacient
1863	barbituric acid	somnifacient
1869	*digitalis nativelle* isolated	heart failure
1874	salicylic acid synthesized	pain, fever
1886	acetanilide	pain, fever
1887	phenacetin	pain, fever
1890	diphtheria antitoxin	diphtherin
1894	tetanus antitoxin	tetanus
1907	salvarsan	syphilis
1915	indirect blood transfusion	blood loss
1916	diphenyl ethyl hydantoin	epilepsy
1920	mercurial diuretics	edema
1921	insulin	diabetes
1921	plasmoquin	malaria
1924	parathyroid extract	tetany
1926	liver extract	pernicious anemia
1927	vitamin D	rickets
1929	estrogens	replacement
	adrenal extracts	replacement

based in observation and reason rather than in all-embracing systems of ultimate causes. Sydenham was Hippocratic in his insistence on observation of individual cases. But he sought, in addition, to group cases with similar symptoms into classes, creating identifiable clinical entities. He believed therapy could be improved by careful observation of patients' responses to treatment, thus leading to the discovery of specific remedies.

> In the first place it is necessary that all diseases be reduced to definite and certain species, and that, with the same care which we see exhibited by botanists in their phytologies; since it happens, at present, that many diseases, although included in the same genus, mentioned with a common nomenclature, and resembling one another in several symptoms are, notwithstanding, *different in their natures, and require a different medical treatment.* [4]

	Agent	Use
1930	oxytocin	labor
1932	plasma	shock
1933	riboflavin	deficiency
1934	sulfonamides	pneumonia, gram$^+$ infection
	cyclopropane	anesthesia
	thiamin	deficiency
1935	testosterone	replacement
1937	niacin	pellagra
1938	pyrodoxine	replacement
1939	sulfadiazine	pneumonia, gram$^+$ infection
1940	sulfathiazole	pneumonia, gram$^+$ infection
1941	penicillin	gram$^+$ cocci
	coumadin	anticoagulant
1942	heparin	anticoagulant
1943	folic acid	anemia (megaloblastic)
1944	streptomycin	tuberculosis gram$^-$ infection
1947	chloramphenicol	typhoid, gram$^-$ infection
1948	vitamin B$_{12}$	megaloblastic anemia
	ACTH	replacement
	corticosteroids	replacement
1951	chlorpromazine	psychopharmacy
1950s–1975	tranquilizers, antidepressants, oral contraceptives, antihypertensives, oral diuretics, antithyroid agents, radioactive isotopes, antineoplastic agents, prostaglandins, new antibiotics, antiparasitic agents.	

Figure 1. Discreteness and Specificity in Medical Theory

Clinical Entity; Case and Fact	Diseased Organ, Seat of Disease	Diseased Tissue	Diseased Cell	Diseased Molecule
T. Sydenham 1624–89	G.B. Morgagni 1682–89	M.F.X. Bichat 1771–1802	A. Virchow 1821–1902	L. Pauling (1901–)

Bacterial Cause	Immunologic Specificity	Genetic Specificity
L. Pasteur 1822–95 R. Koch 1843–1910	E. Von Behring ⎫ S. Kitasato ⎬ 1894 K. Landsteiner 1900 ⎭	G. Mendel 1822–84 A. Garrod 1819–1907

Active Principles of Medicinals	Active Principles Synthesized	Chemotherapy	Antibiotics
"Alkaloid" Chemists 1805–20	"Coal Tar" Chemists 1860	P. Ehrlich Theory "Side-chain" Theory 1890 Salvarsan 1905	A. Fleming (1881–1955)

Specific ⟶ Radical Diagnosis
Specific ⟶ Radical Therapeutics

Sydenham held firmly to the traditional doctrine of the four humours and an elaborate theory of epidemics and constitutions. However, he reestablished the Hippocratic tradition of careful observation of specific clinical events.[5] This emphasis, and the concept of disease localization, is at the heart of modern clinical medicine and especially pertinent to clinical pharmacology. Sydenham set the stage for objectively recorded criteria of effectiveness, measured against the natural history of specific, untreated diseases, rather than conforming to the broader theory of disease as a whole-body phenomenon. Protesting against untested remedies, he asked:

> Where is the particular importance in just telling us that once, twice, or even oftener, this disease has yielded to that remedy? We are overwhelmed as it is with an infinite abundance of vaunted medicaments, and here they add new ones. Now, if I repudiate the rest of my formulae, and restrict myself to this medicine only, I must try its efficacy by innumerable experiments, and I must weigh, in respect to both the patient and the practice, innumerable circumstances, before I can derive any benefit from such a solitary observation.[6]

However, Sydenham never elaborated a totally satisfactory classificatory system of his own. Neither did his successors Boissier de Sauvages (1707–67) or Linnaeus (1707–78), although they did focus sharply on discrete symptoms and proximate manifestations, rather than on distant causes of illness.[7]

A very great impetus to localization of disease, and the second conceptual thread leading to discreteness and specificity, was G. B. Morgagni's detailed descriptions of organs as the "seats" of disease. Morgagni (1682–1771) wrote his great treatise *De sedibus et causis morborum per anatomen indagatis* almost a century after Sydenham. It provided tangible evidence that clinical illness could be anatomically localized, and that the symptoms which manifested an illness externally were often caused by lesions in specific organs. This concept of anatomical discreteness was extended to specific tissues by Xavier Bichat (1771–1802) and his followers in the Paris school, and then to specific cells by Rudolf Virchow (1821–1902). The modern concepts of molecular, subcellular, and biochemical pathology are extensions of this search for morphological substrata for the symptomatic manifestations and natural histories of disease.

Specificity in therapeutics was suggested, well before disease localization, by Paracelsus (1493–1541). The search for a connection between symptom and remedy had also inspired the "doctrine of signatures," by which plant remedies were selected on the basis of the similarity in appearance to the affected organ.[8] Infusions of heart-shaped foxglove for heart failure was a classic example, yet, the first of its active principles was not isolated until 1869.

But the relationship of medication to symptoms did not have a convincing basis until the early years of the nineteenth century. Then, the close association between chemistry and medicine, with chemists often serving as teachers of materia medica, eventuated in the isolation of the active principles of plant medicinals. In just the first two decades (1805–20), such potent alkaloids as morphine, colchicine, strychnine, and quinine were isolated, and their effects on man and animals studied.

Even more significant was the chemical synthesis of some of these active principles, as well as of a growing number of organic molecules, by the nascent azo dye and coal tar industry, after 1860.[9] Such useful chemicals as salicylic acid, acetanilde, chloral hydrate, barbituric acid, and chloroform were synthesized, and found a place in therapy. They were forerunners of the massive outpouring of synthetic molecules into twentieth-century pharmacies—each inspired by the frequent hope, and less frequent actuality of a specific therapeutic action.

At the end of the nineteenth century and the early part of the twentieth, Paul Ehrlich provided the most powerful intellectual stimulus for the notion of pharmacological specificity with his work on trypanocidal dyes, his synthesis of salvarsan (1905), and most of all, by his "side-chain theory" (1890), which postulated specific binding of active agents to tissue sites. He thus opened the era of chemical agents consciously designed to act with molecular and cellular specificity.

Modern microbiology added two additional dimensions to the expanding concepts of specificity in disease and treatment. Toward the latter part of the nineteenth century, Pasteur and Koch demonstrated that identifiable microorganisms (certain bacteria) could be primary causative agents of certain categories of illness. Their students and followers, shortly thereafter, showed that the chemical toxins produced by these bacteria elicited specific responses in the sera of animals to which they were administered. In 1891, the antitoxin produced in the serum of the horse by E. Von Behring and S. Kitasato was used to treat a child with diphtheria, opening up the whole era of specific immuno- and serotherapy. Immunology and immunochemistry have turned out to be among the most productive explanatory and therapeutic modalities available to medicine. There were only a very few years between Landsteiner's discovery, in 1900, of the specificity of blood types, which made blood transfusion a safe possibility, to the eradication by immunization of numerous infectious diseases, and finally, to the explanation of the mechanisms of hypersensitivity in the pathogenes of many diseases.

Even more startling and pregnant with possibility is the fruition in the twentieth century of the careful demonstrations of the specificity of the laws of heredity by Mendel. The most delicate and exquisitely specific relationships between genes and particular proteins and enzymes have been uncovered. Verifiable explanations were provided for A. Garrod's clinical observations of the ways in which metabolic disorders may be inherited. Linus Pauling's discovery, in the 1950s, of the biochemical defect which causes sickle cell disease brought genetic, morphological, and chemical specificities dramatically together. The therapeutic potentialities, as well as the dangers of gene manipulation, synthesis, and recombination are among the most urgent scientific and moral problems which we face today.[10]

A new dimension was added to the emerging concept of specificity of therapeutics by the discovery of sulfonamides, in the late thirties, and of penicillin, in the early forties. Not only could treatment be directed against particular symptoms, but for the first time, therapeutics could become radical—that is, it could eradicate the primary cause of an illness, in this case, particular micro-organisms. Chemical and antibiotic therapy matched the curative power of the surgeon's knife, which, during the same period was repairing, replacing, and excising every conceivable diseased organ. The surgeon's domain, which had always been specific, now extends beyond the imagination and capabilities of even his boldest predecessors of fifty years ago.

Though not entirely radical, since they do not entirely remove the primary cause of a disease, hormone and vitamin therapy have permitted specific replacement of crucial molecules in the body. Some of these natural substances have even been synthesized or improved, so that physiology can be restored to normal; some inherited or acquired hormone deficits can be compensated for completely, if not eliminated.

A mere listing of the chronology of the development of therapeutic specificity is sufficient to demonstrate how long the concept has incubated, as well as the exponential nature of its growth in the last fifty years (see table 1). The sheer number, and the impressive effectiveness of agents aimed at specific elements in the disease process have almost completely overcome the dominant views of the previous century. No longer is illness conceived of primarily as an imbalance in the body's input or output, or therapeutics as an enterprise directed at restoring the balance of total body economy upset by disease. Diseases are now seen as discrete entities, with discrete causes; medications are selected for specific, not generic actions; therapy is aimed at removing causes, if at all possible, and genuine cure is, in many diseases, a very realistic objective; the measure of effectiveness, as it was in the nineteenth century, is not a predictable physiological response, but a predictable alteration in the expected evolution of the disease.

Figure 2 shows how very recent have been the developments in specific therapy. For most of the long history of medicine, physicians relied on magico-religious rituals or empirical remedies. Quite late in the modern era, the first active principles of some of the oldest useful botanicals were isolated, and later some of them were synthesized. The even more highly specific measures, such as the use of antisera, the isolation of blood fractions, and the synthesis of polypeptide hormones, are products of the last few decades. They confer on therapeutics the capability of effecting cure at the molecular loci of disease. The era of specific and radical therapeutics has really only begun, and its future can scarcely be predicted with any accuracy. What seems certain is that the trend toward ever greater specificity will continue, with profound effects on the medical profession and upon society.

THE EFFECT OF THE NEW THERAPEUTICS ON MEDICINE AND THE MEDICAL PROFESSION

It has taken time for the full force of these characteristics of contemporary therapeutics to modify the thinking and behavior of physicians. Even now, the responses have not been uniform. Nonetheless a twentieth-century

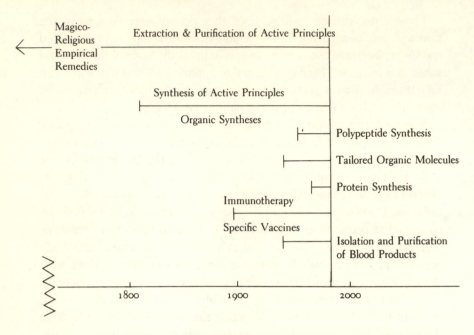

Figure 2. Developments in specific therapy.

medical ethos, a dominant spirit, has emerged which is substantially different from that of the nineteenth century.

This ethos has several clearly defined characteristics directly related to the power and specificity of contemporary therapeutics. The physician has become a specialist, the master over certain limited domains defined by disease, organ system, therapeutic technique, or institutional requirements. Specific treatments and diagnostic procedures require special mastery. The rapid rate of appearance of new knowledge in each field requires a limitation of the domain to be mastered. Specific therapies demand use of the hospital, which has become the center of the physician's interest and activities. The more arcane the knowledge, the more difficult the technique, the longer the training period, and the more scientific the language required for its mastery, the more highly regarded the specialty will be.

Medicine is rapidly becoming identified with its technical armamentarium; whatever lies outside the domain of specific diagnosis or treatment is considered by increasing numbers of physicians as outside the domain of medicine itself. The recent renaissance of "family medicine" as a specialized field has been generated by public pressures outside of the establishment of medical education. Its lack of a specific subject matter and special techniques place it at a conceptual disadvantage in medical schools and hospitals where medicine is identified with specialism. So much is this the case that family medicine has been forced to describe the generalist as a specialist in order to survive academically.[11]

In deference to this spirit of equating medicine with specific treatments, some of our wisest essayists decry the expenditure of our national resources on "halfway" technologies—those which only palliate or contain disease, rather than radically curing it.[12] They express the not unjustifiable hope that sooner or later our most devastating diseases will be conquered by research and technology. As a result, medical students are selected for their performance in the sciences, and impressed with the extreme importance of the basic and clinical sciences.

According to this view, cure by specific therapy becomes the only really proper sphere for the physician. Care, helping the patient to cope, reassuring, educating, and relieving worry, while not directly deprecated, nonetheless become less than honourable endeavours, not requiring a high level of sophistication. Doctor and patient share less of a common concern—the patient seeking to be well, the physician to diagnose and cure a specific illness over which he has mastery.

Physicians, too, become increasingly alienated from each other, since each specialist uses a different language, and commands a different body of knowledge or set of techniques. The physician identifies with his specialty rather than with the profession of medicine. The sense of corporate professional responsibility for the health of society is lost. Rather, the physician becomes a technician superbly capable of healing a discrete portion of the patient's anatomy. He leaves the remaining "nonspecific" elements of care and treatment to others, or he may insist that the patients are, after all, "fundamentally tough" and very well able to get along quite well on their own.[13]

The physician easily develops an inflated estimation of the value of his own expertise or special therapeutic maneuver. The tendency to overutilize the techniques with which he identifies is frequently manifest. Given the nature of the dominant professional ethos, once a patient has come to him, the physician feels useless unless he "rules out" every possibility of a disorder in his domain before releasing the patient to another specialist. The undiagnosed patient who has seen several specialists customarily has a long list of diseases which have been ruled out, at considerable expense and loss of time. He knows what he does not have, but is little enlightened on what his trouble may be in the first instance.

Interestingly, the vaunted scientific spirit of modern therapeutics has not resulted in the therapeutic nihilism and noninterventionism which nineteenth-century physicians feared from too large an infusion of science. We have only to contemplate the 1.5 billion prescriptions written yearly outside the hospital to see that possession of specific therapy does not ensure therapeutic parsimony.[14] Rather it seems to stimulate an excess zeal for one's new, particular, pharmacotherapeutic panaceas.

The objectivity of science upon which progress in therapeutics so heavily depends, paradoxically, is suppressed when the physician confronts the patient's need to "take something" and his own urge to "do something." The modern therapist, no less than his colleagues of centuries past, often uses the symbolic power of medication for essentially nonpharmacologic purposes.[15] The prescription still seals the transaction, serves as a substitute for conversation, terminates the interview, and provides a means of getting the patient to return.

Modern therapeutics is frequently classified as "rational," in contrast to the nonspecific remedies and untested, multi-ingredient prescriptions of years past. But strictly speaking, every medical system is "rational," in that its conclusions proceed more or less logically from its premises. All treatment systems are directed at the presumed causes of illness. As Fabrega, Ackerknecht, and others have shown in their ethnomedical studies, most cultures entertain some theory of disease.[16] Whether disease is thought to be due to object intrusion, breaking a taboo, loss of the soul, or demonic possession, the therapeutic ritual is rationally justified. Chant, dance, ritual sacrifice, or herbal potion—all are directed at reaching the presumed cause of the disease. The medical systematists of the nineteenth century were all highly rationalistic, fitting observations into their speculative schemata in highly formal fashion, with influences in society going well beyond the confines of medicine.[17]

What distinguishes modern therapeutics is not its superior rationality, but its scientific epistemology. Effectiveness is judged by the tests of scientific evidence, not by conformity to an all-encompassing theory, the details of a preset ritual, or the exhibition of some physiological response like emesis, diuresis, or catharsis. Effectiveness in modern therapeutics is defined as the capability of an agent, demonstrably and measurably, to alter the statistically predictable natural history of the disease. The very criteria of effectiveness which Sydenham hoped for in the seventeenth century are at last attainable. The truly effective agent either eliminates the primary cause, replaces some deficient vitamin or hormone, or ameliorates symptoms, thus altering unmistakably the natural history of a clinical entity in predictable ways.

Modern therapeutics is therefore not simply *rational,* but in its most complete expression it is scientifically *radical*—that is, it can completely remove the primary cause of a disease. This is the ultimate aim of therapeutic specificity. Even today, it is achieved by only a few therapeutic agents —notably the effective antimicrobial agents (penicillin, streptomycin, sulfonamides, and their cogeners and successors), as well as antimalarial and antiprotozoan agents.

Less radical, but highly specific, are those agents which alter the natural history of disease by specific reversal of some pathophysiological accompaniment of disease—digitalis glycosides acting on myocardial contractility, diuretics enhancing sodium excretion in heart failure, thyroid hormone replacement in hypothyroidism, insulin in diabetes, or vitamin B_{12} in magaloblastic anomia. Hope is high that further extensions of radical therapeutics will yield agents which can act effectively against the causes of the remaining unconquered disorders such as cancer, vascular disease, viral infections, and the diseases of the nervous system.

The effectiveness of modern therapeutics adds a powerful strain of positivism and reductionism to the twentieth-century medical ethos. Ultimate explanations for disease are sought in chemistry and physics. The success of these efforts has revived the dreams of the seventeenth-century Cartesians—the iatrochemists and iatrophysicists—who first sought ultimate explanations for disease in mathematical and scientific terms.

These attitudes of mind have been and continue to be useful in seeking out radically effective medical treatments. When they are universalized, however, to all realms of medical practice, they become impediments to the fulfillment of the more sensitive moral and social responsibilities of medicine. The less palpable, nonmensurable questions of value which color medical decisions are, as a result, approached uncritically, and even superficially. The unavoidable hubris which follows on the successes of scientific therapeutics leads subtly to the assumption that moral, as well as technical authority are vested in the physician.

But as Alasdair MacIntyre has forcefully argued, and legal opinion sustains, the patient has become his own moral agent.[18] His moral beliefs and values demand consideration in any medical decision. There is a growing disquietude among patients and public, who perceive a widening gap between the patient's interest and the interests of medicine. Much of the demand for government regulation and legal constraints, and for institutional monitoring of medical decisions is rooted in the public perception that the physician assumes moral as well as technical authority in the care of patients, and that his conscious or unconscious positivism makes him oblivious to the sensitivities of moral and value conflict with his patient.

This concern is heightened by a greater public awareness of the dominant values in medical education. Its positivist bias depreciates discourse about such nonobjective matters as values. We seem to be preparing a future generation of physicians out of tune with the requirements of critical moral discourse. Medical education has yet to strike the right balance between scientific objectivity as a means to advance medical knowledge and its limitations in making decisions for particular patients.[19] Making a right and good decision for *this patient* involves a value decision only partly justified on scientific grounds.

The dominant educational ethos has been challenged largely by a call for a new model of medicine based in the behavioral sciences.[20] The recent growth of interest in family medicine, primary care, and "humanistic" medicine are likewise reactions to the positivism of medical education.[21]

As in the nineteenth century, physicians and educators are paradoxical in their response to the scientific character of contemporary medicine. Practitioners decry the conversion of medicine to science, while enthusiastically exploiting the wonders of pharmaceutical chemistry; academicians adhere to scientific canons in their investigations, yet lapse into therapeutic enthusiasm in their practices.

Therapeutic enthusiasm and the pharmacological "imperative" are attractive to many physicians in academia, as well as to those in in practice. Therapeutic parsimony, which would conceptually be most consistent with the canons of scientific therapeutics, is still the doctrine of a few, who are often upbraided by colleagues and patients for their "Calvinistic" scruples in distributing the benefits of the pharmaceutical cornucopia.

EFFECTS OF THE NEW THERAPEUTICS ON
SOCIETY AND THE PHYSICIAN-PATIENT
RELATIONSHIP.

The maturation of the concepts of the discreteness of disease processes and the specificity of therapeutic agents has impressively and irrevocably transformed the whole ethos of the medical profession. We have examined some of these transformations as they affect the physician's perceptions of himself, and his intellectual attitudes. Their impact on society and the relationship between patient and physician has been equally profound.

It is difficult to imagine any human activity that has more materially altered the conditions of human existence than medicine. Therapeutics, as a conscious and specific attempt to control human disease, is little more than a century old. Its polemical detractors of present and previous times notwithstanding, the net effect has been beneficial for mankind. This is so, even when we acknowledge that the enormous range of therapeutic capabilities raises valid questions concerning their human purpose and value.

We now take for granted the conquest of infectious disease, the primary prevention of epidemic infections, the care of trauma, the control of metabolic and deficiency disorders, the ability of surgeons to cope with so many previously disastrous emergencies, the virtual elimination of puerperal sepsis, the decline in infant mortality, and such mundane, but qualitatively important things as control of tooth decay, visual and auditory aids, and the like. We must credit modern therapeutics with making contributions to many facets of human life.

The physician is highly regarded today as a wonder-worker who mediates between the patient and the mysterious forces of science and technology. He is master of the instruments and techniques which can cure illness and save lives. He is the immediate embodiment, for most people, of the vaunted powers of science. All seek access to his special expertise and want the most specialized knowledge brought to bear on their own problems.

In contrast with his professional predecessors, today's physician is no longer the mediator in a generally accepted cultural value system. He deals in a language foreign to the patient; he often is not a member of the same community; he knows little of the patient's lifestyle or family, and the patient knows less about his. When patient and physician meet, stranger meets stranger. The bond between patient and physician is fashioned by the physician's special knowledge, not by his role as a delegated interpreter of a commonly held set of beliefs about health, illness, and their place in human existence. Indeed, in a pluralistic society, the possibility of such a commonly held set of beliefs is increasingly remote.

Previously, the physician could offer few specific remedies, so that the "will of God" or of "nature" would take its course. The physician might assist that course, but he was not in control, as he is today. With power so clearly in the doctor's hands, the patient wonders whether his physician has access to "all" the knowledge necessary, and whether it is, in fact, being used to the patient's advantage. When the physician's remuneration was meager, and he was a member of the community, the question of his using his power in his own self-interest might arise, but with far less force. Today, when the doctor is a stranger, the patient is caught in a fearful dilemma: he must trust the physician, because of his power to heal, but that trust is undermined by the fear of the physician's economic self-interest.

The strength of this ambivalence is evident in the series of measures initiated by the public, which aim, directly or indirectly, at limiting the physician's "discretionary space"—the region within which he can exert his expertise without outside interference. The Patients' Bill of Rights, the legal concern with informed consent and proper disclosure, the regulation of experimentation on human beings, the institutionalization of peer, and quality control for physicians, and the malpractice crisis speak eloquently to the wide disparity between the physician's and the patient's expectations of each other.

This new tension in the therapeutic encounter is puzzling to physicians, as well as to patients. The doctor believes he is acting in the age-old paternalistic relationship in which the physician determines what is "good." With his expanded therapeutic powers, he feels better qualified than ever to decide what the patient needs, not realizing that these very powers can, in themselves, create mistrust. The tensions between patient and doctor become most acute when moral values are at issue, as they are in cases requiring decisions about prolongation of life, abortion, care of the aged, or the treatment of infants with multiple congenital malformations.

A further dilemma marks the relationships of patients with physicians: the conflict between medicalization and demedicalization.[22] Those who are impressed with the capabilities of modern therapy would extend the medical model to disorders not yet susceptible to its methodology: according to this view, criminal behavior, alcoholism, drug abuse, smoking, and almost every sort of personal disaffection can all be "treated," as illness. Others call, instead, for a restriction of the domain of medicine to the strictly organic and obvious situations approachable by treatment modalities already in hand. Still others favor demedicalization, to the point of returning more responsibility and initiative to patients for their own health and healing.[23]

The attractions and the dangers of the power of medicine confuse legislators, as well. Some believe the health of the nation depends upon more physicians, hospitals, expanded diagnostic testing, and freer access to medication; others, with equal vigor, would redirect our resources to self-care, patient education, and prevention aimed at changing lifestyles with respect to exercise, diet, drinking, reckless driving, and the like.

While granting high status and financial return to the specialists, more patients than ever are distressed with the fragmentation and disorganization of care that specialization produces. Their distress is especially great when the patient's problem is relatively simple, requiring reassurance, counseling, or simple symptomatic remedies. The specialist's lack of interest is decried, and demands are made within the profession, and without, for the return of the physician to a hieratic role. He is urged to become again the counselor, advocate, and friendly healer he is thought to have been in times past.

Yet even when the physician offers help of this kind, he encounters the universal expectation that a drug will accompany even the simplest transaction. The effectiveness of modern treatment raises public expectation that there is a drug for every indisposition. The chemical agent becomes the symbol of the doctor's concern and power, and without it the transaction is considered ineffective. The physician is accused of merely "talking" to the patient. Physicians respond to this disappointment by prescribing too many drugs. The result is an overmedicated society, expending billions of dollars for medicines which fail utterly to satisfy the very criteria of effectiveness in which scientific therapeutics took its origin.[24]

Only one or two more examples are needed to underscore how much change the physician's relationship to patients and society is undergoing. For example, American society expresses an intense desire to exploit all the marvels of modern pharmacotherapeutics, while fearing the mounting danger and cost of unfavorable side effects. The government is urged, on the one hand, to increase the powers of the Food and Drug Administration, and on the other, to liberalize the range of drugs which can be self-prescribed and purchased. Likewise, we know that to gain the benefits of the stringent criteria for effectiveness which distinguish scientific therapeutics requires extensive use of the method of randomized clinical trials in humans, yet, there is a growing move to severely limit the circumstances and conduct of these trials. Indeed it is being argued, and not altogether illogically, that the randomized clinical trial is ethically questionable, and that a more acceptable mode of investigation would be the retrospective study.[25] Public desire for new pharmaceuticals is matched by increasing regulatory control over the introduction of all new agents, and there is some evidence that these regulatory moves have delayed and impeded the testing and utilization of new therapeutic agents in this country.

In another paradox, modern therapeutics, which owes its accomplishments to science and technology, has induced a new surge of belief in the magical. The powers of the few really specific agents are transferred to all chemical agents. Drugs take on mystical qualities as avenues to human desires for tranquility, intelligence, better memory, aphrodisia, weight reduction—the whole list of human yearnings for a "better" life. Chemical salvation exists side by side with scientific pharmacology. In the popular media, the two are fused into a new magico-religious value system as powerful as any to be encountered in primitive societies.

Contemporary therapeutics has thus transformed our ideas and attitudes about illness, health, happiness, and satisfaction. Its sociocultural influence extends well beyond the physician's office and the hospital corridors.

THE NEXT QUARTER OF A CENTURY

The dilemmas raised by the achievements and the potential of contemporary therapeutics are destined to become more complex and more acute in the remaining years of the twentieth century. Serious social issues will be raised by the need for society to respond to this dilemma, resolve the paradoxes which we have outlined, and possibly alter traditional values. Whatever the dangers inherent in a future expansion of the capabilities of therapeutics, its obvious benefits, or promise of benefits, are not likely to be given up. The quest will continue to receive strong social sanction. This means that some central questions must be more consciously faced.

The first of these is to decide more explicitly what society wants medicine to be, and what span of functions it wishes to assign to physicians. It is clear that specialization, the expansion of media technology, and the search for ever more specific and radical modes of scientific treatment will continue to be the responsibility of physicians. What, then, will happen to the traditional Aesculapian powers or hieratic functions of the physician? Are we to follow the course suggested by the more ardent proponents of technological medicine who would exclude the caring, sustaining, and reassuring functions from any association with medicine?

This is not a realistic eventuality, even if it were desirable. The more affluent a society becomes, the lower is its threshold for discomfort, and the greater the demands for relief of even the most minor indispositions.[26] The need therefore, for nonradical therapy, and, hopefully, for therapy avoiding the use of drugs but involving human interaction—counseling, explaining, reassuring, assisting the patient to cope—are sure to persist and increase.[27] Hopefully, the shortsightedness of chemical "coping" will be appreciated and the myth of salvation through the pharmacy will be dispelled.

In addition, society and physicians must also deal with the residuum of patients not completely healed, and perhaps even made a little worse, by partially effective chemotherapy for cancer, or cardiovascular disorders. The human and personal consequences of living with illnesses in which drastic treatments prolong life without curing is already a dominant concern.

Much of the discontent with medicine today arises from the disjunction patients feel between the doctor's technical role and the hieratic role which he formerly performed. We shall have to accept a fact (an unpalatable fact, for many) that the ideal of reuniting these two radically different functions may become impossible. The attitudes of mind, the motivations, and the education of the technical specialist are fundamentally different from those of the Aesculapian physician. If we are to optimize the utility of both, we shall be forced to think of two different kinds of physicians performing two fundamentally different kinds of therapy.

One kind of physician (and these will be in the minority) will be educated specifically to develop and practice radical therapy, employing high technology. Society must demand of them rigorous standards of technical competence. Caring and humaneness are not excluded, but they can be exercised over a limited range of problems. It is uneconomical to expect the technomedical physician to spend much time in explanation and education except in respect to his technical operations. To relate these to the patient's whole life situation will ordinarily be beyond the capacities and inclinations of this kind of physician. This will be particularly true with the patients who are not cured by technology and who then become, in some ways, the victims of the imperfections of that technology.

The majority of physicians should be educated to perform the hieratic and Aesculapean functions—those needed for the majority of human needs of the more ordinary kind, and for those patients with complex disorders who are not "cured" by radical therapeutics. Whether these caring functions are performed, in the future, by family physicians or by "extending" the roles of physician's assistants, nurse practitioners, or psychologists, some fusion of these professions, at least functionally, is to be expected.

It is essential that society have access to the undeniable benefits of high technology in medicine provided by physicians educated to provide such services competently. Equally essential is avoidance of a theory of medicine which excludes those human needs not susceptible to technological solution which require personal interactions, or a more general integration of psychological and physical measures in healing. Two organizing principles —one scientific and radical, and one human and personal—are required, and the central issue is not to exclude one or the other, but to enable them to interact synergistically.

Similar difficulties attend the resolution of the other dilemmas which I have sketched. How far into human life should we extend the medical model? Granting its effectiveness in curing discrete diseases, with discretely defined causes, is it likely that the same model will cure most of our social disabilities and pathologies, as some suppose? Much depends upon a clearer idea of what we wish to define as health and disease—and this is, above all, a question of values.

Is it healthy or desirable, for example, to live in a society in which every household, every handbag, every schoolbag or attaché case is outfitted with specific drugs to counteract the indispositions of the day—anxiety, depression, disappointment, poor-tasting food, a dull novel, a nasty boss, unsatisfying sex, or fear of the upcoming examination in mathematics? Or, must we look to a better educated, more prudent public, able to make a more restrained use of specific chemical agents and to respond to the tensions of ordinary living with greater emotional maturity?

These questions are the practical expressions of a deeper cultural and philosophical dilemma. The fragmentation of therapy which the discreteness and the radicalness of today's therapeutics fosters atomizes our view of health and illness, and even of daily life. Philosophers, moralists, and others search for a way to reassemble the multitudinous centrifugal forces in the medical encounter. Can we recapture something of the kind of congruence between the physician's and patient's view of health and life which the medicine man shares with his client, or which the patient shared with his physician, according to Professor Rosenberg, in the nineteenth century? Is it desirable? Is it necessary?

Or, is it more mature to assign medicine a limited role in our lives, so that we do not look for more than it can offer? Its domain could be limited to those disorders susceptible to specific therapy. On this view, the hieratic, personal and supportive functions could be assigned to people outside the medical profession altogether—to the patient himself, his family, friends, or a new set of therapists whose training would not be technical.

In a pluralistic society, we can expect no uniform answer to such questions. There is no universally held world view to call upon for answers. Somewhere between the extremes of the conflicting attitudes I have described lies some common set of values yet to be defined. The first step in their definition is a far more intensive engagement of medicine with the humanities, and with those who make public policy. This is a difficult discourse to initiate and to sustain, yet it is precisely this diversity in viewpoints which must be reconciled in some realistic way. The dilemmas of modern therapeutics are simply subsets of the wider problems which man's technological achievements will continue to create.

What will "post-modern medicine," as Renee Fox has called it, look like? She has suggested that the medicine of the future might combine technological skill with the best elements in archaic and modern medicine.[28] The new amalgam would allow for greater sensitivity to mystery, to the existential situation of modern man, to the social and historical forces which can affect his well-being, and to the limitations of technology. How feasible such an amalgam might be is surely problematic at this moment.

Clearly the unprecedented accomplishments of twentieth-century therapeutics have forced us to confront the recurrent challenge of mankind—to define what it is to be human. The task is assuredly more difficult for each successive era, and, just as assuredly, inescapable.

NOTES

1. I have paraphrased Rosenberg's analysis in the next several paragraphs to contrast it with the notions of discreteness and specificity which succeeded the nineteenth-century views.

2. Pedro Lain-Entralgo, "The Health and Perfection of Man," *Diogenes* 31 (Fall 1960): 1–18, reviews the notion of disease as imbalance and disharmony historically and relates it to contemporary personalist medicine, which aims at restoring health by enabling the patient to restore a balance of all elements in his life.

3. The sketch of the early history of the ideas of specificity and radical therapy is based on inferences drawn from several accounts of the history of medicine in the sixteenth through the eighteenth centuries. Especially helpful are the following: Lester S. King, *The Philosophy of Medicine: The Early 18th Century* (Cambridge: Harvard University Press, 1978); Lester S. King, *A History of Medicine, Selected Readings* (Penguin, 1971); Fielding H. Garrison, *An Introduction to the History of Medicine* (Philadelphia: W. B. Saunders, 4th ed., reprinted 1966); Arturo Castiglione, *A History of Medicine*, trans. and ed. E. B. Krumbhaar (New York: Knopf, 1941); Michel Foucault, *The Birth of the Clinic, The Archaeology of Medical Perception* (New York: Pantheon, 1973).

4. Thomas Sydenham, *The Works of Thomas Sydenham, trans. from the Latin by Dr. Greenhill, with a Life of the Author,* by R. G. Latham, cited in King, *History of Medicine,* pp. 117–18.

5. Kenneth Dewhurst, *Thomas Sydenham (1624–1688): His Life and Original Writings* (Berkeley: University of California Press, 1966).

6. Sydenham, *Works,* cited in King. We are not yet free of this fallacy, as the distended size of our modern pharmacopeias and formularies vividly attest.

7. Inci Bowman, "Classification of Diseases, Part I: Thomas Sydenham (1624–1689) and Principles of Classification," *The Bookman* 3:6 (June 1976): 1–10. See this, together with three subsequent parts in *The Bookman*, vol. 3, nos. 7, 8, 10, for July, August, October 1976.

8. Scott Buchannan, *The Doctrine of Signatures: A Defense of Theory in Medicine* (London: Kegan Paul, 1938).

9. William N. Hubbard, Jr., *The Origins of Medicinals. Advances in American Medicine: Essays at the Bicentennial,* vol. 2.

10. See Stanley N. Cohen, "Recombinant DNA: Fact and Fiction," *Science* 195 (February 1977): 654–57, for a particularly good summarization of the possibilities of developing specific biological strains tailored to produce specific antibodies, hormones, or vitamins with therapeutic usefulness—as well as potential dangers.

11. Edmund D. Pellegrino, "Academic Viability of Family Medicine: A Triad of Challenges," Paper presented at the University of Maryland Family Medicine Conference, 5 March 1977 (in press).

12. Lewis Thomas, "On the Science and Technology of Medicine," *Daedalus* (Winter 1977): 37–38.

13. Ibid., p. 46.

14. "The Top 200 Drugs, 1974 vs. 1975: Generics Rise by 3.2% Despite 1% Dip in Total Rx Volume," *Pharmacy Times* (April 1976): 37.

15. Edmund D. Pellegrino, "Prescribing and Drug Ingestion Symbols and Substances," *Drug Intelligence and Clinical Pharmacy* 10 (November 1976): 624–30.

16. Erwin H. Ackerknecht, *Medicine and Ethnology, Selected Essays* (Bern:

Verlag Hans Huber, 1971); Horacio Fabrega, Jr., and Daniel B. Silver, *Illness and Shamanistic Curing in Zinacantan: An Ethnomedical Analysis* (Stanford, Ca.: Stanford University Press, 1973).

17. David Musto, "Therapeutic Intervention and Social Forces: Historical Perspectives," in *American Handbook of Psychiatry,* ed. Daniel X. Freedman and Jarl E. Dyrud (New York: Basic Books, Inc., 1975), vol. 5, *Treatment,* pp. 37–38; Joseph F. Kett, *The Formation of the Medical Profession: The Role of Institutions, 1780–1860* (New Haven: Yale University Press, 1969), pp. 97–101, pp. 132–64. The professional and cultural influences of Thomsonianism and homeopathy in nineteenth-century medicine are well documented.

18. Alasdair MacIntyre, "Patients as Agents," in S. Spicker and T. Engelhardt, Jr., eds., *Philosophical Medical Ethics: Its Nature and Significance,* Philosophy and Medicine, vol. 3 (Dordrecht, Holland: D. Reidel Publ., in press).

19. Edmund D. Pellegrino, "The Anatomy of Clinical Judgement: Right Reasons and Right Action," ibid.

20. George L. Engel, "The Need for a New Medical Model: A Challenge for Biomedicine," *Science* 196 (April 1977): 129–36.

21. See Mary M. Belknap, Robert A. Balu, Rosalind N. Grossman, *Case Studies and Methods in Humanistic Medical Care: Some Preliminary Findings.* (San Francisco: Inst. for the Study of Humanistic Medicine, 1975). This work interprets medical humanism largely in terms of the need for humanistic psychology in the education of physicians. The breadth of interpretations of the seductive term "medical humanism" is outlined in my own paper, "Educating the Humanist Physician: An Ancient Ideal Reconsidered," reprinted in *Musings Quarterly* (Jour. of Medical Undergraduate Society, U. of Brit. Columbia) 1 (Fall 1974).

22. Renee C. Fox, "The Medicalization and Demedicalization of American Life," *Daedalus* (Winter 1977): 9–22.

23. See Rick Carlson, *The End of Medicine* (New York: John Wiley and Sons, 1975); Ivan Illich, *Medical Nemesis: The Expropriation of Health* (New York: Pantheon, 1976).

24. Edmund D. Pellegrino, "Prescribing and Drug Ingestion Symbols."

25. See Charles Fried, *Medical Experimentation, Personal Integrity, and Social Policy* (New York: North American Elsevier, 1974), pp. 157–60.

26. See Pierre Cornillot, "The Ambiguities of the Health Concept in Industrialized Societies," in *Health, Higher Education and the Community: Towards a Regional Health University,* ed. Pierre Duquet (Paris: Organization for Economic Cooperation and Development, 1977), p. 105.

27. See Pedro Lain-Entralgo, *The Therapy of the Word in Classical Antiquity.* ed. and trans. L.J. Rather and John M. Sharp (New Haven: Yale University Press, 1970).

28. Renee C. Fox, "Medical Evolution Explorations in General Theory," in *Social Science,* vol. 2 (New York: The Free Press,) pp. 785–86.

SUGGESTIONS FOR FURTHER READING

The past dozen years have seen an increasing interest in the history of medicine and especially its social aspects. A number of textbooks and collections have been published in response to this demand; one of these, *Sickness and Health in America* (Madison: University of Wisconsin Press, 1978), edited by Judith Walzer Leavitt and Ronald L. Numbers, contains an excellent annotated bibliography at pp. 433–41. This contains references to most of the more important recent works on medicine in America. There is no recent survey of the history of medicine generally. Fielding H. Garrison's *An Introduction to the History of Medicine,* 4th ed. (Philadelphia and London: W. B. Saunders, 1966; originally published, 1929) remains a reliable and comprehensive but now much dated survey. Henry Sigerist's great synthesis of medical history was never to reach beyond his first two projected volumes: *A History of Medicine. Volume I: Primitive and Archaic Medicine* and *Volume II: Early Greek, Hindu, and Persian Medicine* (New York: Oxford University Press, 1951, 1961). Richard H. Shryock's *Development of Modern Medicine,* 2d ed. (New York: Knopf, 1947) is an important pioneering attempt to place the history of medicine in general social history; it is now more than thirty years old and should be used with care. A useful inventory of approaches to the history of medicine is Edwin Clarke's *Modern Methods in the History of Medicine* (London:

University of London, 1971). Richard H. Shryock's *Medicine and Society in America, 1660–1860* (New York: New York University Press, 1960) remains a useful overview. For another approach to the place of medicine in nineteenth-century American society, see Charles E. Rosenberg, *The Cholera Years: The United States in 1832, 1849 and 1866* (Chicago: University of Chicago Press, 1962). Erwin H. Ackerknecht has written a number of incisive studies of various aspects of medical history: Erwin H. Ackerknecht, *A Short History of Medicine* (New York: Ronald Press, 1955); *A Short History of Psychiatry,* 2d ed. rev. (New York: Hafner, 1968); *Therapeutics from the Primitives to the 20th Century* (New York: Hafner, 1973); *History and Geography of the Most Important Diseases* (New York: Hafner, 1965). Owsei Temkin is possibly the most broad-ranging of living medical historians; no one interested in the field should be unaware of his major works. These include *The Falling Sickness: A History of Epilepsy from the Greeks to the Beginnings of Modern Neurology,* 2d ed. rev. (Baltimore: Johns Hopkins University Press, 1971); *Galenism: Rise and Decline of a Medical Philosophy* (Ithaca, N.Y.: Cornell University Press, 1973); and *The Double Face of Janus and Other Essays in the History of Medicine* (Baltimore: Johns Hopkins University Press, 1977).

CONTRIBUTORS

GERALD L. GEISON, associate professor of the history and philosophy of science at Princeton University, is the author of *Michael Foster and the Cambridge School of Physiology: The Scientific Enterprise in Late Victorian Society.* His teaching and research interests include the historical relationship between medical theory and medical practice. He is currently at work on a projected book, *The Private Science of Louis Pasteur.*

GERALD N. GROB, professor of history at Rutgers University, has written extensively about the history of American psychiatry, mental hospitals, and medicine. His books include *Mental Institutions in America: Social Policy to 1875; The State and the Mentally Ill; Edward Jarvis and the Medical World of Nineteenth-Century America;* and *Workers and Utopia.* He is currently working on the second volume of *Mental Institutions in America,* covering 1875–1940.

JANET WILSON JAMES, formerly director of Radcliffe's Schlesinger Library on the History of Women in America, is associate professor of history at Boston College. She was associate editor of *Notable American Women, 1607–1950.*

ROBERT E. KOHLER is assistant professor of the history and sociology of science at the University of Pennsylvania. He has been researching the history of American scientific institutions and disciplines since the Civil War, and is writing a book on the history of medical reform and biological chemistry in America from 1875 to 1940.

RUSSELL C. MAULITZ, author of a number of articles on nineteenth- and twentieth-century scientific medicine, is assistant professor of the history of medicine in the Department of History and Sociology of Science and in the Department of Medicine at the University of Pennsylvania. He is working on studies of European pathology in the early nineteenth century, and of twentieth-century internal medicine.

RONALD L. NUMBERS teaches the history of American science and medicine at the University of Wisconsin-Madison, where he is chairman of the Department of the History of Medicine. His publications include *Prophetess of Health: A Study of Ellen G. White; Creation by Natural Law: Laplace's Nebular Hypothesis in American Thought; Almost Persuaded: American Physicians and Compulsory Health Insurance, 1912–1920; Sickness and Health in America: Readings in the History of Medicine and Public Health*, edited with Judith Walzer Leavitt; and *The Education of American Physicians: Historical Essays*. His current research focuses on the history of health and lifestyle in America.

EDMUND D. PELLEGRINO, president and professor of philosophy and biology at the Catholic University of America, has written extensively on mineral metabolism, and on the philosophy and ethics of medicine. He is founding editor of the *Journal of Medicine and Philosophy* and director of the Institute for Human Values in Medicine. His books include *Humanism and the Physician* and a newly completed manuscript, *The Philosophical Basis of Medical Practice*.

JAMES REED, associate professor of history at Rutgers College, is the author of *From Private Vice to Public Virtue: The Birth Control Movement and American Society since 1830*. He is completing an anthology of interviews with women activists in the birth control movement, and has begun a study of the career of the Yale psychobiologist, Robert M. Yerkes.

CHARLES E. ROSENBERG is professor of history at the University of Pennsylvania. He is the author of *The Cholera Years: The United States in 1832, 1849 and 1866; The Trial of the Assassin Guiteau: Psychiatry and Law in the Gilded Age;* and *No Other Gods: On Science and Social Thought in America*, as well as a contributor to scholarly journals in the history of science and medicine. He is currently at work on a study of medical care in America from 1800 to 1920.

MORRIS J. VOGEL is associate professor of history at Temple University. He has studied the American hospital as a social institution, and is the author of a forthcoming book on that subject, *The Invention of the Modern Hospital: Boston, 1870–1930*. His current work is on morbidity experience in the nineteenth-century city.